Complementary and Alternative Medicine for Older Adults

A Guide to Holistic Approaches to Healthy Aging

About the Editors

ELIZABETH R. MACKENZIE, PHD, has been a researcher and educator in the field of complementary and alternative medicine for two decades. Dr. Mackenzie completed her doctoral dissertation on health belief systems and community-based healthcare at the University of Pennsylvania in 1994, whereupon she joined the Institute on Aging at the University of Pennsylvania Health System and conducted research on cultural issues in health and healthcare. As a Research Assistant Professor in the division of geriatric medicine, she was the principal investigator of a study on aging, mental health, and prayer. Dr. Mackenzie currently teaches courses on humanistic medicine in the School of Arts and Sciences at the University of Pennsylvania, where she is a Senior Fellow in the Writing Center, a Lecturer in the History and Sociology of Science department, and an Associate Fellow of the Institute on Aging. Dr. Mackenzie is the author of *Healing the Social Body: A Holistic Approach to Public Health Policy,* numerous journal articles, and several book chapters. In addition to her academic work, Dr. Mackenzie is a long-time student of yoga, qigong, and body psychotherapy.

BIRGIT RAKEL, MD, earned her medical degree from the Freie University of West Berlin, Germany in 1988. Dr. Rakel completed her internship before moving to England, where she received her General Practitioner (GP) training. She worked as a GP in London, where she also completed a fellowship at the Royal London Homoeopathic Hospital. Dr. Rakel relocated to the U.S. in 1996, where she completed a residency and became board certified in Family Medicine. Since 2001, Dr. Rakel has been on the faculty of the Jefferson Myrna Brind Center for Integrative Medicine at Thomas Jefferson University Hospital in Philadelphia PA, one of the first academic medicine centers in North America that integrates CAM into patient care, teaching, and research. Dr. Rakel was recently awarded a Bravewell Fellowship, an appointment that allows her to further her training at the University of Arizona's Program in Integrative Medicine under the direction of Andrew Weil, MD. She presents nationally on topics related to aging and integrative medicine.

Complementary and Alternative Medicine for Older Adults

A Guide to Holistic Approaches to Healthy Aging

Edited by
Elizabeth R. Mackenzie, PhD
Birgit Rakel, MD

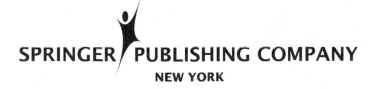

SPRINGER PUBLISHING COMPANY
NEW YORK

Springer Publishing Company, Inc.
11 West 42nd Street
New York, NY 10036

Acquisitions Editor: Helvi Gold
Production Editor: Jeanne Libby
Cover design by Joanne Honigman
Typeset by Daily Information Processing, Churchville, PA

07 08 09 10 / 5 4 3 2

Library of Congress Cataloging-in-Publication Data

Complementary and alternative medicine for older adults : a guide
    to holistic approaches to healthy aging / [edited by] Elizabeth
    Mackenzie, Birgit Rakel.
        p. ; cm.
    Includes bibliographical references and index.
    ISBN 0-8261-3805-5
    1. Alternative medicine. 2. Holistic medicine. 3. Older people—
Diseases—Alternative treatment. I. Mackenzie, Elizabeth R.,
    1961–   . II. Rakel, Birgit.
    [DNLM: 1. Complementary Therapies—methods—Aged.
    2. Health Promotion—methods—Aged. 3. Holistic Health—Aged.
    WB 890 C73667 2006]
    R733.C65284 2006
    613'.0438—dc22

2005031316

Printed in the United States of America by Bang Printing.

Contents

Contributors

Elaine Abbott, MMT, MT-BC, is a board-certified music therapist, with over 7 years of experience working with the elderly in continuing care retirement communities and skilled nursing facilities. She has a master's degree in music therapy and is currently working on her PhD in music therapy at Temple University.

Amy L. Ai, PhD, is an associate professor of social work at the University of Washington in Seattle and serves as a principal or co-investigator for several large NIH-funded studies pertaining to spirituality and health, and integrative medicine. Dr. Ai is a fellow of the National Institute on Aging and a John A. Hartford Faculty Scholar.

Kathleen Avins, MMT, MT-BC, is pursuing her PhD in music therapy at Temple University, where she also teaches. A board-certified music therapist who has more than 12 years of clinical experience with a variety of populations; she is currently working with the Hospice of New Jersey.

Michael J. Baime, MD, is the founder and director of the Penn Program for Stress Management and is clinical assistant professor at the University of Pennsylvania Health System. He is an expert in the efficacy of mindfulness meditation–based stress management and is nationally recognized for his adaptations of mindfulness meditation techniques for use in widely varied settings, including schools, hospitals, businesses, and government. Dr. Baime is the University of Pennsylvania site director and co-principle investigator of the parent grant. Dr. Baime began the practice of meditation in 1969 and is currently a senior meditation teacher in the Karma Kagyu lineage of Tibetan Buddhism.

Michael Briggs, PharmD, is an expert in phytomedicine in private practice and a freelance medical writer.

Robert Butera, MDiv, PhD, is the director of the YogaLife Institute in Devon, Pennsylvania. Dr. Butera is the publisher of a local holistic magazine, *Yoga Living,* and runs numerous educational and training programs in the Philadelphia area. He studied classical yoga with Dr. Jayadeva and Hansaji Yogendra at the Yoga Institute in Bombay, India, and is author of *Classical Yoga Study Guide.*

Jack Carman, ASLA, is a landscape architect and the president of Design for Generations LLC, a company devoted to therapeutic gardening. He has over 18 years' experience in the analysis, planning, design, and management of therapeutic outdoor environments for senior communities, health care facilities, schools, and places of worship.

Cheryl Chapman, RN, HNC, NCTMB, is a massage therapist in private practice in New Jersey who specializes in geriatric massage. Ms. Chapman is a continuing education provider for the National Certification Board for Therapeutic Massage and Bodywork (NCTMB) and has been nationally certified since 1992. She is a board member of the American Massage Therapy Association and past president of the New Jersey chapter of the AMTA.

Kevin Chen, PhD, MPH, is an associate professor of psychiatry in the Robert Wood Johnson Medical School at UMDNJ, with a doctorate degree in social psychology and statistics and a master's degree in public health. His major research interests include research methodology, epidemiology of substance use/abuse, sociology of mental health, and medical applications of qigong and mind–body interaction. His current research includes the study of qigong therapy for addiction, arthritis, cancer, and other health conditions.

Mari Clements, MS, DAy, is an Ayurvedic practitioner in private practice at the Media Wellness Center in Media, Pennsylvania. Ms. Clements is a board-certified diabetes educator, a certified Jin Shin Do acupressure therapist, and an experienced wellness counselor. She has served as a holistic counselor and therapist to students at Swarthmore College and the University of Pennsylvania.

Ara DerMarderosian, PhD, is a professor of pharmacognosy and medicinal chemistry at the University of the Sciences in Philadelphia. For over 3 decades, Dr. DerMarderosian has taught and conducted research in pharmacology and phytochemistry, and serves as the science adviser to the Philadelphia District FDA Laboratories. He has over 100 publications in journals and books.

Joel S. Edman, DSc, FACN, CNS, is a clinical assistant professor and clinical nutritionist at the Myrna Brind Center for Integrative Medicine at Thomas Jefferson University. Dr. Edman is a nutritional counselor, educator, and researcher. He has 15 years of experience as a nutritionist in an integrated medicine setting.

Joyce Frye, DO, FACOG, MBA, is an NIH-NCCAM research fellow in the Center for Clinical Epidemiology and Biostatistics at the University of Pennsylvania School of Medicine in Philadelphia and the president of the American Institute of Homeopathy. Dr. Frye has been a homeopath in private practice for many years. Her current research agenda focuses on homeopathy and reproductive health.

Master FaXiang Hou, is the founding director of the Qigong Research Society in Mt. Laurel, New Jersey, where he holds private consultations and teaches a hereditary form of qigong passed down to him through his familial lineage (Ching Loong San Dian Xue Mi Gong Fa). Master Hou was designated a certified master by the International Qigong Science Association. He is the author of *Qigong for Health and Well-Being and Unleashing the Power of Food.*

Eileen Kennedy, MA, NCTMB, APP, CIMI, is a nationally certified massage therapist. She has additional certification in geriatric, cancer, and mastectomy massage. Ms. Kennedy has published in numerous professional massage journals and shares a private practice with Cheryl Chapman in New Jersey.

Marc Micozzi, MD, PhD, is a leader in the field of integrative medicine. He is the founding editor-in-chief of the *Journal of Complementary and Alternative Medicine: Research on Paradigm, Practice and Policy.* He is also the editor of the first U.S. textbook on complementary and alternative medicine, *Fundamentals of Complementary and Alternative Medicine.* In 2002, he became the founding director of the Policy Institute for Integrative Medicine in Philadelphia and Washington, DC, working to educate policymakers, the health professions, and the general public about integrative medicine.

Caroline Peterson, MA, ATR, is a registered art therapist and mindfulness meditation–based stress reduction teacher with the Myrna Brind Center of Integrative Medicine at Thomas Jefferson University in Philadelphia. Ms. Peterson coordinates clinical research there in mindfulness-based art therapy and is also on the staff of the Wellness Community of Philadelphia, where she leads Open Studio groups for persons with cancer.

Sandy Ransom, RN, MSHP, is the director of the Texas Long Term Care Institute in the College of Health Professions of Southwest Texas State University in San Marcos, Texas. Ms. Ransom has published widely and has presented nationally on innovations in nursing home care. She presented testimony to the U.S. Senate Special Committee on Aging regarding Eden Alternative outcomes and has traveled as far as Australia to teach providers about the Eden Alternative.

James K. Rotchford, MD, MPH, is a physician in private practice in Washington State and the founding president of the Washington chapter of the American Academy of Medical Acupuncture. Dr. Rotchford is a fellow of the American Academy of Medical Acupuncture, a fellow of the American College of Preventive Medicine, and is board certified in public health and general preventive medicine. He has numerous publications in peer-reviewed journals and edits *Acubriefs,* a newsletter devoted to medical acupuncture.

Elaine J. Yuen, PhD, is a research assistant professor of family medicine in the Center for Research in Medical Education and Health Care at Thomas Jefferson University in Philadelphia. Dr. Yuen is a meditation teacher in the Shambhala and Tibetan Buddhist traditions, as well as an interfaith hospital chaplain. She is currently pursuing research in the field of spirituality and health.

Preface

This book is a compilation of chapters written by experts in their field on various modalities and dimensions of holistic health care and aging. We envision the book to be a compendium of reliable and authoritative information on complementary and alternative therapies that health professionals may use as they seek to improve the health and quality of life of those in their care.

Because the field is changing rapidly as *complementary and alternative medicine* translates itself into *integrated medicine,* and many modalities undergo scientific evaluation while others remain largely unexplored, any book on holistic health care is but a snapshot of a moving target. A generation ago, chiropractic was still on the fringes of acceptability, whereas now it is considered routine in most communities. Some of the modalities included here are well known, whereas others are more obscure. But they are all holistic in that they address the mind, emotions, and spirit as well as the body, and each has significance for an aging population.

It is difficult, if not impossible, to cover all holistic modalities in a single book. CAM modalities have a way of producing new variations at a considerable rate as practitioners experiment and recombine forms. A comprehensive treatise on bodywork alone, in addition to covering the myriad forms of massage (e.g., Swedish, shiatsu, deep tissue, and myofascial release), would require chapters on the Feldenkrais method, the Alexander technique, chiropractic, Network Spinal Analysis (NSA), zero balancing, Trager, Rolfing, craniosacral therapy, and reflexology. This is only a partial list and does not include the growing field of body psychotherapy or modalities that use energy medicine in conjunction with bodywork (e.g., polarity therapy). Rather than produce an encyclopedic collection of every conceivable modality (these already exist), what we have done here is to present an introduction to those modalities that may be of most use in the care of the aged, and are relatively easy to integrate into a conventional model of care or self-care. Most importantly, each chapter concludes with a list of resources that the reader can use to explore the topic further. If, for example, a geriatrician is caring for a patient who expresses an interest in taking valerian for her insomnia, the physician can refer to the chapter on herbs to learn more about it and can gather even more information by following the resources listed in the back, thereby gaining the ability to advise knowledgably. Or, if a social worker is concerned about one of his clients' mild depression, he can peruse this book for information on yoga, meditation, or acupuncture to get a sense of what might be of help and how to access classes or practitioners.

We begin the book with chapters on nutrition, herbs and supplements, and homeopathy. These are modalities that can be integrated into a medical practice or a program of guided self-care. Although physicians and nurses learn more about nutrition than formerly, most of us could always use more information on the healing properties of foods, especially as this topic relates to aging. Closely related to nutrition is the topic of herbs and supplements. Older adults can purchase all manner of substances over-the-counter, and sales of supplements such as melatonin, DHEA, and omega-3 fatty acids are brisk. Health care professionals who know something about the herbs and supplements that their patients are already taking are better equipped to deliver high-quality care, as are those who can advise patients on what to add (or not to add) to their regimen. Despite the fact that the therapeutic mechanism underlying homeopathy is controversial and not well understood by the biomedical community, we have included it here because homeopathic remedies are readily available over-the-counter and easily incorporated into conventional or self-care. Properly used, they also could serve as an important, inexpensive, and safe adjunctive therapy for many of the chronic conditions common among older adults.

The next chapters cover music, art, and massage therapies, services that require trained practitioners. Music and art therapies are most often found in institutionalized settings such as hospitals and nursing homes, where they are used to complement conventional care. People typically find massage therapists on their own, although holistic physicians frequently employ such therapists in their practices. It is one of the holistic modalities most underutilized by older adults, with numerous possible health benefits.

We grouped together the chapters dealing with Asian perspectives on health and healing, chiefly Chinese and Indian. Traditional Chinese medicine and Ayurveda are complex, cosmopolitan systems rooted in millennia of research and practice in their countries of origin. We chose to give the reader some sense of the underlying philosophy of the East, with chapters introducing some of the most accessible aspects of these systems (i.e., yoga, acupuncture, and qigong).

Next, we included chapters on spirituality and meditation, as well as two chapters that pertain most closely to improving the quality of life in long-term care. We feel that it is crucial for professionals to consistently consider the emotional and spiritual dimensions of health, especially when caring for persons who may be approaching the end of their lives.

This is purposefully not an "antiaging" book. In truth, the only remedy for growing older is death, for as long as we live, we age. Instead, we view this book as a collection of information on how to age healthfully by employing modalities that consider the whole person—body, mind, and spirit—in their approach, thus maximizing opportunities for the older adult to live his or her life to its fullest, as vibrant and vigorous as possible.

We hope this book will find its way into private practices, public clinics, hospitals, skilled nursing facilities, senior centers, anywhere health professionals are busy serving the "young-old," the "old-old," or even those on the threshold of becoming "old." Information within may inspire doctors, nurses, gerontologists, and social workers to learn more about integrated medicine, helping them include some of these approaches into their practices or giving them the necessary information so that they can confidently refer their clients and patients to holistic practitioners or activities. The more we know, the better we can serve the older adults who look to us for advice, relief, information, and care. May you enjoy this book in excellent health.

ELIZABETH R. MACKENZIE AND BIRGIT RAKEL

Acknowledgments

Books, especially ones like this, are the product of many persons' efforts, and the editors would like to thank those who contributed to its completion. Obviously, the chapter authors deserve the lion's share of thanks. We are profoundly grateful for their expertise and their willingness to pour their knowledge into this book.

ERM: In addition, I would like to thank Helvi Gold who initially approached me with the concept for the book and who (with her colleagues at Springer Publishing) waited patiently while it coalesced. Birgit Rakel's impeccable understanding of the practice of holistic medicine has been immensely valuable in shaping the content and contours of this book. I am also grateful to the following friends and teachers who have deepened my understanding of how holistic principles apply to health: Ute Arnold, Carrie Demers, MD (of the Himalayan Institute), Master FaXiang Hou, Bernardo Merizalde, MD, Deborah and Patrick Redmond, Suzanne Richman (Goddard's Health Arts and Sciences Program), and Joan White. Finally, I would like to express my gratitude to my academic mentors David J. Hufford, PhD and Risa Lavizzo-Mourey, MD, MBA for all their advice and help over the years.

BR: This book would not have been possible without Elizabeth Mackenzie's endurance, enthusiasm, and expertise. Thank you to everyone at Springer Publishing, but especially to Helvi Gold who supported us through the editing process. Thank you to my family and friends in Germany and the U.S. for all their encouragement, and to Jon Kabat-Zinn, PhD and Robert T. Sataloff, MD, DMA for inspiring me to reach beyond my limitations.

Foreword

Some years ago, I was participating in a review session for the *Healthy People 2000 Report,* in which national public health goals were articulated for the coming decade.

Among five "flagship" goals, there were two that literally didn't add up: to increase the average longevity and to increase the average number of years of healthy life span. There was a marked discrepancy in these goals for longevity and for healthy life span, with the latter being several years shorter than the former. My prediction for the headline in the *Washington Post* was "Government Says Alright to Be Ill the Last Several Years of Life."

Today, there is increasing concern that longevity not outdistance healthy life span and increasing evidence that therapies classified as holistic, alternative, and complementary may provide benefit. Most diseases and disorders are age-related. Age is the largest single risk factor for most cancers and many chronic diseases.

Utilization of complementary and alternative medicine (CAM) is widespread and increasing among adults in the United States (Micozzi, 2001). A recent survey showed that two thirds of adults show lifetime use of CAM by age 33 (Kessler et al., 2001), Further, CAM use is highest among post–baby boomers (7 out of 10), with only 5 out of 10 boomers and 3 out of 10 preboomers. These trends may represent an openness to CAM that has more to do with managing medical conditions than with lifelong attitudes inclusive of "holistic" healing.

In addition, two thirds of health maintenance organizations offered at least one type of alternative therapy as of 1999, (Wootton & Sparber 2003) with acupuncture, massage, and nutritional therapy the most likely modality to be added. The best predictor of CAM use is higher education, perhaps reflecting disposable income as well as knowledge, awareness, and attitudes.

Regional variations are quite consistent, with such diverse areas as South Carolina, Northern California, Florida, and Oregon all registering in the range of one half to two thirds of respondents to a survey using CAM (Wootton & Sparber 2003). Up to half of all clients do not tell their physicians, indicating that much additional work on integration of CAM into the continuum of care is needed.

A high proportion of adults with cancer utilize CAM. Several surveys found rates of 80% or higher. In one study, 40% of CAM users abandoned conventional care after adopting CAM. (Wooton & Sparber 2003) For breast cancer, despite the relative effectiveness of conventional care, CAM use was as high as 74%.

CAM use is also marked in neurological diseases, psychiatric disorders, physical disabilities, psoriasis, diabetes, and other disorders (Wootton & Sparber, 2003). The range of CAM modalities utilized are well reflected in the topics covered in this volume.

In addition to the management of medical conditions, CAM therapies have gained increasing attention in chronic disease prevention. Although CAM is often thought of as more related to healthy lifestyle and the prevention of disease, in fact, there has been more evidence about the effectiveness of CAM in treatment. Clinical trials on CAM are increasing in number, while prevention trials are larger, longer, more costly, more complex, and ultimately more rare (Moon & Micozzi, 1989).

Nonetheless, the article "Vitamins for Chronic Disease Prevention in Adults" by Fairfield and Fletcher in June 2002 in the *Journal of the American Medical Association* documented the importance of nutrition and finally provided substantiation for the role of dietary supplementation in light of the typical U.S. diet and nutrient composition of foods. Dietary supplement use is already prevalent among older Americans. In addition, efforts are under way to provide older Americans with dietary supplementation by the Healthy Foundation, with support from U.S. Senator Tom Harkin (D-Iowa) and by the Dietary Supplements for Senior Health Program with support from U.S. Senator Larry Craig (R-Idaho), who chaired the Senate Special Committee on Aging. In 2001, the Committee on Aging commissioned a report on the use of dietary supplements in older Americans by the General Accounting Office. The GAO report documented the problems associated with this practice but did not address the evidence of benefits; the Committee on Aging has promised to revisit the issue.

Because the interest and investment in CAM have broadened and deepened among health professionals, policymakers, and the public, this text is a timely addition to the literature on complementary and alternative medicine. It has been edited by two highly skilled and knowledgeable professionals in CAM research and practice, with contributions from a national sample of recognized experts in relevant fields. This important topic should be given a wide audience.

MARC MICOZZI, MD, PHD
Director, Informatics Institute for
Complementary and Integrative Medicine
Bethesda, MD

REFERENCES

Fletcher, R. H., & Fairfield, K. M. (2002). Vitamins for chronic disease prevention in adults. *Journal of the American Medical Association, 287*, 3127–3129.

Kessler, R. C., Davis, R. B., Foster, D. F., et al. (2001). Long term trends in the use of CAM therapies in the US. *Annals of Internal Medicine, 135*(4), 262–268.

Micozzi, M. S. (2006). *Fundamentals of complementary and alternative medicine* (3rd ed.). Philadelphia: Saunders

Moon, T. E., & Micozzi, M. S. (1989). *Nutrition and cancer prevention: Investigating the role of micronutrients*. New York: Marcel Dekker.

Wooton, J. C., & Sparber, A. (2003). Surveys of complementary and alternative medicine usage. *Seminars in Integrative Medicine, 1*(1), 10–24.

CHAPTER ONE

Holistic Approaches to Healthy Aging

Elizabeth R. Mackenzie and Birgit Rakel

Two large demographic realities of the contemporary United States are about to converge: The "baby boomer" generation now sits on the threshold of old age (defined as 65 and over), and use of complementary and alternative medicine (CAM) continues to increase, especially among those over age 40. One recent survey found that among the factors associated with the highest rates of CAM use was being age 40 to 64 (Tindle, Davis, Phillips, & Eisenberg, 2005). A survey of California seniors found that 41% of the older adult population uses CAM (Astin, Pelltier, Marie, & Haskell, 2000). Most national surveys show CAM use hovers around 30% to 60% of the adult population, and the trends point to increasing use.

The field of CAM and aging is likely to experience an explosion of growth in the next few years. Yet research into CAM applications to aging, per se, has just begun, and the health professionals who care for older adults typically receive no special training in CAM and aging.

As scientific advances shed increasing light on the effectiveness of specific treatments for certain conditions common in this population, older adults and the health professionals who serve them need an authoritative source in which reliable information is gathered. At present, the majority of older adults who use CAM do not discuss this use with their doctors (Astin et al., 2000), and few doctors raise the subject with their patients (Sleath, Rubin, Gwyther, & Clark, 2001). It is a de facto "don't ask, don't tell" policy. Yet the National Center for Complementary and Alternative Medicine (NCCAM) at the National Institutes of Health

(NIH) states, "Most importantly discuss all issues concerning treatment and therapies with your health care provider, whether a physician or practitioner of CAM. Competent healthcare management requires knowledge of both conventional and alternative therapies for the practitioner to have a complete picture of your treatment plan" (http://nccam.nih.gov/health/). To enhance communication, health professionals need a reliable source of information about CAM and aging, and older adults themselves need to be better informed about current scientific research on CAM.

The NIH's NCCAM defines CAM as "those treatments and health care practices not taught widely in medical schools, not generally used in hospitals, and not usually reimbursed by medical insurance companies." This covers a wide array of modalities. However, most have some underlying assumptions or perspectives in common. Very often, CAM differs from conventional medicine (or biomedicine) because it is "holistic" in that it acknowledges physical, mental, emotional, energetic, and spiritual dimensions of the individual in a way that conventional approaches typically do not. Although there is a growing interest in biopsychosocial approaches to health among practitioners and researchers, academic convention has typically compartmentalized the study of health into distinctly separate fields and subspecialties. Generally speaking, "holism" is one way to differentiate CAM from conventional medicine. A corollary to this is that CAM tends to seek healing the *person* rather than curing the *disease*. Another characteristic of holistic approaches is that they tend to focus on prevention and health promotion, rather than on treating symptoms after they have arisen. (Although many patients turn to CAM modalities for relief or cure, the basic philosophy of CAM is to pay attention to diet, lifestyle, thoughts, emotions, relationships, and even energetic imbalances before disease manifests.)

Because CAM modalities tend to be holistic in perspective, they generally do not categorically distinguish between mind and body, the physical and the mental. For this reason, they are ideally suited to patients with mental health problems, particularly those that are chronic or are related to other chronic conditions such as arthritic pain and fibromyalgia. Anxiety, depression, substance abuse, cognitive decline, and dementia are all conditions with complex etiologies that are treatable with CAM modalities. Chronic conditions have not responded as well, by and large, to conventional biomedicine as have acute conditions.

It may be that as specific CAM techniques continue to be tested and proven effective, integrating CAM modalities into regular treatment will become the standard of care for certain conditions. For example, a treatment protocol for cognitive decline has been developed and tested by the Alzheimer's Prevention Foundation that includes nutritional modification, nutrient supplementation, herbs (ginkgo biloba), medication, hormone replacement therapy, and mental training (e.g., headline discussion, music, and art) (Khalsa, 1998).

Massage, music therapy, and visualization have been shown to be effective in reducing anxiety and depression (Field, Quintino, Henteleff, Wells-Keife, & Delvecchio-Feinber, 1997), dietary factors have been implicated in mental health (Miller, 1996), and homeopathy has shown some intriguing promise in treating depression and anxiety (Davidson, Morrison, Shore, Davidson, & Bedayn, 1997). Furthermore, due to compatibility with nature and natural systems, CAM practices and substances are less likely to produce side effects and contribute to problems of polypharmacy than conventional pharmaceutical preparations.

Older adults tend to suffer from chronic conditions, many of which have a psychological or behavioral component. It is precisely for these types of ailments that CAM modalities are ideal. Biomedicine has been more successful in curing acute conditions than in treating chronic disease. This may be due in part to a failure to treat the whole person, including all biopsychosocial dimensions of the individual. Most CAM approaches simultaneously consider physical, mental, emotional, and energetic or spiritual factors of health and disease. In fact, a truly holistic approach does not make categorical distinctions among these dimensions. For an older adult experiencing depression, low back pain, arthritis, and social isolation, for example, conventional biomedical interventions (e.g., pain medication, antidepressants, and anti-inflammatory agents) tend not to address the root cause of these conditions, may create a chemical dependency, and may contribute to polypharmacy problems.

CAM approaches, such as regularly attending yoga classes, could help in all these areas. Yoga has been shown to be effective in reducing anxiety, controlling pain, and improving flexibility, and attending any class will diminish social isolation. Furthermore, for older adults at risk for polypharmacy problems, CAM modalities are potentially of great importance. If one or two medications could be reduced or eliminated as the result of some CAM intervention, the dangers of harmful drug interactions could be diminished while improving the individual's quality of life.

A review of the medical literature on CAM and conditions common among older adults suggests that there are alternative approaches to treating these conditions that have scientific merit but that are not yet widely prescribed (or even understood) by physicians. Moreover, few patients who are utilizing these remedies discuss this with their doctors (Astin et al., 2002). Some examples of CAM treatment for which there is good scientific evidence for effectiveness are glucosamine sulfate, acupuncture, and transcutaneous electrical nerve stimulation (TENS) for arthritis; meditation and biofeedback for hypertension; and exercise for depression.

ARTHRITIS

There is good scientific evidence that at least the following three CAM modalities are effective approaches to treating arthritis: glucosamine sulfate, acupuncture, and TENS. The nutrient glucosamine sulphate has been shown in several clinical trials to be an effective treatment for osteoarthritis (Bruyere et al., 2004; Cohen, Wolfe, Mai, & Lewis, 2003; Reginster et al., 2001). Although the exact mechanism of action is not known, one hypothesis is that glucosamine and chondroitin may have chondroprotective (cartilage-protecting) actions (Brief, Maurer, & DiCesare, 2001). Despite the uncertainty about the mechanism of action, the evidence is convincing enough to prompt the *Journal of the American Medical Association* to publish a meta-analysis of studies that concluded that glucosamine and similar substances probably are efficacious in the treatment of osetoarthritis (McAlindon, LaValley, & Felson, 2000). A 2001 article in *Current Rheumatology Reports* flatly states that the "documented efficacy of glucosamine for pain relief and function improvement in patients with knee osteoarthritis" requires that the American College of Rheumatology reassess their official recommendations with regard to first-line treatments for osteoarthritis (Hochberg, 2001). A systematic review of seven clinical trials found that acupuncture shows promise as a treatment for osteoarthritis of the knee (Ezzo et al., 2001). Among the randomized clinical trials is a 1999 study of 73 patients with osteoarthritis of the knee that found that acupuncture is an effective treatment (Berman et al., 1999). A subsequent study (also randomized) with 570 patients confirmed these results (Berman et al., 2004). Transcutaneous electrical nerve stimulation is another CAM intervention with scientifically backed claims to efficacy for arthritis. A systematic review of seven clinical trials found that TENS was more effective than placebo for pain control in arthritis patients (Osiri et al., 2000).

HYPERTENSION

Hypertension (or high blood pressure) is the most common cardiovascular risk factor in the United States; approximately 60% of adults have hypertension or prehypertension (Wang & Wang, 2004). Meditation and biofeedback have both been found to be useful in treating chronic hypertension. It has been well known for over 20 years that biofeedback can play a therapeutic role in the treatment of hypertension. One of the first trials of biofeedback for hypertension was conducted in 1976 and found positive results (Patel & Datey, 1976). Since that time, several trials have produced similar results (Henderson, Hart, Lal, & Hunyor, 1998;

Nakao, Yano, Nomura, & Kuboki, 2003), although others have yielded contradictory findings (Hunyor et al., 1997). There is also evidence that meditation is a useful practice for hypertensives. Several recent clinical trials published in major medical journals have shown that transcendental meditation (TM) produces a reduction in hypertension among various populations (Barnes, Treiber, & Davis, 2001; Castillo-Richmond et al., 2000; Schneider et al., 2005). A recent pilot trial of a form of Ayurvedic medicine (Maharishi Vedic medicine) among older adults found that this approach was useful in reducing the risk for coronary heart disease (Fields et al., 2002).

DEPRESSION

It is estimated that 15% to 20% of older adults experience symptoms of depression (Gallo & Lebowitz, 1999), which may not be adequately treated due to the stigma of receiving psychotherapy and the side effects associated with antidepressants. Many studies have shown that aerobic exercise decreases depressive symptoms (Kritz-Silverstein, Barrett-Connor, & Corbeau, 2001; Lane & Lovejoy 2001; Moore & Blumenthal 1998). Attending religious services likewise appears to improve mood (McCullough & Larson, 1999), and there is some evidence that prayer may reduce symptoms of depression and anxiety (Rajagopal, Mackenzie, Bailey, & Lavizzo-Mourey, 2002). There is also limited evidence that diet (Miller, 1996) and homeopathy (Davidson et al., 1997) can be useful adjunctive therapies in the treatment of depression.

The modalities discussed above are just the tip of the iceberg regarding holistic health care and aging. This brief review, however, shows that there is already scientific evidence for CAM use that is not yet thoroughly disseminated among health professionals or their elderly patients. In fact, some commentators have noted that the potential benefits that CAM modalities have to offer older adults mandate their exploration and, when appropriate, their integration.

INEFFECTIVE, CONTRAINDICATED, DANGEROUS, OR UNPROVEN THERAPIES

It should be noted that not all CAM therapies are always effective, benign, appropriate, or properly understood. Several herbal remedies are contraindicated for certain patients, for example. Licorice root tends to raise blood pressure and should not be used by hypertensives, and ginkgo biloba is a blood thinner that can adversely interact with antithrombotic drugs or even aspirin. The antianxiety herb kava kava has been implicated in liver toxicity (Russmann, Lauterburg, & Helbling, 2001), and some herbs commonly used in traditional Chinese medicine may be harmful (Chang, Wang, Yang, and Chiang, 2001).

Despite the NCCAM's increased funding for the scientific assessment of CAM, many remedies fall under the category "unproven." It is worth noting that this merely indicates that no definitive scientific research has yet been conducted. An unproven intervention or treatment may well turn out to be effective once the research findings are complete. However, without proof, caveat emptor. The intervention could also turn out to be harmless but ineffective, or (rarely) harmful. Normally, the less invasive the treatment, the lower the probability of risk. Because so many CAM treatments are not invasive relative to conventional medicine, the risk tends to be low. Although there may be no large-scale clinical trials of massage therapy for fibromyalgia to prove its effectiveness, for example, receiving regular treatments from a practitioner licensed in therapeutic massage is unlikely to harm. On the other hand, a more invasive intervention such as chelation therapy (itself not a holistic therapy per se, but a medical procedure first developed to treat heavy metal toxicity) may pose some health risks, has little scientific data to back its claims, and is quite costly. The three most important questions to ask about an unproven treatment are What is its potential to do harm? What will it cost? and What does the anecdotal evidence say?

CONCLUSION

Educating consumers and providers of health care about CAM in all its dimensions and manifestations is critically important at this juncture. Persons over 85 are the fastest growing age segment of the U.S. population, and with this trend comes increased numbers of persons managing the chronic ailments and diseases of old age (Dossey, 2002). It is inevitable that large numbers of persons will turn to CAM to seek treatments for some of these conditions, and the more accurate information about this topic available to them and their caregivers, the better off they will be. This book will help deliver reliable information about CAM and aging on which older adults and the persons who care for them can rely.

REFERENCES

Astin, J. A., Pelltier, K. R., Marie, A., & Haskell, W. L. (2000). Complementary and alternative medicine use among elderly persons: one-year analysis of a Blue Shield Medicare supplement. *Journal of Gerontology A, 55*(1), M4–9.

Barnes, V. A., Treiber, F. A., & Davis, H. (2001). Impact of transcendental meditation on cardiovascular function at rest and during acute stress in adolescents with high normal blood pressure. *Journal of Psychosomatic Reseach*, *51*(4), 597–605.

Berman, B. M., Lao, L., Langenberg, P., Lee, W. L., Gilpin, A. M., & Hochberg, M. C. (2004). Effectiveness of acupuncture as an adjunctive therapy in osteoarthritis of the knee: A randomized, controlled trial. *Annals of Internal Medicine, 141*(12), 901–910.

Berman, B. M., Singh, B. B., Lao, L., Langenberg, P., Li, H., Hadhazy, V., Bareta, J., Hochberg M. (1999). A randomized trial of acupuncture as an adjunctive therapy in osteoarthritis of the knee. *Rheumatology, 38*(4), 346–354.

Brief, A. A., Maurer, S. G., & DiCesare, P. E. (2001). Use of glucosamine and chondroitin sulfate in the management of osteoarthritis. *Journal of the American Academy of Orthopedic Surgeons, 9*(2), 71–78.

Bruyere, O., Pavelka, K., Rovati, L. C., Deroisy, R., Olejarova, M., Gatterova, J., et al. (2004). Glucosamine sulfate reduces osteoarthritis progression in postmenopausal women with knee osteoarthritis: Evidence from two 3-year studies. *Menopause, 11*(2), 138–143.

Castillo-Richmond, A., Schneider, R. H., Alexander, C. N., Cook, R., Myers, H., Nidich, S., et al. (2000). Effects of stress reduction on carotid atherosclerosis in hypertensive African Americans. *Stroke, 31*(3), 568–573.

Chang, C. H., Wang, Y. M., Yang, A.H., & Chiang, S. S. (2001). Rapidly progressive interstitial renal fibrosis associated with Chinese herbal medications. *American Journal of Nephrology, 21*(6), 441–448.

Cohen, M., Wolfe, R., Mai, T., Lewis, D. (2003). A randomized, double blind, placebo controlled trial of a topical cream containing glucosamine sulfate, chondroitin sulfate, and camphor for osteoarthritis of the knee. *Journal of Rheumatology, 30*(3), 523–528.

Davidson, J. R., Morrison, R. M., Shore, J., Davidson, R. T., & Bedayn, G. (1997). Homeopathic treatment of depression and anxiety. *Alternative Therapies in Health and Medicine, 3*(1), 46–49.

Dossey, L. (2002). Longevity. *Alternative Therapies in Health and Medicine, 8*(3), 12–16, 125–134.

Ezzo, J., Hadhazy, V., Birch, S., Lao, L., Kaplan, G., Hochberg, M., & Berman, B. (2001). Acupuncture for osteoarthritis of the knee: A systematic review. *Arthritis Rheum, 44*(4), 819–825.

Field, T., Quintino, O., Henteleff, T., Wells-Keife, L., & Delvecchio-Feinber, G. (1997). Job stress reduction therapies. *Alternative Therapies in Health and Medicine, 3*(4), 54–56.

Fields, J. Z., Walton, K. G., Schneider, R. H., Nidich, S., Pomerantz, R., Suchdev, P., et al. (2002). Effect of a multimodality natural medicine program on carotid atherosclerosis in older subject: A pilot trial of Maharishi Vedic medicine. *American Journal of Cardiology, 89*(8), 952–958.

Gallo, J. J., & Lebowitz, B. D. (1999). The epidemiology of common late-life mental disorders in the community: Themes for a new century. *Psychiatric Services, 50*(9), 1158–1166.

Henderson, R. J., Hart, M. G., Lal, S. K., & Hunyor, S. N. (1998). The effect of home training with direct blood pressure biofeedback of hypertensives: A placebo-controlled study. *Journal of Hypertension, 16*(6), 771–778.

Hochberg, M. C. (2001). What a difference a year makes: Reflections on the ACR recommendations for the medical management of osteoarthritis. *Current Rheumatology Report, 3*(6), 473–478.

Hunyer, S. N., Henderson, R. J., Lal, S. K., Carter, N. L., Kobler, H., Jones, M., et al. (1997). Placebo-controlled biofeedback blood pressure effect in hypertensive humans. *Hypertension, 29*(6), 1225–1231.

Khalsa, D. S. (1998). Integrated medicine and the prevention and reversal of memory loss. *Alternative Therapies in Health and Medicine, 4*(6), 38–43.

Kritz-Silverstein, D., Barrett-Connor, E., & Corbeau, C. (2001). Cross-sectional and prospective study of exercise and depressed mood in the elderly: The Rancho Bernardo study. *American Journal of Epidemiology, 153*(6), 596–603.

Lane, A. M., & Lovejoy, D. J. (2001). The effects of exercise on mood changes: The moderating effect of depressed mood. *Journal of Sports Medicine and Fitness, 41*(4), 539–545.

McAlindon, T. E., LaValley, M. P., & Felson, D. T. (2000). Efficacy of glucosamine and chondroitin for treatment of osteoarthritis. *Journal of the American Medical Association, 284*(10), 1241.

McCollough, M. E., & Larson, D. B. (1999). Religion and depression: A review of the literature. *Twin Research, 2*(2), 126–136.

Miller, M. (1996). Diet and psychological health. *Alternative Therapies in Health and Medicine, 2*(5), 40–48.

Moore, K. A., & Blumenthal, J. A. (1998). Exercise training as an alternative treatment for depression among older adults. *Alternative Therapies in Health and Medicine, 4*(1), 48–56.

Nakao, M., Yano, E., Nomura, S., & Kuboki, T. (2003). Blood pressure-lowering effects of biofeedback treatment in hypertension: A meta-analysis of randomized controlled trials. *Hypertension Research, 26*(1), 37–46.

Osiri, M., Welch, V., Brosseau, L., Shea, B., McGowan, J., Tugwell, P., & Wells, G. (2000). Transcutaneous electrical nerve stimulation for knee osteoarthritis. *Cochrane Database Systematic Review, 4,* CD002823.

Patel, C., & Datey, K. K. (1976). Relaxation and biofeedback techniques in the management of hypertension. *Angiology, 27*(2), 106–113.

Rajagopal, D., Mackenzie, E., Bailey, C., & Lavizzo-Mourey, R. (2002). The effectiveness of a spiritually-based intervention for relieving subsyndromal anxiety and minor depression in older adults. *Journal of Religion and Health, 41*(2), 153–166.

Reginster, J. Y., Deroisy, R., Rovati, L. C., Lee, R. L., Lejeune, E., Bruyere, O., et al. (2001). Long-term effects of glucosamine sulphate on osteoarthritis progression: A randomized, placebo-controlled clinical trial. *Lancet, 357*(9252), 251–256.

Russmann, S., Lauterburg, B. H., & Helbling, A. (2001). Kava hepatotoxicity. *Annals of Internal Medicine, 135*(1), 68–69.

Sleath, B., Rubin, R. H., Campbell, W., Gwyther, L., & Clark, T. (2001). Ethnicity and physician—older patient communication about alternative therapies. *Journal of Alternative and Complementary Medicine, 7*(4), 329–335.

Tindle, H. A., Davis, R. B., Phillips, R. S., & Eisenberg, D. M. (2005). Trends in use of complementary and alternative medicine by US adults: 1997–2002. *Alternative Therapies in Health and Medicine, 11*(1), 42–49.

Wang, Y., & Wang, Q. J. (2004). The prevalence of prehypertension and hypertension among US adults according to the new joint national committee guidelines: New challenges of the old problem. *Archives of Internal Medicine, 164*(19), 2126–2134.

CHAPTER TWO

Healthy and Therapeutic Diets That Promote Optimal Aging

Joel S. Edman

Good nutrition is an important foundation for optimal aging. This chapter will focus on the major concerns that occur with aging, such as cardiovascular disease, cancer, osteoporosis and cognitive dysfunction. Other aspects of diet and dietary guidelines as they relate to aging also will be discussed. Information about other aging-related diseases may be obtained from the resource list provided at the end of this chapter.

Although this chapter will focus on dietary approaches, it is important to realize that diet is closely linked with nutritional supplementation for several reasons. First, therapeutic levels of many nutrients often cannot be achieved by diet alone. Second, if dietary guidelines are too difficult for patients to follow, it can be a relief to patients to recommend a less stringent diet that is complemented by nutritional supplementation. Third, it is important to appreciate that the basis of good nutrition is an effective dietary regimen and that nutritional supplementation can add to significant therapeutic effects. Some people focus on nutritional supplementation, believing that it can overcome a poor diet; in my experience, this is usually not successful.

HOW DIETS AND DIETARY GUIDELINES DIFFER IN AN INTEGRATIVE MEDICAL SETTING IN COMPARISON TO A DIETETICS SETTING

There are a few key differences between medical nutrition therapy practiced in an integrative or complementary and alternative medicine (CAM) clinic in comparison to a dietetics clinic. One primary difference is that integrative nutritionists are much more likely to recommend therapeutic

11

diets for all symptoms or disorders. For example, the avoidance or limitation of refined sugars and flour products is considered very important, as is the recommendation for more fresh and better quality foods such as those that are organically grown. Integrative nutritionists are also more likely to recommend more extreme therapeutic diets, such as a vegan or vegetarian diet, an elimination diet, a macrobiotic diet, the Ornish diet, the Gerson diet, or the Atkins diet. Elimination diets are often recommended for irritable bowel syndrome (IBS), inflammatory bowel disease (IBD), migraines, allergy/sensitivity, and other disorders. Another important distinction is that nutritionists and integrative medical practitioners are much more likely to prescribe nutritional supplements to go along with therapeutic diets, whereas most dietitians are often not trained in the use of nutritional supplements and have little experience with their use.

CARDIOVASCULAR DISEASE

Important Dietary Guidelines for Preventing Cardiovascular Disease

Perhaps the most important factors contributing to cardiovascular disease (CVD) are insulin resistance and the development of insulin resistance syndrome, metabolic syndrome, or dysmetabolic syndrome. One study estimated the prevalence of metabolic syndrome in the United States at 47 million people (Ford, Giles, & Dietz, 2002). The characteristics of metabolic syndrome have been well described (Reaven, 1995) and are presented in Figure 2.1. It clearly illustrates that environmental factors (diet, exercise, stress, etc.) and genetic influences can contribute to insulin resistance as the central characteristic that appears to cause a variety of cardiovascular risk factors.

Obesity, especially central obesity, is thought to be the primary cause of insulin resistance and metabolic syndrome; however, this does not always appear to be true. For example, 50% of patients with essential hypertension are believed to have insulin resistance, and obesity is not always present (Feldstein et al., 2002).

A good review of diet and CVD prevention can be found in Hu and Willett (2002). The review suggested that convincing evidence supports three dietary strategies: in Figure 2.1:

1. Substituting nonhydrogenated unsaturated fat for saturated and trans fats
2. Increasing intake of omega-3 fatty acids from fish, flaxseeds, soy, nuts, and green leafy vegetables
3. Consuming a diet high in vegetables, fruits, nuts, and whole grains, and low in refined grain products

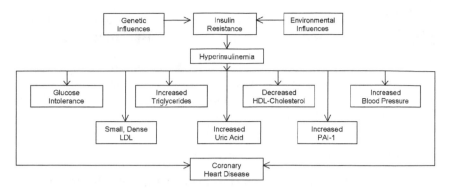

FIGURE 2.1 Metabolic syndrome and insulin resistance. (From G. M. Reaven, *Physiology Review, 75,* **473–486.)**

HDL, high-density lipoprotein; LDL, low-density lipoprotein; PAI-1, plasminogen activator inhibitor.

Incorporating Dietary Fat Guidelines Into Practical Dietary Suggestions

The first step outlined above refers to decreasing saturated fat and trans fat in the diet. Saturated fat is found in animal products, such as red meat and whole-milk dairy. These should be reduced in the diet and replaced by proteins such as fish high in omega-3 fatty acids (e.g., salmon, sardines, tuna, and mackerel) and beans or legumes, including soy and soy products. Trans fats are present in hydrogenated oils found in many refined grain and flour products, such as cookies, crackers, and cakes. These should be minimized or avoided. Increasing monounsaturated fat in the diet would come from nuts and seeds, avocado, olive oil, and foods or dressings made with these ingredients.

Benefits

There are three main benefits from these guidelines:

1. Increasing food nutritional value from
   - Vitamins
   - Phytochemicals—flavanoids, carotinoids, lignans, etc.
   - Minerals
   - Healthy fatty acids (monounsaturated and omega-3s)
   - Fiber
2. Low glycemic index/glycemic load foods: These produce a slower increase in blood glucose that positively influences insulin levels and insulin resistance. More recent research suggests that

glycemic load may be a better indicator because it assesses glycemic index plus the carbohydrate quantity, although more studies are needed.
3. Decreasing the intake of refined foods that are often of poor nutritional value and high in calories: This is especially effective when healthy snacks (fruit, nuts and seeds, vegetables, etc.) can be consumed in place of high sugar and fat snacks.

Individualizing Diets

It is essential to individualize diets to maximize the benefit to patients and have patients effectively comply with recommendations. For example, the primary feature of insulin resistance and metabolic syndrome is central obesity. If patients can successfully lose weight, they can greatly reduce their risk for CVD. However, there are many that do well with a balanced calorie deficit diet such as Weight Watchers, and others that do well with a lower carbohydrate approach such as the Carbohydrate Addict's diet or the Atkins diet (dietary carbohydrate limited to 15–100 g per day). More research is needed, however, to determine the optimal type and amount of protein, carbohydrate, and fat for each person, with the understanding that restrictive diets are very difficult to maintain over the long term. Therefore, lifestyle approaches that provide guidelines for diet and exercise are important for both weight loss and maintenance of weight loss.

An integrative medicine setting would also be much more likely to encourage and support a lifestyle approach that includes regular exercise, stress management techniques, and other approaches that may be specifically needed by individual patients. For example, emotional eating and sugar cravings are often challenges that need to be effectively addressed in order to lose weight and control blood sugar and cholesterol over the long term. These issues also need to be addressed for patients with IBS, IBD, rheumatoid arthritis, cancer, and other disorders in which diet has an important therapeutic role.

Recommended Diet for Cholesterol Reduction

The guidelines described above to include more vegetables, fruit, whole grains, and nuts for reducing CVD risk are also suggested for cholesterol reduction. This was the gist of the Adult Treatment Panel (ATP III) recommendations from the National Cholesterol Education Program (NCEP) (Pasternak, 2003). However, the role of glycemic regulation or control in influencing triglyceride and cholesterol levels is underappreciated. This is one of the main reasons for the improvement of lipids on a low carbohydrate diet, although there are many important factors (Foster et al., 2003; Westman et al., 2002).

Approaches to Help Reduce or Control Hypertension

There has been an interesting progression of dietary research that has been done to examine blood pressure. This research has reflected four phases:

1. Sodium restriction: This has been very controversial, with advocates and detractors staking out very firm positions (Luft & Weinberger, 1997). Some people are salt sensitive, whereas others are not, but the prudent approach would suggest some limits, with the broader approach recommended here.

2. Dietary Approaches to Stop Hypertension (DASH): This showed a significant influence of a diet high in whole grains, vegetables, and fruit, with other guidelines producing an improvement in blood pressure that was greater for hypertensives and African Americans (Appel et al., 1997).

3. Sodium restriction and DASH: Sodium restriction had an additive beneficial effect to the DASH diet (Sacks et al., 2001).

4. Diet and comprehensive lifestyle: Lifestyle factors (weight loss, sodium restriction, increased physical activity, and limited alcohol) were combined with DASH and found to reduce blood pressure in those with above-optimal blood pressure and those with stage 1 hypertension (Appel, 2003).

Specific mention should also be made regarding dietary magnesium effects because there is evidence that magnesium supplementation can reduce blood pressure (Witteman et al., 1994). This probably occurs because magnesium produces a vasodilating effect. Magnesium also has important influences on glucose tolerance and diabetes (Paolisso et al., 1989).

Dietary Influences on Newer Risk Factors for Cardiovascular Disease

There are dietary influences on newer risk factors for CVD, such as high-sensitivity C-reactive protein (hs-CRP) and homocysteine.

High-Sensitivity C-Reactive Protein

More recent research suggests that hs-CRP is an independent risk factor for CVD and may be the single best predictor of future cardiac events (Ridker et al., 2003). Two recent studies have shown that dietary guidelines can reduce hs-CRP levels. One study showed beneficial effects for a lower glycemic load diet (Liu et al., 2002). Another recent investigation showed that a vegetarian dietary portfolio reduced hs-CRP significantly, and it was comparable to the reduction produced by a statin (Jenkins et al., 2003). The diet portfolio was high in plant sterols, viscous fiber (from oats, barley, and psyllium), soy, almonds, and other specific foods.

Homocysteine

Dietary folate does correlate with homocysteine levels; however, it is important to remember a few issues. First, dietary adjustments are helpful for reducing CVD risk, but supplementation is appropriate to reduce homocysteine levels. Also, an important cause of elevated homocysteine is that there are two common genetic polymorphisms/single nucleotide polymorphisms (SNPs) that reduce the activity of the primary enzyme that metabolizes homocysteine, methyltetrahydrofolate reductase (MTHFR). Again, this suggests that diet has an important role, but supplemental folate may be necessary to compensate for this genetic influence.

Relationship Between Antioxidants and Cardiovascular Disease

The investigations of the relationship between antioxidant nutrients and CVD have largely been disappointing. There are, however, several factors that complicate this relationship, including the following: (1) the oxidation of low-density lipoprotein (LDL) cholesterol is one of the earlier steps in the atherosclerosis process that may make it more difficult to assess; (2) many of the studies have looked only at vitamins C and/or E, whereas there are many more potent phytonutrients (some known and perhaps some still to be identified) that may need to be evaluated either individually or in combination; and (3) there are no good clinical measures of oxidative stress that have been found to be effective in human research in that they correlate with clinical outcomes.

CANCER

Important Dietary Guidelines for Preventing Cancer

Some of the most important guidelines for preventing cancer are the following:

1. The National Cancer Institute's Five-a-Day program for vegetables and fruit: This is largely the effort to promote a natural healthy diet rich in vitamins, minerals, phytonutrients, fiber, and other factors. Added to this are recommendations for beans or legumes and whole grains, which are also good sources of health-promoting nutrition.

2. Maintaining healthy weight: Although more research is needed to understand the mechanisms, increased weight and insulin resistance appear to increase the risk for colon cancer, breast cancer, prostate cancer, and other types of cancer. Therefore, in addition to encouraging foods listed in point 1, as well as including healthy fats such as omega-3 fatty acids and monounsaturated fats, limiting highly processed and refined foods, or "junk food," is important.

3. Recommendations for specific types of cancer: Lycopene (mostly from tomato products) and soy products (containing isoflavones), for example, have been shown to be protective of prostate cancer (Giovannucci, 1999; Messina, 2003). Also, having more than five servings of alcohol per week appears to increase the risk of breast cancer (Li et al., 2003).

Conflicting or Inconclusive Study Results in Cancer Research

There are several problems and challenges in conducting nutrition and cancer research:

1. Many dietary factors are interrelated: For example, if a cancer patient is encouraged to change from a typical American diet to a vegetarian-based diet, the recommended diet will likely be higher in fiber, phytochemicals, unsaturated fats, vitamins, and minerals, and lower in saturated fats and animal proteins. It is therefore difficult to evaluate the influence of one or two specific factors.

2. Quantifying dietary intake is imprecise: Food records and food frequency questionnaires provide estimates of nutritional content, especially when considering that foods grown in different environments or soils can have different nutritional contents. There can also be differences in nutrient loss based on manufacturing and distribution factors. Finally, there are concerns about the accuracy of describing meal composition and quantifying portion sizes.

3. There are many different types and stages of cancer that have varying influences: These include immune factors, genetics, emotional or psychological factors, and environmental factors. Sometimes only the most powerful influences are identified through current research models.

Relationship Between Dietary Fat and Cancer

The relationship between dietary fat and cancer is controversial because there are studies showing that higher fat diets increase the risk of some cancers, whereas other studies have shown that they do not. The reason for these conflicting results, in addition to the problems described previously, is probably that it is important to look at the types and amounts of different fats. For example, fats are categorized as saturated, monounsaturated, and polyunsaturated, and the optimal balance for immune function, cancer prevention, and/or cancer treatment is unknown. Fat intake may be further categorized by the omega-3/omega-6 fatty acid ratio. This could have effects on cancer-related issues such as immune function, inflammation, and hormonal balance.

Dietary fat intake is also associated with choices for dietary proteins. With regard to protein foods and the types of fat associated with them, fish consumption and associated omega-3 fatty acids appear to decrease prostate cancer risks, whereas red meat and cooking effects increase the risk of some cancers. Most nutritionists would generally agree, however, that dietary saturated fat and trans fats should be reduced, and dietary omega-3 fatty acids and monounsaturated fats should be increased.

Anticancer Phytochemicals

Table 2.1 shows the foods and food groups that contain phytonutrients, which may influence cancer risk.

Relationship Between Antioxidants and Cancer

As described in Table 2.1, many foods contain antioxidant phytonutrients that may be beneficial for cancer prevention. Numerous studies have found an inverse association between diets high in vegetables and fruit and cancer risk. Despite this evidence, the specific cause or mechanism that underlies this relationship has not been definitively shown. The most likely antioxidant mechanisms are protection from free radical damage to tissues and/or preservation of immune function. As mentioned previously, however, diets higher in vegetables and fruit have other differences that may influence risk, such as altered fatty acid composition and increased fiber intake.

Antioxidant influence and use during cancer treatment are very controversial, although this is mainly concerned with antioxidant nutritional supplements that may interfere with chemotherapy and radiation therapy effectiveness. Most nutritionists would agree to recommend a diet as healthy as possible that would contain significant amounts of antioxidant nutrients and phytonutrients. Nutritional guidelines for cancer patients and cancer survivors remain one of the most important areas for future research.

Effects of Refined or Nutrient-Poor Diets on Nutritional Deficiency and Cancer Risk

Deficiencies of micronutrients such as folate, vitamin B_{12}, vitamin C, vitamin E, iron, and zinc can mimic radiation damage by producing

TABLE 2.1 Examples of Anticancer Phytochemicals

Phytochemical	Actions	Sources
Carotenes	Antioxidants Enhance immune functions	Dark-colored vegetables such as carrots, squash, spinach, kale, tomatoes, yams, and sweet potatoes; fruits such as cantaloupe, apricots, and citrus fruits
Coumarin	Antitumor properties Enhance immune functions Stimulate antioxidant mechanisms	Carrots, celery, fennel, beets, and citrus fruits
Dithiolthiones, glucosinolates, and thiocyanates	Block cancer-causing compounds from damaging cells Enhance detoxification	Cabbage family vegetables: broccoli, Brussels sprouts, kale, etc.
Flavonoids	Antioxidants Direct antitumor effects Immune-enhancing properties	Fruits, particularly richly colored fruits such as berries, cherries, and citrus fruits; also tomatoes, peppers, and greens
Isoflavonoids	Block estrogen receptors	Soy and other legumes
Lignans	Antioxidants Modulate hormone receptors	Flaxseed and flaxseed oil; whole grains, nuts, and seeds
Limonoids	Enhance detoxification Block carcinogens	Citrus fruits and celery
Polyphenols	Antioxidants Block carcinogen formation Modulate hormone receptors	Green tea, chocolate, and red wine
Sterols	Block production of carcinogens Modulate hormone receptors	Soy, nuts, and seeds

From Murray, M., Birdsall, T., Pizzorno, J. E., et al. (2002). *How to prevent and treat cancer with natural medicine.* New York: Riverhead Books.

chromosomal deoxyribonucleic acid (DNA) single- and double-strand breaks and/or oxidative lesions. Ames (2001) found that the level of folate deficiency that may cause DNA damage was present in approximately 10% of the U.S. population and that it was much higher in poor Americans.

Obesity and Cancer

A 16-year study by the American Cancer Society found that overweight and obesity increases the risk of many types of cancers, and increases the death rate from several forms of cancers (Calle et al., 2003). This was true for almost all cancers. The potential mechanisms include

1. Higher levels of sex hormones such as estrogens
2. Higher levels of insulin and growth factors, such as insulin-like growth factors
3. Pro-inflammatory activity

Dietary Guidelines for Treating Cancer

This research is just beginning in earnest. It is fairly difficult research to do because there are so many variables to control, and the methods for dietary analysis are not very precise. Therefore, most practitioners largely recommend the same diets for primary and secondary prevention. A good discussion of nutritional guidelines for cancer survivors has been presented in *CA: A Cancer Journal for Clinicians* (2001; Vol. 51, No. 3).

Therapeutic Diets as Adjuvant Cancer Therapy

Very little controlled research has been done on therapeutic diets, such as the macrobiotic and Gerson diets, as a treatment for cancer, and most of the reports are anecdotal. One particular case series of 23 pancreatic cancer patients who followed a macrobiotic diet showed a significant improvement in length of survival (Carter et al., 1993). With regard to the Gerson diet, there is a report that suggests that this approach may increase 5-year survival rates for melanoma (Hildenbrand et al., 1995).

It is okay to recommend these diets until more objective data are collected. Caution should be exercised, however, to monitor these patients carefully, as all cancer patients should be monitored. Also, consideration must be given to the difficulty of these kinds of restrictive diets. Therefore, these programs should be available to those who are most interested in making the kinds of dietary and lifestyle changes that are required, but they should not be promoted through tactics that draw on feelings of fear or guilt.

Future Research on the Relationship Between Diet/Nutrition and Cancer

Although there are many ongoing areas of research that are important, perhaps the most important research that is needed will more specifically examine cancer survivorship and diet/nutrition. In addition, information will emerge about the specific phases of cancer and mechanisms of pathology, such as cancer initiation, angiogenesis, apoptosis, and inflammation, that may be influenced by diet and nutritional supplementation. Finally, other miscellaneous issues that are more specifically considered by integrative medicine practitioners will be examined, including

1. Dietary quality: organic versus nonorganic foods
2. Environmental toxicity influence on immune function and susceptibility to cancer
3. Detoxification methods for cancer prevention and treatment

Recommendations for Patients With Cancer

It is very important for patients with cancer to follow as healthy a diet as they can. This would include eating a vegetarian-based diet, incorporating specific cancer-fighting foods, and avoiding or minimizing refined sugars, refined flour products, and other unhealthy foods. In fact, diet should be considered a foundation approach that is combined in an integrative model that addresses regular exercise, stress management techniques, dietary supplements, psychosocial-spiritual support, and other CAM modalities.

A healthy diet is important because it

1. Provides important vitamins, minerals, fatty acids, and phytochemicals
2. Helps people feel better physically and emotionally on a day-to-day basis
3. Encourages patients' participation in their care and healing, and provides a measure of control
4. Gives patients hope

OSTEOPOROSIS

Important Dietary Guidelines for Preventing and Treating Osteoporosis

Dietary guidelines are very important for preventing osteoporosis. These guidelines need to be part of an integrative program that addresses sunlight exposure (for vitamin D status), exercise, and factors that contribute to excessive calcium excretion (protein, caffeine, soda and alcohol intake, and smoking).

The most important dietary guideline involves the intake of calcium. Although this mineral is found in the highest levels in dairy products, there are many other foods that contain calcium, such as specific types of fish, dark green leafy vegetables, soy/tofu, nuts and seeds, dried fruits, kelp, and sea vegetables.

There are also studies supporting the influence of magnesium on bone density and strength (Stendig-Lindberg, Tepper, & Leichter, 1993). Magnesium is also found in many of the foods listed above, but another good source is whole grains.

In most cases, however, calcium, magnesium, and vitamin D intake should be complemented by nutritional supplementation to ensure that appropriate levels of these nutrients are obtained. As described below, there are often many problems in the elderly that may contribute to poor intake, absorption, and/or utilization of nutrients. Finally, these guidelines should be recommended based on objective findings established through bone densitometry testing.

Malnutrition and Nutritional Deficiency in the Elderly

Some of the general issues that contribute to malnutrition and nutritional deficiency in the elderly are the following:

- Depression
- Chronic or intercurrent diseases
- Disability, loss of independence
- Loss of a spouse, bereavement
- Financial problems, poverty
- Alcohol abuse
- Polypharmacy
- Visual impairment
- Mental impairment, confusion
- Surgery

Aging and Adequate Levels of Calcium, Magnesium, and Vitamin D

There are several specific problems related to aging that may make it more difficult to get adequate levels of calcium, magnesium, and vitamin D. Many older patients, for example, may have difficulties with dental problems that make chewing difficult or painful. Still others may have gastrointestinal disorders such, as hypochlorhydria or atrophic gastritis, which impair the digestion of foods and absorption of important dietary nutrients. Another important problem is lack of sunlight for producing vitamin D.

Vitamin D Deficiency in the Elderly

As many as 50% of institutionalized and free-living elderly may have vitamin D hypovitaminosis (Holick, 2003). Although much of this prevalence may come from inadequate sunlight, especially for the elderly who live in higher latitude climates, vitamin D–fortified foods (e.g., milk, bread, and cereal) have previously been found to contain variable levels of vitamin D.

Green Leafy Vegetables and Osteoporosis

Green leafy vegetables contain a variety of minerals and vitamins that have a central role in maintaining bone health. The two most important, calcium and magnesium, have been discussed above. However, two other nutrients found in green leafy vegetables are being shown to have significant influences:

1. Vitamin K_1 (the form of vitamin K found in plants): Vitamin K_1 helps to convert osteocalcin to its active form. Osteocalcin constitutes a major portion of the noncollagen protein matrix in bone and helps to hold calcium molecules in place.
2. Boron: Boron appears to function as a cofactor for the conversion of vitamin D to its active form, 1,25-dihydroxy D_3.

COGNITIVE DYSFUNCTION

There are several studies that support a relationship between diet and memory problems, or cognitive dysfunction. In the Rotterdam study, for example, a higher saturated fat and cholesterol diet was found to increase the risk of dementia, whereas dietary fish consumption was found to decrease risk (Kalmijn et al., 1997). A more recent study supported this finding when it reported that eating fish once per week or more was associated with a 60% reduced risk of developing Alzheimer's disease (AD) (Morris et al., 2003). This study also found that total intake of omega-3 fatty acids correlated with reduced risk. Other sources of omega-3 fatty acids include nuts and seeds (especially flaxseeds), dark green leafy vegetables, and soy products.

A recent study of antioxidant vitamin intake did not show a relationship between dietary, supplemental, or total intake of carotenes and vitamins C and E and risk of AD (Luchsinger et al., 2003). However, it is well accepted that oxidative stress is involved in the pathogenesis of AD.

Although there is some research suggesting that antioxidants are protective (Tabet et al., 2002), the data are currently weak.

Cardiovascular Disease and Dementia

There is a clearer relationship between diet and cardiovascular disease that in turn contributes to the second leading cause of dementia, multi-infarct dementia. As described in the section on cardiovascular disease, therapeutic dietary guidelines are beneficial for improving cholesterol levels, hypertension, type 2 diabetes, and overweight and obesity.

Research has also shown that impaired glucose tolerance is associated with poor memory and hippocampal atrophy in a healthy elderly population (Convit et al., 2003). Although diet can influence glucose tolerance, the relationships are more complex because it is well known that chronic stress can cause hippocampal atrophy and contribute to glucose intolerance.

Another risk factor that is important to CVD and dementia is hyperhomocysteinemia. Elevated homocysteine, an independent risk factor for CVD and dementia (Seshadri et al., 2002), is influenced by dietary and supplemental folate, vitamin B_{12}, and vitamin B_6.

Recommended Dietary Guidelines for Prevention of Cognitive Dysfunction

The diet should be similar to that which was recommended previously:

1. A nutrient-rich diet so that there is adequate protein (with amino acids) that contain precursors of specific neurotransmitters, as well as B complex vitamins and magnesium that are important cofactors for their synthesis
2. Healthy fats for healthy cell membranes that depend on an optimal ratio of omega-3 to omega-6 fatty acids, and good quantities of protective antioxidants. Dietary fish is a good source of omega-3, as is flaxseed and flaxseed oil. Minimizing or limiting animal fats with saturated fat and omega-6 fatty acids is also generally recommended.
3. Antioxidants found in vegetables, fruit, and, to a degree, whole grains. The range of antioxidants helps protect membranes from damage and rigidity that over time can impair nerve cell functions

Role for Dietary Guidelines in the Treatment of Dementia

There is little evidence to base recommendations for treating dementia; however, diet can significantly impact nutritional intake, cell membrane fatty acid composition, and general well-being, so it should always be addressed. Dementia is a good example of a condition that illustrates the importance of combining diet with nutritional supplementation. It would not be wise to believe that diet alone could have enough of an influence to improve cognition function. Core supplements could include B complex vitamins, magnesium, omega-3 fatty acids, and antioxidants. There is also research supporting the use of ginkgo biloba (Le Bars, 2003).

Two additional important issues are

1. Intervening as early as possible in the pathogenesis
2. Using other integrative medicine techniques, such as stress management, and developing a social or support network

LONGEVITY

A chapter on aging would not be complete without asking the question Is increased longevity possible?

Although this is a difficult and complicated question to answer, most people are aware that caloric restriction in several animal models is the only known reproducible method shown to significantly increase longevity. The efforts under way to investigate this relationship in humans have been reviewed recently (Heilbronn & Ravussin, 2003). The review discussed the mechanisms for this relationship:

- Reduced metabolic rate
- Oxidative stress
- Insulin resistance
- Altered neuroendocrine function
- Altered sympathetic nervous system function

Because the level of caloric restriction (about 30%) is relatively severe, it is unlikely that this approach will have adequate compliance by a significant number of people or for a significant period of time.

Other Ways to Extend Life Span Besides Caloric Restriction

Probably the most viable approach to extending life span besides caloric restriction is pursuing a more moderate caloric restriction while at the same time addressing the mechanisms of aging that have been identified. From a methodological standpoint, an integrative health care approach is ideal to most effectively address these factors. For example, reduced metabolism could be addressed through various forms of exercise, oxidative stress can be prevented with appropriate dietary guidelines and targeted nutritional supplementation, and altered neuroendocrine and sympathetic nervous system function could be influenced by stress management techniques. Although this may sound like a simple approach, the challenge will be to identify the most important factors involved, to determine the most effective therapeutic approaches that are required, and to design an overall program that will produce significant benefit. This may be further complicated by a need to address biological individuality.

~ CONCLUSION

The information presented in this chapter describes how diets have an important and foundation role in preventing and treating common disorders associated with aging. The core dietary recommendations for the disorders described are very similar and include an emphasis on vegetables, fruit, whole grains, healthy proteins (fish, beans or bean products, and lean meats), healthy fats, and healthy snacks. With regard to cardiovascular disease, dietary approaches have been shown to reduce weight, hypertension, hyperlipidemia, blood glucose and insulin levels, and possibly inflammation. The influence of dietary guidelines and dietary components on cancer and cognitive dysfunction are less well understood, but as research on diet and nutrition and these disorders progresses, more clear preventive and therapeutic guidelines will emerge.

Interestingly, there are dietary issues or patterns and physiological mechanisms that are consistently present across a range of disorders that have been described in this chapter. Examples include the following:

- Obesity: This contributes to CVD and cancer risk, as well as cognitive decline, through cardiovascular and other mechanisms.
- Insulin resistance: A feature of overweight and obesity, insulin resistance is also caused by chronic diseases such as cancer and inflammation.
- Oxidative stress: The research results examining antioxidants and CVD have been disappointing, but antioxidants do play a role in cardiovascular disease, at least in the early stages. Oxidative stress effects on aging, immune function, cancer, and cognitive decline are important and have been found in various research models.
- Healthy fatty acids and healthy fats: Omega-3 fatty acids and monounsaturated fat help to reduce circulating lipids, regulate immune function, and influence nerve cell membrane composition and function. This is an area for significant future research and development, in which cell membrane omega-3/omega-6 fatty acid

ratios are correlated with various disorders, and dietary guidelines and nutritional supplementation recommendations are designed to optimize fatty acid balance.

- Dietary magnesium: Magnesium is often inadequate in the diet, but it has been shown to influence many bodily functions, including blood sugar regulation, hypertension and cardiovascular activity, bone density, and nervous system function.

Other areas are just beginning to be explored or need significantly more research. These include

- Phytonutrients and phytochemicals: Thousands of biologically active components have been identified and investigated. However, there are still probably thousands remaining to be identified that may have important biological effects and require specific dietary guidelines to produce therapeutic benefit.
- Diet/nutrient and gene interactions: With completion of the human genome project and the identification of the entire genetic code, there will be a clearer understanding of dietary relationships to genetic transcription markers as well as genetic polymorphisms that may suggest modifying dietary guidelines for specific individuals.
- Complementing dietary guidelines with nutritional supplementation: Diet clearly needs to be the foundation of a good nutritional approach; however, prudent and effective recommendations for nutritional supplements can maximize the potential benefit to patients.

With the aging population, there will be increasing pressure to address many of the important issues that have been presented in this chapter. Effectively meeting the challenges described here will undoubtedly lead to an improved quality of life and most likely increased longevity. An integrative medicine model is also an ideal approach to explore these issues and develop solutions because the issues are multifactorial and interrelated and require the expertise of an interdisciplinary clinical and research collaboration.

RESOURCES

American College of Nutrition, 300 S. Duncan Ave., Suite 225, Clearwater, FL 33755; voice line: (727) 446-6086; fax: (727) 446-6202; Web site: http://www.am-coll-nutr.org/

DrWeil.com and Weil A. Eating Well for Optimum Health. New York: Alfred A. Knopf, 2000.

Institute for Functional Medicine, 4411 Pt. Fosdick Drive NW, Suite 305, P.O. Box 1697, Gig Harbor, WA 98335; telephone: (800) 228-0622; fax: (253) 853-6766; Web site: http://www.functionalmedicine.org

Jean Mayer USDA Human Nutrition Research Center on Aging, Tufts University, 711 Washington Street, Boston, MA 02111-1524; telephone: (617) 556-3000; fax: (617) 556-3344; Web site: http://hnrc.tufts.edu/

Life Extension Foundation, Life Extension Foundation, P.O. Box 229120, Hollywood, FL 33022; telephone: (800) 226-2370; fax: (954) 761-9199; Web site: http://www.lef.org

National Institute on Aging, Office of Nutrition, National Institutes of Health; Building 31, Room 5C27, 31 Center Drive, MSC 2292, Bethesda, MD 20892; telephone: (301) 496-1752; Web site: http://www.nia.nih.gov/

REFERENCES

Ames, B. N. (2001). DNA damage from micronutrient deficiencies is likely to be a major cause of cancer. *Mutation Research, 475,* 7–20.

Appel, L. J. (2003). Lifestyle modification as a means to prevent and treat high blood pressure. *Journal of the American Society of Nephrology, 14,* S99–S102.

Appel, L. J., Moore, T. J., Obarzanek, E., Vollmer, W. M., Svetkey, L. P., Sacks, F. M., et al. (1997). A clinical trial of the effects of dietary patterns on blood pressure: DASH Collaborative Research Group. *New England Journal of Medicine, 336,* 1117–1124.

Calle, E. E., Rodriguez, C., Walker-Thurmond, K., & Thun, M. J. (2003). Overweight, obesity, and mortality from cancer in a prospectively studied cohort of U.S. adults. *New England Journal of Medicine, 348,* 1625–1638.

Carter, J. P., Saxe, G. P., Newbold, V., Peres, C. E., Campeau, R. J., & Bernal-Green, L. (1993). Hypothesis: Dietary management may improve survival from nutritionally linked cancers based on analysis of representative cases. *Journal of the American College of Nutrition, 12,* 209–226.

Convit, A., Wolf, O. T., Tarshish, C., & de Leon, M. J. (2003). Reduced glucose tolerance is associated with poor memory performance and hippocampal atrophy among normal elderly. *Proceedings of the National Academy of Sciences USA, 100,* 2019–2022.

Feldstein, C. A., Akopian, M., Renauld, A., Olivieri, A. O., Cauterucci, S., & Garriolo, D. (2002). Insulin resistance and hypertension in postmenopausal women. *Journal of Human Hypertension, 16*(Suppl. 1), S145–150.

Ford, E. S., Giles, W. H., & Dietz, W. H. (2002). Prevalence of the metabolic syndrome among US adults: Findings from the third National Health and Nutrition Examination Survey. *Journal of the American Medical Association, 287,* 356–359.

Foster, G. D., Wyatt, H. R., Hill, J. O., McGuckin, B. G., Brill, C., Mohammed, B. S., et al. (2003). A randomized trial of a low-carbohydrate diet for obesity. *New England Journal of Medicine, 348,* 2082–2090.

Giovannucci, E. (1999). Tomatoes, tomato-based products, lycopene, and cancer: Review of the epidemiologic literature. *Journal of the National Cancer Institute, 91,* 317–331.

Heilbronn, L. K., & Ravussin, E. (2003). Calorie restriction and aging: Review of the literature and implications for studies in humans. *American Journal of Clinical Nutrition, 78,* 361–369.

Hildenbrand, G. L., Hildenbrand, L. C., Bradford, K., & Cavin, S. W. (1995). Five-year survival rates of melanoma patients treated by diet therapy after the manner of Gerson: A retrospective review. *Alternative Therapies in Health Medicine, 1,* 29–37.

Holick, M. F. (2003). Vitamin D: A millenium perspective. *Journal of Cellular Biochemistry, 88,* 296–307.

Hu, F. B., & Willett, W. C. (2002). Optimal diets for prevention of coronary heart disease. *Journal of the American Medical Association, 288,* 2569–2578.

Jenkins, D. J., Kendall, C. W., Marchie, A. , Faulkner, D. A., Wong, J. M., Emam, A., et al. (2003). Effects of a dietary portfolio of cholesterol-lowering foods vs lovastatin on serum lipids and C-reactive protein. *Journal of the American Medical Association, 290,* 502–510.

Kalmijn, S., Launer, L. J., Ott, A., Witteman, J. C., Hofman, A., & Breteler, M. M. (1997). Dietary fat intake and the risk of incident dementia in the Rotterdam Study. *Annals of Neurology, 42,* 776–782.

Le Bars, P. L. (2003). Magnitude of effect and special approach to ginkgo biloba extract EGb 761 in cognitive disorders. *Pharmacopsychiatry, 36*(Suppl. 1), S44–449.

Li, C. I., Malone, K.E., Porter, P. L., Weiss, N. S., Tang, M. T., & Daling, J. R. (2003). The relationship between alcohol use and risk of breast cancer by histology and hormone receptor status among women 65–79 years of age. *Cancer Epidemiology Biomarkers Prevention, 12,* 1061–1066.

Liu, S., Manson, J. E., Buring, J. E., Stampfer, M. J., Willett, W. C., & Ridker, P. M. (2002). Relation between a diet with a high glycemic load and plasma concentrations of high-sensitivity C-reactive protein in middle-aged women. *American Journal of Clinical Nutrition, 75,* 492–498.

Luchsinger, J. A., Tang, M. X., Shea, S., & Mayeux, R. (2003). Antioxidant vitamin intake and risk of Alzheimer disease. *Archives of Neurology, 60,* 203–208.

Luft, F. C., & Weinberger, M. H. (1997). Heterogeneous responses to changes in dietary salt intake: The salt-sensitivity paradigm. *American Journal of Clinical Nutrition, 65,* 612S–617S.

Messina, M. J. (2003). Emerging evidence on the role of soy in reducing prostate cancer risk. *Nutrition Review, 61,* 117–131.

Morris, M. C., Evans, D. A., Bienias, J. L., Tangney, C. C., Bennett, D. A., Wilson, R. S., et al. (2003). Consumption of fish and n-3 fatty acids and risk of incident Alzheimer disease. *Archives of Neurology, 60,* 940–946.

Murray, M., Birdsall, T., Pizzorno, J. E., Passariello, N., Varricchio, M., & D'Onofrio, F. (2002). *How to prevent and treat cancer with natural medicine.* New York: Riverhead Books.

Paolisso, G., Sgambato, S., Pizza, G., et al. (1989). Improved insulin response and action by chronic magnesium administration in aged NIDDM subjects. *Diabetes Care, 12*, 265–269.

Pasternak, R. C. (2003). Report of the Adult Treatment Panel III: The 2001 National Cholesterol Education Program guidelines on the detection, evaluation and treatment of elevated cholesterol in adults. *Cardiology Clinics, 21*, 393–398.

Reaven, G. M. (1995). Pathophysiology of insulin resistance in human disease. *Physiology Review, 75*, 473–486.

Ridker, P. M., Buring, J. E., Cook, N. R., & Rifai, N. (2003). C-reactive protein, the metabolic syndrome, and risk of incident cardiovascular events: An 8-year follow-up of 14,719 initially healthy American women. *Circulation, 107*, 391–397.

Sacks, F. M., Svetkey, L. P., Vollmer, W. M., Appell, L. J., Bray, G. A., Harsha, D., et al. (2001). Effects on blood pressure of reduced dietary sodium and the Dietary Approaches to Stop Hypertension (DASH) diet: DASH-Sodium Collaborative Research Group. *New England Journal of Medicine, 344*, 3–10.

Seshadri, S., Beiser, A., Selhub, J., Jacques, P. F., Rosenberg, I. H., D'Angostino, R. B., et al. (2002). Plasma homocysteine as a risk factor for dementia and Alzheimer's disease. *New England Journal of Medicine, 346*, 476–483.

Stendig-Lindberg, G., Tepper, R., & Leichter, I. (1993). Trabecular bone density in a two year controlled trial of peroral magnesium in osteoporosis. *Magnesium Research, 6*, 155–163.

Tabet, N., Mantle, D., Walker, Z., & Orrell, M. (2002). Endogenous antioxidant activities in relation to concurrent vitamins A, C, and E intake in dementia. *International Psychogeriatrics, 14*, 7–15.

Westman, E. C., Yancy, W. S., Edman, J. S., Tomlin, K. F., & Perkins, C. E. (2002). Effect of 6-month adherence to a very low carbohydrate diet program. *American Journal of Medicine, 113*, 30–36.

Witteman, J. C., Grobbee, D. E., Derkx, F. H., Bouillon, R., deBruijn, A. M., & Hofman, A. (1994). Reduction of blood pressure with oral magnesium supplementation in women with mild to moderate hypertension. *American Journal of Clinical Nutrition, 60*, 129–135.

CHAPTER THREE

Supplements and Herbs

Ara DerMarderosian and Michael Briggs

The percentage of the population of the United States over the age of 65 is predicted to dramatically increase as the baby boomer generation reaches 65 starting in 2010 (Eisenberg et al., 2001). By 2020, more than 1 billion people worldwide will be age 60 or over. Aging is associated with the occurrence of chronic conditions, such as arthritis, diabetes, and heart disease, and declines in the activities of daily living. The aging process itself cannot be stopped; however, the rate at which aging occurs can be slowed through a comprehensive program of exercise, nutrition, stress reduction, and dietary supplementation. New research and progressive therapies (i.e., herbal medicine) are more readily available to combat these common ailments. It is expected that health care costs will increase exponentially in the United States and worldwide due to the increase in the aging population.

The herbal market in the United States has reached unprecedented growth, with nearly $5 billion spent per year on herbal supplements (Eisenberg et al., 2001). Sales have increased nearly 20% annually in recent years (Eisenberg et al., 2001; Kessler et al., 2001). A survey in 2000 revealed that many patients incorporate complementary and alternative medicine (CAM) with conventional medicine (Blumenthal, 1995; Brevoort, 1996; Eisenberg et al., 2001; Kagan, 2000; Kessler et al., 2001). Herbal medicine is often perceived as a more natural approach to health, and some patients may view this form of therapy as safer than conventional drug therapy. However, all health professionals should be aware that herbs can have numerous adverse effects and can interact negatively with drugs (Boullata & Nace, 2000; Ernst, 1998; Klepser & Klepser, 1999; Lambrecht et al., 2000; Miller, 1998).

In order to advise and counsel patients on the safe and proper use of herbs and nutritional supplements, providers should become educated on the numerous therapeutic uses of herbal products (Bauer, 2000; National Institutes of Health, 1997; Winslow & Kroll, 1998). Unfortunately, much of the scientific literature on herbal medicine suffers from flaws in product quality, statistical analysis, small population size, study design, and bias (Barnes et al., 1999; Talalay & Talalay, 2001), so it is important to read the literature with a critical eye.

HISTORICAL PERSPECTIVE OF HERBAL MEDICINE

Herbal medicine is considered to be one of the oldest forms of health care. Historically, evidence exists from almost every culture around the world about individual cultural contributions to pharmacognosy. Some of the oldest prescriptions are documented on Babylonian clay tablets, and the hieretic (priestly) writing of ancient Egypt on papyrus records hundreds of ancient pharmaceutical and medicinal uses for botanicals or phytomedicinals, including olive oil, wine, opium, castor oil, garlic, grapes, and onion. Many plants also served multiple functions, such as in foods and spices. This botanical abundance represents a collection of the most reliable early medicines that are still used today (DerMarderosian, 1996, 1998).

Plants account for nearly 25% of conventional drug therapies (Goldman, 2001; Vickers & Zollman, 1999). In several third world countries, the World Health Organization records that nearly 75% of traditional medical practices use phytomedicines, including morphine and related opium derivatives, colchicine (from autumn crocus), cocaine (from coca), vincristine and vinblastine (from the catharanthis or vinca plant), reserpine (from Indian snakeroot), etoposide (from mayapple), and taxol (from yew) (Croon & Walker, 1995; Goldman, 2001; Gruber & DerMarderosian, 1996a,b). As we learn more about the historical and folkloric use of botanicals around the world, ethnobotanical and rigorous scientific studies may offer an abundance of new herbal medicines, nutritional supplements, and synthetic derivatives.

We are now in an era of increasing interest in using natural medicines. Science has taught us repeatedly that all things recycle, and herbal medicines are not themselves new but have been in use since the dawn of ancient civilizations (Gruber & DerMarderosian, 1996a). It is as though we are going "back to the future" to the old pharmacopoeias to update previous attempts of standardizing botanical medicines through modern chemical procedures, such as nuclear magnetic resonance spectroscopy, chromatography, and mass spectrometry. The structures of many compounds are virtual modern chemical "molecular keys" that help us elucidate structure–activity relationships of any botanical. This knowledge allows us to fully understand the complexities involved in plant collection, storage, processing, and extraction to prepare uniform, stable dosage forms. Finally, even though we may know the mechanism of action of a single compound, the fact that plants contain mixtures of complex compounds clouds the picture pharmacologically and chemically from the product standardization point of view.

Through the study of structure–activity relationships, natural product research has led to new physiological and pharmacological relationships. Classic examples include morphine (the chemical basis for natural and synthetic opioid analgesics), cocaine (the chemical basis for synthetic local anesthetics like procaine), and ephedra (the chemical basis for central nervous system (CNS) stimulants like the amphetamines and the decongestants, such as pseudoephedrine). Even capsaicin from hot peppers has been reintroduced as a topical analgesic via a new understanding of the release of substance P, which is involved in pain transmission Croon & Walker, 1995; Gillespie, 1997; Gruber & DerMarderosian 1996a,b; Tyler, 1994).

With the discovery of new and resistant organisms each year, natural product research may again lead to new antimicrobials. Resistant forms of bacteria have taught us the importance of new approaches to stimulating and protecting our immune system in the fight against such diseases. The use of immune stimulants, phytochemicals, and nutraceuticals (food as medicine) is beneficial to the human body's defenses and thus may help prevent or even treat various conditions (Gillespie, 1997; Gruber & DerMarderosian, 1996a,b; Vickers & Zollman, 1999).

CURRENT REGULATORY STATUS: DIETARY SUPPLEMENT AND HEALTH EDUCATION ACT OF 1994

According to the Dietary Supplement Health and Education Act (DSHEA) of 1994, a dietary supplement includes any product, excluding tobacco, that contains a vitamin, mineral, herb, or amino acid that is intended as a supplement to the normal diet. Therefore, dietary supplements marketed before October 15, 1994, are considered safe unless they "present a significant or unreasonable risk of illness or injury under conditions of use recommended or suggested in [the] labeling . . . under ordinary conditions of use." (However, the secretary of Health and Human Services is granted emergency powers to remove any dietary supplement from the market if it poses an imminent health hazard.) DSHEA permits "structure or function" (e.g., enhances immune system functioning) claims and warnings and dosage recommendations on various product labels. Prior to this act, these "structure or function" claims would cause the product to be misbranded and removed from the market. A dietary supplement also is considered misbranded if it claims to conform to but does not meet the specifications of an official reference. All claims on a dietary supplement must also include a notice on the label indicating "This product is not intended to diagnose, treat, cure or prevent any disease." The notice also must include a statement that "the product has not been evaluated by the Food and Drug Administration [FDA]." The term *dietary supplement* also must be included on the label with a list of each ingredient by name, quantity, total weight, and identity of any plant parts or ingredients used to derive the product (Food and Drug Administration, 1994; Hathcock, 2001).

DSHEA also permits articles on health advertising (e.g., clinical efficacy claims), which must appear physically separate from the botanical product. All the articles must be truthful and not promote the use of a particular brand of herbal or nutritional supplement. The FDA is responsible for evaluating any false or misleading scientific claims on the botanical ingredient. Prior to DSHEA, such health advertising would have provided the basis for judging the product "misbranded." DSHEA also stipulates that these requirements "shall not apply to or restrict a retailer or wholesaler of dietary supplements in any way whatsoever in the sale of books or other publications as a part of the business of such retailer or wholesaler" (FDA, 1994; Hathcock, 2001).

Scientific study on the usefulness of dietary supplements has been entrusted to the Office of Dietary Supplements, which is part of the National Institutes of Health. Furthermore, the Commission of Dietary Supplement Labels will provide recommendations and report on any regulations associated with labeling dietary supplements. Pharmacists must continue to be aware of any new DSHEA guidelines and all legal changes in order to evaluate the health advertising (e.g., clinical efficacy claims) for herbal products, as well as to provide proper patient counseling. (These are available through the following national center for complementary and alternative medicine Web site: http://nccam.nih.gov.)

BOTANICAL IDENTITY CONCERNS

It is an absolute necessity in the science of pharmacognosy to identify properly all portions of a plant, particularly those containing the active ingredients.

This process can be very challenging because there is still disagreement among taxonomists on the proper naming of many species. For example, *Foeniculum vulgare,* or fennel, is also known botanically as *Anethum foeniculum* (Tyler, 1994).

Processing of Plant Material

It is obvious that whatever part of the plant (e.g., seeds, flowers, or roots) has been shown to possess the greatest therapeutic should be the component used in dosage forms. This should be accompanied by clinical efficacy and minimal toxicity data. It may be necessary to contact the manufacturer to determine what extract (e.g., water soluble, nonpolar, or lipid extraction) or solvent was used to produce the product. Hence, in order to attain any true clinical efficacy, solvents used for extraction must be uniform in order to complete true comparison studies and to define proper dosage recommendations.

Different solvents extract different constituents. Therefore, herbs or dietary supplements need to be subjected to rigorous quality control procedures. They should be quality controlled, just as over-the-counter (OTC) and prescription medicines are controlled. Many clinical studies have been carried out with proprietary herbal extracts (labeled by code numbers or letters) made by certain companies. Usually, crude plant teas and the like are of no major hazard when they are taken moderately. However, there may be an increased risk of adverse reactions with concentrated extracts. In countries such as the United States where the idea of "more is better" is promoted, a patient may take too much herbal or nutritional remedy.

Herbal products often contain a wide variety of different compounds of various classes (e.g., alkaloids, glycosides, steroids, phenylpropanoids, anthocyanins, and essential oils). These complex structures from the plant world have long been the scientific basis of drugs used in pharmacy and medicine. The combined action of these compounds may lead to numerous therapeutic effects. For example, the primary metabolites are not particularly active pharmacologically, but the secondary metabolites are very active pharmacologically. The pharmacological activity of the plant depends on genetics, environment, and fertilization. For example, selection at different times of the year affects herb quality and clinical effectiveness. It is not uncommon also to see mixed activity, depending on which compounds predominate, (Blumenthal et al, 1998; Murray, 1995; *The review of natural products,* 2002; Schulz, Hansel, & Tyler, 1998; Tyler, 1994).

Increased dosages and long duration of use may potentially increase the risk of toxic effects like hepatotoxicity and carcinogenesis. Whether the toxic effects are expressed is often associated with patient-specific characteristics. Plants such as *Symphytum officinale* (also known as comfrey) contain the externally useful drug allantoin (promotes tissue regeneration) and rosmarinic acid (anti-inflammatory). However, if taken internally, the content of pyrrolizidine alkaloids may be potentially hepatotoxic, mutagenic, and carcinogenic, as seen in in vitro studies with animals. For this reason, most countries have banned or restricted the use of comfrey. Comfrey has remained on the market in the United States because it is marketed as a dietary supplement and not as a drug. Fortunately, most reputable manufacturers and suppliers have withdrawn such products from the market. Most recent warnings on which herbs are most toxic appear in the literature (e.g., hepatotoxic effects with kava kava) (Blumenthal et al., 1998; Murray, 1995; *The review of natural products,* 2002; Schulz et al., 1998).

At times, case reports of unusual toxicities are reported with commercial herbal products. However, upon further investigation, these are often due to accidental contamination of the herbal product with poisonous plants (e.g., belladonna) or purposeful adulteration with synthetic drugs, as seen in certain imported preparations from Hong Kong. Furthermore, one should be aware that many imported products may not be subjected to or adhere to good manufacturing practices (GMPs). Therefore, it is best to use products from reliable sources where rigorous GMPs are observed. (Reference to blind random analysis of products via www.consumerlabs.com will help determine which products are legitimate, based on their analytical results.)

NEEDED CLINICAL STUDIES AND HERB–DRUG INTERACTION PROBLEMS

In order to evaluate the safety and clinical efficacy of herbal preparations, a German federal agency in 1978 (Bundesgesundheitsamt) established the Commission E. The Commission E has produced about 400 monographs on various phytopharmaceuticals and combination products. It has reviewed clinical trials, animal studies, case reports, epidemiological studies, and even experimental and traditional uses, with a particular emphasis on safety. Some of these data include the study of the proper identification, purity, adulteration, phytochemical composition, pharmacological activity, therapeutic activity, contraindications, side effects, and dosages. Some have suggested that these compendia represent the most complete and accurate modern body of scientific information on the topic today. As a matter of fact, it has been suggested that the United States should adopt the German system (Blumenthal et al., 1998).

In Europe, as well as in other parts of the world, the clinical use of herbal and nutritional medicines is remarkably different from the United

States. We have chosen the "high-tech" synthesis and commercialization pathway, whereas the "old world" has continued to study and use its folkloric medicine. In much of Europe and Asia, pharmacists prescribe and dispense many officially approved botanical drugs and receive significant training in the science of pharmacognosy and phytomedicine. The various phytopharmaceutical dosage forms (e.g., herbal teas, various extracts, tablets, and capsules) are provided as standardized products with stated contents and concentrations of active ingredients. Among the top 100 most prescribed drugs in Germany for 1990 were six herbs; nearly 4.23 million prescriptions were written for standardized ginkgo biloba preparations alone.

Several herb–drug interaction studies have been published (Boullata & Nace, 2000; Ernst, 1998; Klepser & Klepser, 1999; Lambrecht et al., 2000; Miller, 1998). However, there are no strict requirements for stating any acute or chronic toxicity because herbs are classified as dietary supplements (Edzard, 2002). (There is a voluntary system for reporting suspected adverse effects (USP at 800-4USP-PRN and Medwatch at 800-FDA-1088). The FDA requires extensive and costly clinical trials to verify and prove the clinical efficacy and safety of synthetic drugs. Unfortunately, most companies cannot afford to invest millions of dollars for studies on natural products, given the lack of proprietary patent protection. This helps explain why the clinical efficacy and safety data of most phytomedicinals remain unavailable in the United States, even though extensive therapeutic data from other parts of the world, such as Europe and Asia, are readily available (Byers, 1999; Cassileth, 1999; Talalay & Talalay, 2001).

PATIENT COUNSELING

Pharmacists and other health care professionals should consider the following basic guidelines when counseling a patient about phytomedicinal and combination products.

1. GMPs (e.g., identity, cleanliness, good quality control) are implicit in the DSHEA guidelines. Unfortunately, products on the market suffer from significant differences in their purity, quality, and potency. Therefore, all phytomedicinal products should be purchased from reliable sources.

2. Botanicals should be dated and thus should be discarded according to the expiration date or if more than 1 year old.

3. At times, patients think they can avoid more potent and effective drugs by using "natural" herbs. Counsel patients on the risk and benefits

of all medical treatments and the adverse effects that can develop if neglected by assuming an herb is harmless.

4. Phytomedicinal products are generally used to treat mild, short-term conditions (e.g., constipation, headaches, insomnia, and dyspepsia). A health care practitioner who is knowledgeable in alternative medicine should supervise ongoing therapy.

5. If any adverse reaction occurs, advise patients to discontinue using the herbal or nutritional supplement causing the undesirable side effects, or consider changing the mode of administration. For example, feverfew may be useful in preventing migraine headaches; however, widespread inflammation of the oral mucosa can result from chewing the leaves. Thus, oral capsules should be taken to avoid this adverse reaction.

6. Most phytomedicinal products, like many prescription and OTC drugs, are contraindicated during pregnancy or lactation and should not be used in young children.

7. Generally, avoid excessive combination products. Past and current clinical research with prescription and OTC medications has taught us those combination products (e.g., more than two or three ingredients) are not always justifiable because doses may be too low, or they may interact.

CLASSIFICATION OF EFFICACY-BASED EVIDENCE OF HERBS BY ORGAN SYSTEM

Nervous System

Feverfew

Botany. The medicinal components of feverfew, or *Tanacetum parthenium,* are contained within the leaves, as well as in the seed. This short, bushy perennial, which is native to Europe and found throughout the United States, has yellow-green leaves, yellow flowers, and grows 15 cm to 60 cm tall (Blumenthal et al., 1998; Heptinstall et al., 1992; McDermott et al., 1998; *The review of natural products,* 2002).

History. This herb has a rich history of use in traditional and folk medicine, particularly among Greek and early European herbalists. Considered an effective preventive treatment for migraine headaches, feverfew has been used to treat menstrual pain and fevers (fever reducer, or febrifuge), as well as respiratory (e.g., asthma), dermatologic (e.g., dermatitis), and musculoskeletal (e.g., arthritis) ailments (Blumenthal et al., 1998; Heptinstall, 1988; *The review of natural products,* 2002).

TABLE 3.1 Popular Herbs and Their Uses

Herb	Primary Use
Black cohosh	Symptoms of menopause
Echinacea	Immune stimulant
Feverfew	Migraines
Gingko	Vascular dementia
Saw palmetto	Enlarged prostate
St. John's wort	Mild depression
Valerian	Insomnia
Ginseng	Immune stimulant
Rhodiola rosea	Stress reduction

This chart lists a handful of the most popular herbs for aging-related conditions; these herbs are reasonably safe for most populations, although each may be contraindicated for specific patients.

Basic medicinal chemistry. The parthenolides comprise up to 85% of the total sesquiterpene lactone content and are considered the principal active ingredient. The Canadian Health Protection Branch recommends a daily dosage of 125 mg of a dried feverfew leaf preparation containing at least 0.2% parthenolide. There are still some disagreements on the active constituents of the plant (Heptinstall et al., 1992).

Pharmacological activity and main therapeutic use. Numerous clinical trials in humans indicate that feverfew may offer relief in patients suffering from migraines. There appear to be multiple mechanisms of action for the pharmacologic activity of feverfew, such as inhibition of prostaglandin synthesis and serotonin release from platelets and polymorphonuclear leukocyte granules. The former offers support for the claimed benefit of feverfew in migraines and arthritis (Blumenthal et al., 1998; Johnson et al., 1985; *The review of natural products,* 2002).

Toxicology. The primary adverse reactions with feverfew are associated with the gastrointestinal system. Feverfew may induce widespread inflammation of the oral mucosa, such as lip swelling, swollen tongue, and oral mucosal ulcerations. It is advised to use oral capsules of feverfew to avoid this adverse reaction. Some patients who abruptly stop taking feverfew complained of a cluster of nervous system reactions, including rebound headaches, insomnia, anxiety, joint pain, and muscle stiffness; therefore, it is recommended to taper off feverfew over several weeks. Due to the lack of clinical studies, use is not recommended during pregnancy

TABLE 3.2 Popular Herbs to Avoid

Herb	Primary Reason
Ephedra	Cardiovascular/nervous system damage
Kava kava	Liver toxicity

This list is by no means exhaustive. Before taking or advising others to take any herb, it is important to educate yourself on its properties and contraindications. *The PDR on Herbal Medicine* is an excellent and authoritative source (see Resources).

and lactation. Use with caution in patients on anticoagulants due to feverfew's action on platelets (Blumenthal et al., 1998; Klepser & Klepser, 1999; *The review of natural products,* 2002).

Gingko

Botany. The medicinal components of ginkgo (*Ginkgo biloba* L.) are contained within the leaves. Ginkgo is considered the world's oldest living tree species and grows to a height of about 125 feet. Ginkgo species are dioecious; in late autumn females trees produce a plumlike gray-tan fruit. The inner seed is edible and resembles an almond. However, the fleshy pulp has a foul and offensive odor and may cause contact dermatitis (Blumenthal et al., 1998; Jacobs & Browner, 2000; *The review of natural products,* 2002; van Beek & Lelyveld, 1992; Victoire et al., 1988.)

History. Traditional Chinese physicians historically have used ginkgo to treat ailments such as asthma and chilblains (swelling of hands and feet due to exposure to damp cold). Ginkgo appeared in the Western world after technological advances in the 1960s made it possible to detect its active constituents. The oral and intravenous dosage form of ginkgo is one of the most widely prescribed medications in Europe (Blumenthal et al., 1998; Jacobs & Browner, 2000; *The review of natural products,* 2002).

Basic medicinal chemistry. The neuroprotective properties are associated with the leaf constituents, which include approximately 40 flavonoids (e.g., bilobetin, ginkgetin, isoginkgetin, and sciadopitysin) and flavonols (e.g., quercetin and kaempferol) and their glycosides. The major terpene molecules (bilobalide and gingolides A, B, C, J, and M) of ginkgo also are postulated to have neuroprotective activity (Blumenthal et al., 1998; Braquet, 1989; *The review of natural products,* 2002; van Beek & Lelyveld, 1992; Victoire et al., 1988).

Pharmacological activity and main therapeutic use. Well-designed clinical studies in humans document the clinical efficacy of ginkgo for

TABLE 3.3 Popular Supplements and Their Primary Uses

Supplement	Primary Use
Coenzyme Q_{10}	Antioxidant
Fish oil	Cardiovascular support; anti-inflammatory
Glucosamine	Osteoarthritis
Ipriflavone	Osteoporosis
Melatonin	Insomnia; jet lag

treatment in cerebral vascular insufficiency, dementia, circulatory disorders, and potentially asthma. As indicated, the plant is an antioxidant and has neurotransmitter/receptor modulatory and antiplatelet activating factor properties (Diamond et al., 2000).

The main therapeutic use of the commercially available ginkgo extract has been in the treatment of cerebral vascular insufficiency. Multiple pharmacological mechanisms have been proposed for ginkgo extract (Egb 761) (Blumenthal, Goldberg, & Brinckmann, 2000; Diamond et al., 2000; Vorberg, 1985). DeFeudis (1991) analyzed nearly 50 double-blind studies involving 9,800 patients on ginkgo biloba extract; the number of side effects was exceptionally low and included mostly gastrointestinal discomfort. The typical daily dose of ginkgo biloba is 120 mg to 160 mg, with CNS symptoms typically improving in about 4 to 6weeks.

A randomized, placebo-controlled, prospective, double-blind, multicenter, 24-month trial investigated the effect on 156 Alzheimer-type patients receiving 240 mg/kg of ginkgo biloba extract (LeBars et al., 1997). Psychopathological assessment evaluating memory, attention, and improvement in activities of daily living resulted in substantiating clinical efficacy of the extract. Other clinical studies (Kanowski et al., 1997; LeBars, Kiese, & Itil, 2000; Logani et al., 2000; Schulz, Huebner, & Ploch, 1997) suggest that ginkgo biloba is effective in treating mild to moderate Alzheimer's dementia. Its mechanism of action is postulated to be similar to second-generation cholinesterase inhibitors (analogous to donepezil, rivastigmine, and metrifonate). In Germany, the majority of prescribers prefer ginkgo biloba to standard antidementia drugs, such as acetylcholinesterase inhibitors (Forstl, 2000), because the active constituents of ginkgo biloba are capable of inhibiting the free radical nitric oxide (NO), which is involved with many CNS disorders (Bastianetto et al., 2000).

Evidence also exists for the clinical efficacy of ginkgo biloba in treating peripheral vascular disorders, such as Raynaud's disease, acrocyanosis, and postphlebitis syndrome. There are several double-blind, multicenter clinical studies that demonstrate statistical and clinical significance for the use of ginkgo biloba in improving pain-free walking in patients who suffer from peripheral arterial disease. For example, patients receiving either 120 mg or 240 mg of ginkgo biloba extract daily for 24 weeks showed a statistically significant improvement in pain-free walking distance, as well as maximum walking distance. Both doses were well tolerated for all patients randomized to either dosing schedule with little to no side effects (Schweizer & Hautmann, 1999).

The ginkgolides also competitively inhibit the binding of platelet-activating factor (PAF) to its membrane receptor. These findings may be useful in treating the symptoms associated with asthma. A double-blind, randomized, crossover human study subjected patients to their specific dust or pollen antigen. The results of the trial demonstrated patients receiving 40 mg three times a day (tid) of ginkgo biloba suffered from less early- and late-phase airway hyperactivity (Braquet, 1987).

Toxicology. Contact or ingestion of the fleshy fruit pulp of ginkgo biloba (seed covering) may produce severe skin irritation and allergic reactions. The seeds contain the ginkgotoxin (4-0-methylpyridoxine), which is recognized in Japan and China for causing food poisoning. If ingested, approximately 50 seeds may cause loss of consciousness and produce tonic/clonic seizures. Despite this case report, the cooked or canned seeds are available commercially in Asian markets. Because of the lack of clinical studies, use is best avoided during pregnancy and lactation (Rosenblatt & Mindel, 1997; Wada et al., 1988).

St. John's Wort

Botany. The medicinal components of St. John's wort (*Hypericum perforatum* L.) are contained within the oval-shaped leaves and the golden yellow flowering buds that bloom from June to September. Although native to Europe, this plant is an aromatic perennial found throughout the United States and parts of Canada. It generally grows to a height of 1 to 5 feet and is considered an aggressive weed found in the dry ground of roadsides, meadows, woods, and hedges (Blumenthal et al., 1998; *The review of natural products*, 2002).

History. Since the Middle Ages, this herbal remedy has been valued for its anti-inflammatory and healing properties. This plant also has been used as an antidepressant, gastrointestinal aide (e.g., gastritis), and diuretic, as well as a sleep aid. There is no scientific evidence to support the folk treatment as an anticancer agent (Blumenthal et al., 1998; *The review of natural products*, 2002).

Basic medicinal chemistry. The flavonoid components include quercetin, kaempferol, amentoflavone, luteolin, and the glycosides rutin and hyperoside. The 10% tannin content may contribute to the astringent effect of St. John's wort.

The phenol components include caffeic, chlorogenic, and p-coumaric acids and hyperfolin. St. John's wort also contains the anthraquinone derivatives of hypericin and pseudohypericin (Blumenthal et al., 1998; *The review of natural products,* 2002).

Previously, hypericin was regarded as the main active constituent for antidepressant activity in St. John's wort (Chatterjee et al., 1998a; Muller et al., 1998). However, hyperforin now is considered the primary active constituent for the plant's antidepressant activity. Hyperforin is a potent lignand for the pregnane X receptor (regulates expression of cytochrome P450 (CYP) 3A4 monooxygenase, which is involved with the oxidative metabolism of > 50% of all drugs), indicating that St. John's wort may interact with the metabolism of more drugs than previously thought (Moore et al., 2000; Obach, 2000; Roby et al., 2000; Vandenbogaerde et al., 2000).

Pharmacological activity and main therapeutic use. Clinical research has focused on the efficacy of St. John's wort in mild to moderate depression; premenstrual syndrome; sleep quality; seasonal affective disorder; and antibacterial, antifungal, and antiviral activity (Blumenthal et al., 1998; *The review of natural products,* 2002).

The antidepressant activity of St. John's wort is considered as efficacious as many serotonin reuptake inhibitors (SSRIs, e.g., fluoxetine), tricyclic (e.g., amitriptyline and imipramine) and tetracyclic (e.g., maprotiline) antidepressants, and benzodiazepines (e.g., diazepam). This activity is strongly supported by multiple clinical controlled trials. Hyperforin, the main active constituent, is an uptake inhibitor of (γ-aminobutyric acid (GABA), dopamine, L-glutamate, norepinephrine, and 5-HT (Chatterjee et al., 1998b; Laakmann et al., 1998; Linde et al., 1996; Philipp et al., 1999; Volz, 1997).

Most clinical studies from 1984 to 1997 evaluated St. John's wort (focusing on activity of hypericin, typically 0.5%) as being clinically efficacious in treating mild to moderate depression (Harrer et al., 1999; Linde et al., 1996; Linde & Berner, 1999; Shelton et al., 2001; Wheatley, 1998). Although most of the studies were of short duration (4–6 weeks), a meta-analysis (Kim et al., 1999; Linde et al., 1996) of 23 randomized trials with a total of 1,757 patients diagnosed with mild to moderate depression concluded that St. John's wort was significantly and clinically superior to placebo and similarly effective to conventional antidepressants.

Several other reviews (meta-analyses) concluded with similar outcomes (Kim et al., 1999).

Recent randomized, double-blind, placebo-controlled trials indicate an increased patient response with hyperforin 5% versus hyperforin 0.5%. One hundred forty-seven patients diagnosed with mild to moderate depression were randomized to receive either one tablet tid of a placebo, 0.5% hyperforin, or 5% hyperforin. The Hamilton Rating Scale for Depression was used to access patient response at the start and end of the study, as well as on days 7, 14, and 28. The study concluded the therapeutic effect was statistically ($p = .004$) and clinically significant for patients receiving the 5% hyperforin (Chatterjee et al., 1998a,b).

The results of a more recent single randomized control trial study declared St. John's wort ineffective in treating patients with severe depression. This 2-month study included 200 patients randomized to receive either placebo or 900 mg four times a day (qid) (dose potentially increased to 1,200 mg qid in week 5) of St. John's wort. Remission of illness was not statistically significant ($p < .02$) for patients receiving St. John's wort. However, St. John's wort is indicated for use in patients suffering from mild to moderate depression (Shelton et al., 2001).

Toxicology. The most common adverse effects are gastrointestinal upset (e.g., nausea, vomiting, and diarrhea) and photosensitivity, purportedly due to hypericin (Duran & Song, 1986; Roots, 1996). Gastrointestinal upset usually occurs at the initiation of therapy and resolves with continued use. Photosensitivity, characterized by inflammation of the skin and mucous membranes, appears more significant in animals that graze on the plant. At least one clinical trial in humans indicated no significant phototoxic effects (Schempp et al., 2001). Other reported adverse effects include anxiety, restlessness, neuropathy, fatigue, and hypomania. The use of St. John's wort is contraindicated during pregnancy and lactation.

Valerian

Botany. The medicinal components of valerian (*Valeriana officinalis* L.) are contained within the roots. This herbaceous perennial is found throughout the temperate regions of North America, Europe, and Asia. The dried rhizome contains a volatile oil that is known for its distinctive and offensive odor (Blumenthal et al., 1998; *The review of natural products,* 2002).

History. Valerian has been used for centuries as a sedative, and its use persists in France, Germany, and Switzerland (Blumenthal et al., 1998; *The review of natural products,* 2002). The plant was considered to be a fragrant perfume during the 16th century.

Basic medicinal chemistry. The valerian root contains three classes of compounds: (1) the volatile oil containing monoterpenes (e.g., borneol) and active sesquiterpenes (e.g., valerenic acid), (2) the valepotriates or nonglycosidic iridoid esters, and (3) a small number of alkaloids. The sedative activity of the plant is believed to be related to the valerenic acid and valepotriate content (Blumenthal et al., 1998; Houghton, 1999, 1999; *The review of natural products,* 2002).

The valepotriates include more than a dozen related compounds and are considered the most important chemical group responsible for the sedative effects of the plant. These compounds are found throughout the plant, but the roots contain the highest concentration (range 0.1–2.0% dry weight). The compounds hydrolyze quickly and are unstable in acid or alkaline environments (Andreatini & Leite, 1994; Houghton, 1988, 1999).

Pharmacological activity and main therapeutic use. The primary therapeutic use of valerian is for mild sleeping disorders. Although most of the pharmacological research confirms the sedative activity of valerian root (perhaps by influencing GABA, serotonin, and norepinephrine levels), most of the clinical studies lack standardization for the valerian extract (e.g., some studies specified, whereas others used unspecified amounts of valerian extract). It is likely the sedative activity of valerian is not from a single component, but rather from multiple components.

One randomized, double-blind crossover design, placebo-controlled study confirmed the sedative/hypnotic effect of valerian when 128 persons were given either 400 mg valerian extract or placebo (Leathwood et al., 1982; Leathwood & Chauffard, 1985). Patients receiving the valerian recorded a statistically ($p < .05$) and clinically significant improvement in sleep quality. Patients recorded no significant effect on night awakenings and somnolence the next morning. The outcomes of this study appeared to be similar to those of short-acting benzodiazepines.

A randomized, double-blind, placebo-controlled, crossover study with 16 patients (4 male, 12 female) with previously established psychophysiological insomnia concluded that treatment with an herbal extract containing valerian proved beneficial in patients with mild psychophysiological insomnia. Furthermore, patients experienced minimal side effects using an herbal extract containing valerian (Donath et al., 2000).

Toxicology. The toxicity of valerian compounds appears to be low. One report of a 58-year-old man showed symptoms similar to benzodiazepine withdrawal upon discontinuation of large dosages of valerian root for several years. Some controlled clinical trials report very few of the following adverse effects: excitability, cardiac disturbances, and headaches.

Avoid long-term use and during pregnancy (Bladerer & Borbely, 1985; Garges et al., 1998; Lust, 1974).

Kava Kava

Botany. The medicinal components of kava kava *(Piper methysticum)* are in the roots of this large shrub indigenous to Oceania (e.g., Fiji). There are more than 20 varieties of the kava plant, with the black and white grades valued the most for social and commercial purposes. The white grades are of higher value, though economically the black grades are preferred by growers because of the short growing season (Blumenthal et al., 1998; *The review of natural products,* 2002).

History. Traditionally, kava drink is prepared from the roots of the plant. It is one of the most common beverages in the islands of the South Pacific used to induce relaxation. The resultant cloudy mixture is often filtered and served at room temperature. For many centuries, the ceremonial preparation and consumption of kava has been used in the Pacific Islands. In this region, the ancient cultural use of kava drinking was confirmed by finding trace amounts of kavalactones through mass spectrometry. Additional folk historic uses of kava include treatment of wounds, inflammation of the uterus, colds, headaches, rheumatisms, and venereal diseases (Blumenthal et al., 1998; *The review of natural products,* 2002).

Basic medicinal chemistry. The central nervous system activity of the kava root appears to be related to the kavapyrones or substituted dihydropyrones, including methysticin, kawain, dihydromethysticin, and yangonin. Pipermethystine is an alkaloid that is a major component of the leaves (Blumenthal et al., 1998; *The review of natural products,* 2002; Singh, 1992; Smith, 1983).

Pharmacological activity and main therapeutic use. Kava kava is mainly used for its sedative properties. The kavapyrones, active constituents found in kava kava, are responsible for reducing tension and excitement. Clinical trials reveal that kava kava appears to contain pharmacological properties similar to taking oxazepam 15 mg/day or bromazepam 9 mg/day. Thus, kava kava may be an alternative to the benzodiazepines, as well as tricyclic antidepressants (Cauffield & Forbes, 1999; Pittler & Ernst, 2000).

Most human clinical trials determine efficacy based on subjective measures used in various psychological tests (e.g., Hamilton Anxiety Scale, Clinical-Global Impression Scale). Empirical data are lacking, and more clinical trials may be warranted. Most trials suffer from a small patient population, but nearly all the outpatient studies indicate the clinical efficacy of kava kava in improving anxiety symptoms (Cauffield & Forbes, 1999; Pittler & Ernst, 2000; Scherer, 1998; Volz & Kieser, 1997).

Toxicology. German Commission E monographs document eye movement disorders, and mydriasis has been reported. Dermatological features ("kawaism"), such as a reversible darkening or yellowing of the skin and flaking, have been observed following chronic ingestion of kava drink. Weight loss has also been recorded with long-term use of high doses of kava kava. Because of the lack of clinical studies, use during pregnancy and lactation is contraindicated (Mathews et al., 1988; Ruze, 1990).

In March 2002, the FDA issued an advisory notice to consumers and health care professionals regarding the risk of rare, but severe, liver injury associated with the use of kava-containing dietary substances. (Additional information regarding this advisory can be obtained at www.cfsan.fdacgov/~dms/ds/warn.html.) Despite this warning, kava kava is still used by many alternative practitioners in the United States. The validation appears to be related to moderation in dosage and acute usage.

Immune System

Echinacea

Botany. The medicinal components of echinacea (*Echinacea angustifolia* D.C.) are found throughout the entire plant. *Echinacea purpurea* L. Monench and *Echinacea pallida* (Nutt.) Britton have also been used in traditional medicine. This perennial plant is indigenous to the central United States (e.g., native to Kansas, Nebraska, and Missouri) and grows to 3 feet in height (Blumenthal et al., 1998; *The review of natural products*, 2002).

History. This plant was used by Native Americans and was adopted quickly by the early European settlers. In the beginning of the 20th century, the extracts were valued for their anti-infective properties; however, use of these products declined upon the discovery of modern antibiotics. Most current research has focused on the immunostimulant properties of the plant and supports its use in oral, topical, and intravenous dosage forms (Blumenthal et al., 1998; *The review of natural products*, 2002).

Basic medicinal chemistry. Echinacea includes a wide array of chemical compounds with various pharmacological activities, including carbohydrates, alkaloids, essential oils, and other chemical constituents. The carbohydrate echinacin may account for wound-healing properties and immunostimulant activity. Antihyaluronidase activity is associated with numerous caffeol conjugates that have been isolated from E. angustifolia (Blumenthal et al., 1998; The review of natural products, 2002).

Pharmacological activity and main therapeutic use. Numerous in vitro and animal studies document the immunostimulant properties of this plant as an antiviral, antifungal, and antibacterial agent. In Europe, echinacea is approved for the prophylaxis and treatment of colds (Bisset, 1994; Parnham, 1996; Percival, 2000). For example, studies reveal that the active constituents of echinacea affect the phagocytic but not the acquired immune system (Percival, 2000). Echinacea plant extracts have been reported to possess phototoxic antimicrobial activity against pathogenic fungi. These effects are attributed to the ketoalkene and ketoalkyne content. Furthermore, an herbal preparation containing echinacea proved to be statistically significant and clinically relevant when used to enhance immune system functioning against acute viral respiratory tract infections (Binns et al., 2000; Wustenberg et al, 1999).

Additional studies introduced a prepared potent nonstandardized extract of echinacea root into the diets of mice for 1 to 2 weeks. The results indicated that the production of natural killer cells and monocytes was significantly increased in both the bone marrow and the spleen. It is believed that one mechanism of action for this herb is to stimulate new production of those cells responsible for nonspecific immunity (Sun et al., 1999).

Nearly all the human clinical trials follow a similar methodology of having patients take a standardized extract and record any change in duration of illness. For example, results from a randomized, double-blind, placebo-controlled study revealed that echinacea reduced cold symptoms within 2 days. Patients consumed commercial product tablets three times a day for 7 to 9 days. Those patients who benefited the most therapeutically started treatment with echinacea at the initial stages of the cold symptoms (Henneicke-von Zepelin et al., 1999). Therefore, it is generally recommended to start echinacea as soon as cold symptoms are evident to obtain the most benefit.

Toxicology. Echinacea is contraindicated in immunosuppressed patients (e.g., those with human immunodeficiency virus (HIV), autoimmune diseases, and tuberculosis) and should be avoided in this population group (Bisset, 1994; Percival, 2000). Use during pregnancy and lactation should be avoided also due to a lack of sufficient data. However, various review studies on the safety and efficacy of echinacea found little to no toxicity with long-term administration (Percival, 2000).

Respiratory System

The Ephedras

Botany. The medicinal components for many members of the genus *Ephedra* are found throughout the plant. The most well known species is *E. sinica Stapf.,* also known as ma huang. These species are found throughout the world and often resemble small evergreen shrubs (Blumenthal et al., 1998; *The review of natural products,* 2002).

History. The ephedras have been used as stimulants, and it is believed these plants have been used by the Chinese to treat asthma and other bronchial disorders for more than 5,000 years. Additional clinical uses in Asian medicine include the treatment of upper respiratory disorders and musculoskeletal disorders (Blumenthal et al., 1998; *The review of natural products,* 2002).

Basic medicinal chemistry. Comprehensive pharmacologic studies of more than 22 *Ephedra* species indicates that 90% of the alkaloid content was made up of ephedrine and pseudoephedrine. Out of the species studied, *E. sinica* contained the greatest alkaloid content. Dried ephedra should contain no less than 1.25% ephedrine (Liu et al., 1993).

Pharmacological activity and main therapeutic use. The central nervous stimulants of ephedrine and its related alkaloids are active in several routes of administration, including oral, parenteral, and ophthalmic (Hardman et al., 1996). Ephedra may affect the cardiovascular system in several ways, including increase in blood pressure and heart rate; constriction of peripheral blood vessels, potentially relieving congestion in mucous tissues; bronchodilation; and diuretic properties. It can also stimulate contraction of the uterus. Several studies also show enhanced weight loss when ephedra is used in combination with methylxanthines (e.g., caffeine) (Brinker, 1998; Gurley et al, 1998).

The primary active constituent of ephedra is ephedrine, and its main therapeutic use is in the treatment of asthma. Overall, several human clinical trials support the use of ephedrine as an effective bronchodilator as assessed through measurements of increased peak expiratory flow rates. It is postulated that the mechanism of action for ephedrine on bronchial dilation and relaxation of respiratory muscles is through the stimulation of both the alpha- and beta-adrenaline-like receptors (Geumei et al., 1975; Tinkelman & Avner, 1977).

Toxicology. Ephedra is contraindicated for use in patients with high blood pressure, diabetes, hyperthyroidism, chronic heart disease, and any hypersensitivity to sympathomimetic amines. Ephedra is also contraindicated in pregnancy and lactation due to its abortifacient properties. Herb–drug interactions may occur with other sympathomimetic nonprescription medications (e.g., antihypertensives and monoamine oxidase inhibitors (MAOIs)). Ephedrine may also cause toxic psychosis. Large doses of ephedrine may affect the nervous system (e.g., nervousness, vomiting, headache, insomnia, anxiety, restlessness, dizziness, and tingling) and the cardiovascular system (e.g., palpitations and tachycardia). Higher doses of ephedrine may also cause nephrolithiasis. Abuse of ephedrine led to restrictions on sales of products containing ephedrine alkaloids (Schuckit, 1996). As of February 6, 2004, the FDA issued a regulation prohibiting the sale of dietary supplements containing ephedrine alkaloids because such supplements pose an unreasonable risk of illness or injury (for more information, see www.cfsan.fda.gov/~lrd/fpephed6.html).

Urinary System

Saw Palmetto

Botany. The medicinal components of saw palmetto *(Serenoa repens)* are in the commercially harvested brownish black berries of the plant. Saw palmetto grows to approximately 10 feet, and its leaf clusters may attain a length of greater than 2 feet. The plant is native to the southeast region of the United States (Blumenthal et al., 1998; Bombardelli & Morrazzoni, 1997; *The review of natural products,* 2002).

History. Saw palmetto has been used as a mild diuretic and for treating prostatic enlargement. It was eventually dropped from the National Formulary because the therapeutic value of the tea came under question (Blumenthal et al., 1998; The review of natural products, 2002).

Basic medicinal chemistry. Investigators believe the lipid-soluble compounds are responsible for the major pharmacological actions of the plant. Fatty acids and high amounts of sterols comprise nearly 90% of the medicinal components. Various extracts, including beta-sitosterol isolated from the berries, demonstrated an estrogenic activity following parenteral administration in mice. Saturated and unsaturated fatty acids and sterols are contained within the 1.5% oil from the dried berries. The oil is commercially available as a purified fat-soluble extract in Europe (Bombardelli & Morrazzoni, 1997).

Pharmacological activity and main therapeutic use. Preliminary studies have demonstrated the antiandrogenic properties of a hexane extract of the berries through direct action on the estrogen receptors and by inhibiting the enzyme testosterone-5-α-reductase. The saw palmetto extract has been shown to increase the metabolism and excretion of dihydrotestosterone (DHT) by inhibiting the conversion of testosterone to DHT and DHT binding to cellular and nuclear receptor sites (Champault, Patel, & Bonnard, 1984).

Most human clinical trials document strong evidence for the therapeutic use of saw palmetto in treating the symptoms of benign prostatic hyperplasia. These include dysuria, nocturia, and daytime urgency. A double-blind, placebo-controlled study evaluated the hormonal effects of saw palmetto extract given to men with benign prostatic hypertrophy for 3 months prior to surgery. The study found that saw palmetto displayed an estrogenic and antiprogesterone effect as determined by estrogen and progesterone receptor activity (Boccafoschi & Annoscia, 1983).

A meta-analysis (Bach & Ebeling, 1996) of 18 randomized controlled studies, involving nearly 3,000 men with symptomatic benign prostatic hyperplasia concluded that available evidence suggests the extracts of saw palmetto may be efficacious in improving symptoms in men with the condition. These symptoms included diminished nocturia, daytime frequency, and dysuria. The results also indicated the extract of saw palmetto compared with finasteride provided similar responses in reducing the symptoms associated with benign prostatic hyperplasia. The German Commission E monograph recommends a daily dose of 1 to 2 g (about one to two dried berries) or 320 mg of a lipid-soluble standardized extract of saw palmetto for treatment of benign prostatic hyperplasia. Current standardization for saw palmetto ranges from 85% to 95% phytosterol content.

Toxicology. The adverse effects of oral saw palmetto are mainly associated with the gastrointestinal system (e.g., diarrhea, nausea, and minor abdominal pain). A dermatological effect (e.g., pruritis) was noted in a case report. However, in most controlled trials, the incidence of side effects was low (Bach & Ebeling, 1996; Marks & Tyler, 1999).

Endocrine System

Black Cohosh

Botany. The medicinal components of black cohosh (*Cimicifuga racemosa* L. Nutt.) are in the roots. This perennial grows up to 8 feet, blooms from June to September, and is indigenous to the rich woods of Ontario to Tennessee and west to Missouri (Blumenthal et al., 1998; *The review of natural products,* 2002).

History. Black cohosh, along with many other natural ingredients, was part of a popular old-time remedy, Lydia Pinkham's Vegetable Compound, in the early 1900s. Traditional uses of the plant include treatment of gynecological disorders, rheumatisms, and dyspepsia. *Cimicifuga* means "bug repellent," and the plant has also been used for this purpose. Native Americans used the plant to treat snakebites, as well as for female problems. Since the mid-1950s, Remifemin (brand name of the standardized extract of black cohosh) has been used in Germany for the management of symptoms associated with menopause (Blumenthal et al, 1998; *The review of natural products,* 2002). Remifemin has been used in the United States for over 2 decades.

Basic medicinal chemistry. The European literature from the late 1960s discusses the contents of black cohosh. Modern research indicates that the key components include the alkaloids (e.g., *N*-methylcysteine), tannins, and terpenoids (e.g., acetin, 12-acetylactein, and cimigoside). Additional chemical constituents of the plant include acetic, butyric, formic, isoferulic, oleic, palmitic, and salicylic acids; recemosin; formononetin (an isoflavone); phytosterols; acteina (resinous mixture); and volatile oil (Blumenthal et al., 1998; *The review of natural products,* 2002).

Pharmacological activity and main therapeutic use. Most double-blind, placebo-controlled, open trials conclude that black cohosh shows good therapeutic efficacy in alleviating menopausal symptoms and may offer patients an alternative to conventional estrogen replacement therapies. Symptoms of hot flashes, vaginal atrophy and dryness, sleep disturbances, and night sweats are relieved by administration of black cohosh. The active constituents of black cohosh are believed to be particularly useful in treating the climacteric symptoms or those symptoms occurring during the transition to menopause (Hardy, 2000; Lieberman, 1998; Liske, 1998). In one study, follicle-stimulating hormone levels were reduced significantly in women treated for 8 weeks with the commercial product Remifemin. As indicated above, this product is used in Germany and the United States for the management of menopausal hot flashes and may offer an alternative to conventional hormone replacement therapy (HRT) (Duker et al., 1991).

In patients with a history of estrogen-dependent cancer, Remifemin exhibited inhibitory versus stimulatory effects on established breast tumor cell lines dependent on estrogen's presence. Conventional HRT exerts an effect on the endometrium, but Remifemin does not. Thus, no opposing therapy with progesterone is necessary. The adverse effects of estradiol include increased risk for breast, ovarian, and endometrial cancers. However, the pharmacologic activity of the plant's extracts is similar to estriol, which exerts its main effects on the vaginal lining, versus estradiol, which exerts its main effect on the uterine lining (Duker et al., 1991).

A randomized, placebo-controlled, double-blind study of 85 patients recorded statistical and clinical significance for the therapeutic use of black cohosh in reducing the intensity and number of menopausal symptoms (particularly night sweats). Critics of the study note the only limitation is its short (2-month) duration (Jackobson et al., 2001).

Toxicology. Larger doses of black cohosh appear to affect the gastrointestinal, nervous, and cardiovascular systems. Symptoms of nausea, vomiting, dizziness, visual disturbances, reduced heart rate, and increased perspiration have been documented with toxic doses of black cohosh. Black cohosh is contraindicated during pregnancy (i.e., risk of premature birth) and during lactation (Baille & Rasmussen, 1997; Gunn & Wright, 1996; Shuster, 1997).

Adaptogen or Performance Enhancer

Ginseng

Botany. The medicinal components of ginseng (*Panax quinquefolium* L. (American), *P. ginseng* CA Meyer (Asian)) are contained within the leaves and roots. Worldwide, there are numerous species of ginseng that are used in local traditional medicine. The roots mature slowly and often are used to distinguish various types or species of ginseng. Ginseng is grown commercially in the United States. This plant bears its red or yellowish fruits from June to July and grows three to seven compound leaves that drop in the fall (Blumenthal et al., 1998; *The review of natural products,* 2002).

History. Various forms of ginseng have been used for more than 2,000 years in medicine. Ginseng root's man-shaped figure, as well as the name *Panax,* meaning "all healing," adds to ginseng's rich history of being viewed as an overall panacea. Numerous purported uses of ginseng include treatment of cardiovascular diseases (e.g., atherosclerosis) and gastrointestinal disorders (e.g., colitis) and relieving the symptoms of aging, cancer, and senility. Today, ginseng is designated as an adaptogen, or stress-protective agent, most likely due to its saponin content (Blumenthal et al., 1998; *The review of natural products,* 2002; Liu & Xiao, 1992).

Basic medicinal chemistry. A saponin called panaquilon was isolated from *P. quinquefolium* in 1854. Most modern chemical analyses of ginseng have focused on a group of compounds known as ginsenosides or panaxosides. There are at least 28 ginsenosides, and the active constituents vary by species, age of the root, location, season, and curing method. Additional pharmacologic effects may be associated with other minor components, which include flavonoids, vitamins, minerals, enzymes, choline, peptides, volatile oils, and beta-elemene (Cui, Eneroth, & Bjoerkhem, 1994; Liu & Xiao, 1992; Shin et al., 1997).

Pharmacological activity and main therapeutic use. On the basis of in vitro experiments, the pharmacological effects of the ginseng saponins may be associated with antimutagenic, anticancer, anti-inflammatory, antidiabetes, and neurovascular activity (Bahrke & Morgan, 2000; Ong & Yong, 2000). For example, ginsenoside Rb-1 protects against the development of certain gastrointestinal disorders (e.g., stress ulcers) and has CNS activity (depressant, anticonvulsant, analgesic, and antipsychotic). The adrenal gland and pituitary gland help the body respond to stress, and ginseng appears to potentiate the normal function of the adrenal gland (Filaretov et al., 1988). Modern research shows some support for the historical use of ginseng as an adaptogen. These effects include the use of ginseng in enhancing immune system response by increasing production of macrophages, B and T cells, natural killer cells, and colony-forming activity of bone marrow (Filaretov et al., 1988).

The results of a multicenter, randomized, placebo-controlled, double-blind clinical trial studied the immune system response in patients receiving an anti-influenza polyvalent vaccination. In patients receiving 200 mg of standardized ginseng extract versus placebo, there was an increase in natural killer cell activity, thus enhancing immune system activity. Other clinical studies conclude with similar results (Scaglione et al., 1990, 1996).

The 1991 Commission E monograph recommends ginseng for the following uses: counteracting weakness and fatigue, restoring declining stamina and impaired concentration, and managing convalescence. Due to potential hormone-inducing effects, it is recommended that treatment be limited to 3 months. The daily recommended dosage is 200 mg to 600 mg qid for standardized extracts or 1 g to 2 g of the crude drug.

Toxicology. MAOI drugs should not be used with ginseng. One controversial report described "ginseng abuse syndrome," manifested by cerebral arteritis in a 28-year-old female consuming more than 3 g qid for up to 1 month. The syndrome may consist of hypertension, nervousness, sleeplessness, nausea, and vomiting. The most commonly reported side effects of ginseng include euphoria, nervousness, and excitation that usually diminish with dosage reduction. Ginseng may lower blood sugar levels due to the saponin content; therefore, diabetic patients should take ginseng with caution (Newall, Anderson, & Phillipson, 1996; Ryui & Chien, 1995; Sotaniemi, Haapakoski, & Rautio, 1995).

NUTRITIONAL SUPPLEMENTS

Rhodiola Rosea

History

Rhodiola rosea is an herbal remedy that is classified as an adaptogen because of its ability to promote tolerance to various chemical, physical, and biological stressors. Chronic stress is thought to contribute to increased oxidation, inflammation, heart disease, and cancer. Rhodiola, also known as arctic root and golden root, is a popular treatment in Europe and Asia for enhancing performance, decreasing fatigue, improving sleep, and improving depression. Other uses have included prevention of high-altitude sickness[1] and nervous system stimulation.

Chemistry

The main constituents found in rhodiola include antioxidants p-tyrosol, flavonoids such as catechins and proanthocyanidins, and organic acids like caffeic, chlorogenic, and gallic acid.[2] The adaptogenic properties of rhodiola are mainly attributed to p-tyrosol and salidroside content.[3] Currently, rosavin is the constituent used in the standardization of rhodiola extracts. Pharmacokinetic studies conducted on rhodiola show that p-tyrosol is readily absorbed following oral administration.[4]

Pharmacology

The adaptogenic and cardioprotective effects of rhodiola have been primarily attributed to its ability to increase the activity of biogenic amines (norepinephrine, dopamine, and serotonin) in the cerebral cortex, hypothalamus, and brainstem.[5] Changes seen in monoamine levels are thought to be due to inhibition of monoamine oxidase enzymes responsible for degradation of neurotransmitters within the brain. Rhodiola's adaptogenic properties may also be related to induction of opioid peptide biosynthesis as well as stimulation of both central and peripheral opioid receptors.[6] Animal studies using rhodiola in rats showed that when rhodiola-treated rats were exposed to acute stress, no observed elevations or decreases in beta-endorphin levels were found.[7] These findings led researchers to conclude that rhodiola can prevent stress-induced fluctuations in the hypothalamic-pituitary-adrenal axis.

Rhodiola has also shown promise as a treatment for enhancing productivity at work and sleep disturbances. A 2-week study conducted on on night-duty physicians showed improved mental performance and decreased fatigue using daily rhodiola supplementation.[8] Studies conducted on students demonstrate rhodiola's ability to improve mental performance, psychomotor function, and overall well-being. Additional effects noted were improved sleep, increased motivation and mood, and decreased mental fatigue. A comparison of average exam scores in students receiving rhodiola extracts versus those receiving placebo showed scores of 3.47 versus 3.20 for placebo ($p < .05$).[9] Anticancer research on rhodiola has only been conducted in animal studies. However, rhodiola has been shown to inhibit tumor growth and decreased metastasis in rats transplanted with solid Ehrlich adenocarcinomas, lymphosarcomas,[10] or Lewis lung carcinomas. Combination studies using rhodiola extract along with cyclophosphamide resulted in enhanced chemotherapeutic efficacy, decreased antineoplastic toxicity, and decreased metastasis.[11] Combined with doxorubicin (Adriamycin), rhodiola extract demonstrated the ability to inhibit tumor dissemination compared to doxorubicin alone.[12] Hepatotoxicity was also prevented in the rhodiola and doxorubicin–treated group compared to doxorubicin alone.

Dosages for rhodiola supplementation vary depending on the standardization of rosavin. For chronic usage, 360 to 600 mg of a rhodiola extract standardized to 1% rosavin, 180 to 300 mg of an extract standardized to 2% rosavin, or 100 to 175 mg of extracts of 3% rosavin or higher has been suggested. Administration is usually started several weeks before a period of increased stress and maintained until after the stressful period ceases. Single doses for acute uses are generally 2 to 3 times the dosage used for chronic administration and depend on standardization of rosavin.

Toxicology

Rhodiola has shown increased irritability and insomnia at dosages above 1.5 to 2.0 g daily in extracts standardized to 2% rosavin. Rhodiola has been safely administered in patients for as little as one dose up to 4 months of daily usage. Until more long-term data are obtained, a dosing regimen utilizing periodic intervals of abstinence in chronic usage seems justified. The safety of rhodiola in pregnancy and lactation has not currently been established.

Coenzyme Q_{10} (Ubiquinone)

History

Ubiquinone was first isolated in laboratory experiments in the late 1950s. It has since been thoroughly investigated in the United States, Japan, and Russia. Ubiquinone is a key intermediate in the electron transport system of mitochondria, making ubiquinone necessary for optimal production of adenosine triphosphate (ATP). Ubiquinone is the drug of choice for the management of cardiovascular diseases in Japan, specifically congestive heart failure, arrhythmias, hypertension, angina, and cardiomyopathy.[13] Other uses include treatment for cancer, immunostimulation, antiaging, periodontal disease, Parkinson's disease, male infertility, thermogenesis, and physical performance enhancement.

Chemistry

Ubiquinone is structurally related to vitamin K and belongs to a larger class of lipophilic benzoquinones that are involved in cellular respiration. Specifically, ubiquinone is extensively involved in redox reactions in the cellular mitochondrial electron transport chain. Exercise-induced increases in ubiquinone have been demonstrated in red muscle of the quadriceps and soleus muscles of rats, but studies have shown no increase in white muscle.[14] This further illustrates ubiquinone's ability to adapt positively to exercise training.

Pharmacological Activity and Main Therapeutic Use

Ubiquinone has been shown to enhance energy production via the electron transport system, improve cardiac muscle contractility, and act as a potent scavenger of free radicals. It is due to these mechanisms that ubiquinone can be used clinically to treat various conditions. Immunostimulation and antioxidation are two mechanisms by which ubiquinone exerts its anticancer properties. A pair of uncontrolled clinical trials using 390 mg/day of ubiquinone showed significant tumor regression and a decreased incidence of metastasis.[15,16] Additionally, ubiquinone at dosages of 100 to 200 mg daily has been shown to prevent doxorubicin-induced cardiotoxicity, without compromising chemotherapeutic efficacy.[17,18] Cardiac disease states that ubiquinone has been shown to benefit include cardiomyopathy, congestive heart failure, angina, arrhythmias, mitral valve prolapse, and hypertension. Individuals with a family history of diabetes mellitus have shown clinical benefit from ubiquinone supplementation. Decreased serum ubiquinone levels in type II diabetic patients may be associated with subclinical cardiomyopathy, which is generally reversible upon supplementation with ubiquinone. Ubiquinone has been shown to enhance aerobic respiration and performance in red muscle but not white muscle.[14] This effect is more pronounced in sedentary individuals compared to professionally trained athletes. Studies using 1,200 mg ubiquinone daily in Parkinson's disease have demonstrated a protective effect by significantly decreasing disease progression compared to placebo.[19] Standard dosages of ubiquinone range from 50 to 200 mg daily; however, dosages of up to 1,200 mg daily have been used.

Toxicology

Hydroxy-3-methylglutaryl-coenzyme A (HMG-CoA) reductase inhibitors, such as pravastatin and lovastatin, have been shown to deplete serum levels of ubiquinone.[20] They achieve this effect by decreasing the endogenous production of ubiquinone and cholesterol. Therefore, it is generally recommended to supplement with ubiquinone upon initiation of statin therapy. Additionally, beta-blockers, phenothiazines, and tricyclic antidepressants have been shown to inhibit ubiquinone-dependent enzymes. Overall, ubiquinone is well tolerated, with nausea, decreased appetite, and skin eruptions being occasionally reported. Use in pregnancy and lactation is not recommended because of insufficient clinical data.[13] Hypersensitive individuals are advised to refrain from ubiquinone usage.

Fish Oil

History

Excessive intake of trans fatty acids, saturated fats, and arachidonic acid have been linked to chronic inflammation and disease. Because the typical Western diet tends to be high in all of these, increased incidences of obesity, insulin resistance, cancer, and heart disease are higher in industrialized nations compared to third world nations. In cultures that consume a high percentage of fish in their diet, like the Eskimos, lower incidences of atherosclerotic and thrombotic conditions have been observed. Fish oils, notably eicosapentaenoic acid (EPA) and docosahexanoic acid (DHA) (mainly found in coldwater fish such as herring, mackerel, bluefish, and salmon) have been shown to decrease systemic inflammation.[21] EPA and DHA are made from the omega-3 fatty acid alpha-linoleic acid, which cannot be made endogenously. Dietary sources include flaxseed oil, wheat germ oil, nuts, seeds, and vegetables. Common uses for fish oils include enhancement of brain function, increasing hormonal production, cardiovascular support, and chronic inflammation.

Chemistry

Fish oils fall into the category of omega-3 fatty acids, which fall under the larger category of polyunsaturated fatty acids (PUFAs). The most common fish oils are EPA and DHA, which derive from alpha-linoleic acid. Alpha-linoleic acid is first converted to EPA, then into DHA through a series of enzyme-mediated reactions. Although consumption of alpha-linoleic acid can lead to increased levels of EPA, it does not automatically increase DHA levels.[22]

Pharmacology

EPA and DHA compete with arachidonic acid for the cyclooxygenase enzyme in the inflammatory cascade. EPA is converted to thromboxane A_3 via platelet cyclooxygenase, which possesses weak vasoconstrictive properties compared to thromboxane A_2, which is a potent vasoconstrictor. Thromboxane A_2 is formed from the interaction of cyclooxygenase and arachidonic acid. Alternately, when prostacyclin A_3 is formed from endothelial EPA, strong vasodilatory effects are noted as well as inhibition of platelet aggregation. Antiatherogenic properties are noted for EPA and DHA through a reduction in 5-series leukotrienes and chemotaxis. Fish oils lower serum triglycerides and very low-density lipoprotein (VLDL) through inhibition of hepatic triglyceride synthesis; however, the majority of studies have been conducted in men only. In one study conducted with postmenopausal women, fish oil showed a 26% reduction in serum triglycerides regardless of hormone replacement status.[23] The estimated effect of coronary heart disease (CHD) risk reduction was 27% for postmenopausal women. Studies also show fish oils to be helpful in the treatment of dysmenorrhea.[24] EPA and DHA supplementation has been shown to suppress tumor growth and metastasis in breast and colon cancers. Anticancer properties of EPA have been mainly correlated with suppression of cell proliferation, whereas those of DHA appear to be related to induction of apoptosis.[25] Observational studies have demonstrated that low concentrations of omega-3 fatty acids are related to greater severity of depression and impulsive behavior.[26] Omega-3 fatty acid deficiencies may be linked to catecholaminergic dysfunction in depressed individuals. Dietary studies found that 5% to 10% of dietary caloric intake from fish oil significantly increased glucose uptake and maintained normal glucose levels even at high levels of fat intake.[27] Fish oil enhances insulin secretion from pancreatic beta cells, regulating glucose metabolism.[28] Common therapeutic dosage for fish oils varies but typically ranges between 1 and 5 g daily.

Toxicology

Fish oil supplementation is generally well tolerated, with few side effects reported. Toxicity studies conducted to determine dose-limiting toxicities of fish oil mainly report gastrointestinal complaints like diarrhea.[29] Other studies have focused on heavy metal contamination of fish, specifically mercury. Dietary intake of fish is the primary source for mercury exposure in the generalized population.[30] Quality control of product and production is essential for consumer safety. To ensure quality of a product, the fish oil should be purified to remove heavy metals, polychlorinated biphenyls (PCBs), and dioxins.

Glucosamine Sulfate

History

Glucosamine is the physiologic substrate required for the biosynthesis of glycosaminoglycans and hyaluronic acid, which together form proteoglycans. Glucosamine is also required for the synthesis of glycolipids, glycoproteins, lubricants, and protective agents like mucin. The role of glucosamine sulfate in retarding joint degradation is directly related to its ability to stimulate endogenous production of proteoglycans found within the structural matrix of articular cartilage. Studies conducted on glucosamine sulfate have demonstrated efficacy in halting the progression of degenerative joint disease and controlling pain associated with osteoarthritis.[31,32]

Chemistry

Glucosamine is primarily found in chitin, which is a major component of the exoskeleton of various invertebrates. Normally chitin is found in shellfish such as lobster, shrimp, and crabs. Chitin is a cellulose derivative where the C-2 hydroxyl groups have been replaced by acetamido moieties.[13] Glucosamine, or 2-amino-2 deoxyglucose, is isolated chemically from chitin or it can be made synthetically. Glucosamine sulfate is the preferred form for treatment of osteoarthritis, despite the existence of other forms such as the hydrochloride salt or N-acetylglucosamine that have not demonstrated clinical efficacy.[33]

Pharmacology

Osteoarthritis is associated with progressive degradation of articular proteoglycans. Glucosamine sulfate is not only capable of increasing proteoglycan synthesis, it also inhibits proteoglycan degradation and stimulates the regeneration of damaged cartilage. It has also been hypothesized that glucosamine sulfate might promote the incorporation of sulfur into articular cartilage. Sulfate concentrations below 0.3 mM are associated with decreased production of glycosaminoglycans as well as increased collagenase activity.

The main therapeutic use of glucosamine sulfate has been in the treatment of osteoarthritis, or degenerative joint disease (DJD). Several double-blind clinical trials have shown that glucosamine sulfate is more effective than NSAIDs like ibuprofen and placebo in relieving pain and swelling associated with osteoarthritis.[31,34] Symptoms like joint pain and tenderness, decreased mobility, and swelling often improve during a brief 6- to 8-week period of glucosamine sulfate therapy. Most patients should expect a reduction of 50% to 70% in their symptoms. These effects are generally sustained for 6–12 weeks following cessation of use. Preliminary evidence indicates that patients with osteoarthritis of the knee, shoulder, or elbow respond best to glucosamine sulfate therapy, while the poorest response is seen in polyarthritic patiens and arthritis of the hip.[35] Other uses for glucosamine sulfate include tempromandibular joint osteoarthritis[36] and gum disease.

The bioavailability of glucosamine sulfate following oral administration is about 90 percent. It is metabolized in the liver then excreted primarily through the urine with a minor percentage eliminated in the feces. Typical dosage is 1500 mg daily in divides doses for non-obese individuals. Higher dosages are used in these individuals since obesity has been associated with below average responses to glucosamine sulfate.

Toxicology

Glucosamine sulfate is safe and generally well tolerated in patients. Commonly reported side effects are mild and involve gastrointestinal complaints (nausea, diarrhea, vomiting, heartburn,etc.), drowsiness, headaches, and skin reactions.[35] Currently, no LD50 has been established for glucosamine sulfate, since even at extreme dosages of 2.7 g/kg, there is no mortality in rats.[37] Although glucosamine sulfate has been used safely in patients with hepatic dysfunction, pulmonary disorders, circulatory disease, and depression, some concern exists over the use of glucosamine sulfate in diabetic patients. Glucosamine sulfate is hypothesized to promote insulin resistance in both type I and II diabetic patients.[38,39]

Patients with active peptic ulcers undergoing treatment show an increased risk of side effects from glucosamine sulfate.[35] The source of glucosamine sulfate in nutritional supplements is shellfish, therefore, individuals with a hypersensitivity to shellfish should avoid glucosamine sulfate, and its relative chondroitin sulfate.

Melatonin

History

The pineal gland has been a source of curiosity since antiquity. The ancient Greeks considered the pineal gland to be the seat of the soul. Melatonin is a hormone that is produced in the pineal gland and also in extrapineal tissues. Its secretion is inhibited by light and stimulated by darkness. Nocturnal secretion usually begins around 9 pm and peaks between 2 and 4 am.[13] Melatonin levels reach their peak in adolescence and gradually decline with age. Modern studies with melatonin demonstrate it ability to regulate circadian rhythms and body temperature, combat insomnia and jet lag, scavenge free radicals, stimulate the immune system, and prevent aging. Melatonin has been classified as an orphan drug since 1993 for the treatment of circadian rhythm sleep disorders although it is not approved for marketing as a drug.[13] Commercially, melatonin is available in synthetic form or animal-derived pineal gland in dosages ranging from 1 to 5 mg. Use of animal-derived pineal extracts should be discouraged to decrease the transmission of BSE and related viral species.

Chemistry

Chemically, melatonin is known as N-acetyl-5-methoxytryptamine. It can be synthesized from 5-methoxyindole or it can be isolated from bovine pineal glands. Melatonin occurs as a pale yellow crystalline material with a molecular weight of 232.27, relatively low for a hormone.[13]

Pharmacology

Melatonin is useful in the treatment of insomnia, jet lag, decreasing estrogen release, and decreasing breast cancer rates.[40] Its exact mechanism of action is not clearly defined, but melatonin is intricately involved in the regulation of hormone secretion. An internal clock that signals the release of various hormones at different times of the day governs regulation of bodily functions.

Decreased serum melatonin levels have been shown in patients of varying age with insomnia. Studies using 0.3 to 6 mg melatonin administered between 9 and 10 pm have produced inconsistent results.[13] The primary effects of nighttime administration are decreased onset sleep latency and decreased latency to stage II sleep.[13] REM sleep was unaffected and there were no hangover effects reported. Several studies using high doses of melatonin (75–100 mg) administered nightly have shown decreased sleep onset, nighttime awakenings along with increases in sleep efficiency and stage II sleep.[13] In a study conducted on 12 elderly subjects with chronic insomnia, melatonin significantly increased sleep efficiency and decreased wake time after onset of sleep compared to placebo.[41] There were no significant differences in total sleep time or onset of sleep. A study using 5 mg melatonin 3–4 hours before sleep for 4 weeks showed decreased onset of sleep but did not affect total sleep time.[42] Pharmacokinetic studies using 2 mg melatonin produced serum levels that were 10 times higher than normal physiologic levels, however, this effect only lasted 3-4 hours.[43] A study in elderly patients with insomnia showed decreased sleep onset in patients using a 1 mg immediate release form or 2 mg sustained released form after 1 week.[44] Decreased sleep onset improved to a greater extent when the sustained release form was continued for 2 months but not with the immediate release form. Hospitalized patients given low doses of melatonin (~6 mg) nightly fell asleep faster and slept longer than their placebo-matched counterparts.[45]

Melatonin has been investigated in several studies for the prevention of jet lag associated with travel. One study examined the effects of 5 mg melatonin daily in 52 aircraft personnel compared to placebo.[46] Subjects were randomized to placebo, early, and late melatonin groups. The early group began melatonin supplementation 3 days before departure and for 5 days after arrival whereas the late group began melatonin the day of arrival and for 4 days after arrival. Compared to placebo, the late melatonin group reported decreased jet lag, fewer sleep disturbances, and decreased time to recover alertness and energy. Early group melatonin users reported similar or worse effects than placebo. Therefore it is generally recommended to begin supplementing with melatonin early evening preflight followed by bedtime administration for 4 days when traveling eastbound and melatonin at bedtime for 4 days when traveling westbound.[13] Several studies investigating the role of melatonin as an adjunctive treatment in malignancy have shown positive partial responses and stabilization of disease. Animal and in-vitro studies further demonstrate the inhibitory effect of melatonin on tumor growth, specifically breast cancer cell lines.[47] Melatonin is theorized to stimulate natural killer (NK) cell lines and enhance antioxidant activity. European studies using a B-oval, a supplement containing melatonin, show that melatonin can slow the growth rate of tumor cells.[13] Additionally, melatonin has been shown to improve 1 year survival rates in metastatic lung cancer patients.

Use of a sustained release formulation, repeated low doses, or high doses of 5 mg or more ensures effectiveness of melatonin supplementation. Most available preparations of melatonin range from 0.5 to 5 mg dosages.

Toxicology

A randomized, double-blind, placebo-controlled study was conducted to evaluate the effect of melatonin supplementation on nifedipine Gastrointestinal Therapeutic System (GITS, trade name Procardia).[48] Forty-seven mild to moderately hypertensive patients were evaluated and compared to placebo, the melatonin treated group showed an increase in blood pressure throughout the 24-hour period (6.5 mmgHg in systolic and 4.9 mmHg in diastolic pressure). Systolic increases were mainly noted in the afternoon and early evening while diastolic increases were found mainly in the morning. Additionally, an increased chronotropic effect of 3.9 bpm was noted in melatonin-treated subjects.

Few short-term and no long-term safety studies have been conducted on melatonin. Researchers administering 6 g of melatonin nightly for 1 month failed to show any major problems beyond stomach upset and residual drowsiness.[13] Toxicology studies have been unable to determine the LD_{50} even at extreme dosages. Other studies with melatonin have shown no statistical differences between adverse effects reported by patients or in lab results compared to placebo.[49] Minor side effects noted with melatonin dosages <8 mg include headache, transient depression, and "heavy head".[13] Caution should be exercised when using melatonin during the daytime as excessive drowsiness may occur. People who operate heavy machinery or drive for employment should avoid using melatonin while working. Melatonin should be avoided in pregnancy and lactation due to a lack of clinically relevant safety data.

Ipriflavone (Ostivone')

History

Ipriflavone was first discovered in the 1930s but only in the last decade has it been thoroughly investigated by researchers. Over 150 studies have been conducted on the safety and efficacy of ipriflavone in Japan, Italy, and Hungary. Preliminary evidence shows great promise for ipriflavone in the prevention and treatment of osteoporosis along with other bone diseases. 1997 data on ipriflavone showed 2769 patients had been treated in 60 studies for a total of 3132 patient years.[50] Ipriflavone is classified as an isoflavone and is synthesized from dadzein, another isoflavone found in soy.

Chemistry

Chemically ipriflavone is known as 7-isopropoxyisoflavone. It is also known as 7-isopropoxy-3-phenylchromone, 7-isopropoxy-3-phenyl-4H-1-benzopyran-4-one, and 7-(1-methylethoxy)-3-phenyl-4H-1-benzopyran-4-one. It occurs as a solid and is almost completely insoluble in water.

Pharmacology and Therapeutic Use

Ipriflavone and its metabolites work by several mechanisms in the treatment of osteoporosis. In vitro studies demonstrate ipriflavone's ability to stimulate the proliferation of osteoblast-like cell lines and enhance collagen formation.[51] Animal studies have shown that ipriflavone inhibits parathyroid hormone-, vitamin D-, PGE2-, and IL1(-stimulated bone resorption.[52] Additionally, a study conducted to evaluate the interaction of ipriflavone and proosteoclastic cell lines found that it is not mediated by estrogen receptors.[53] Ipriflavone may also increase the sensitivity of the thyroid gland to estrogen-stimulated calcitonin secretion.[54] The lack of estrogenic effects of ipriflavone is best illustrated by a study conducted in 15 postmenopausal women who were given a single dose of 600 mg or 1000 mg daily for 7–21 days.[55] LH, FSH, prolactin, and estradiol were measured after the first and last doses and found to have no change compared to placebo.

Ipriflavone dosed at 200 mg three times daily along with 500–1000 mg calcium significantly improved bone mass compared to placebo in several 2 year studies.[56,57] An Italian study investigated 600 mg ipriflavone and 1 g calcium daily vs. placebo in 112 patients and found a 4–6% increase in bone density along with decrease in fracture rates (2 vs. 11).[58] A recent study published in *JAMA* found no significant change in women taking 200 mg ipriflavone 3 times daily compared to women taking placebo.[59] Bone density did not improve in the treated patients but it did not worsen either. A 12 month open label trial compared ipriflavone with calcitonin (salmon) in 40 postmenopausal women found a 4.3% increase in bone mineral density (BMD) compared to 1.9% increase in the calcitonin-treated group.[60] Ipriflavone has also been reported to be beneficial in Paget's disease, parathyroid dysfunction, and renal osteodystrophy.

Toxicology

Ipriflavone is a safe and generally well tolerated nutritional supplement. In the various human studies conducted on ipriflavone, the incidence of adverse effects was 14.5% for ipriflavone vs. 16.1% for placebo.[50] Common side effects include stomach discomfort, nausea, heartburn, skin rash, headaches, drowsiness, tachycardia. Leukopenia has been reported in patients but occurs rarely.[59] Patients put on long-term ipriflavone therapy should be monitored periodically for white blood cell counts to assess hematologic suppression. Dosages for ipriflavone vary depending on the condition being treated but most studies have used 200 mg 3 times daily. Dosages as high as 1200 mg daily have been used for other disease states of the bone.

Ipriflavone has been shown to increase serum theophylline levels by decreasing theophylline metabolism in pharmacokinetic studies.[61,62] Ipriflavone is metabolized primarily through cytochrome p450 enzymes in the liver. Additionally, ipriflavone acts synergistically with estrogen to normalize calcitonin levels.[54]

Aromatherapy

Aromatherapy is a form of phytotherapy that is growing in popularity. Aromatherapy uses the essential oils from plants for their therapeutic properties. Essential oils are the volatile oils that give plants their distinctive aromas and tastes. Most essential oils—the essence of the plant—are not viscous in texture like olive oil, but rather more volatile in structure like water or alcohol. Essential oils have long been used in cosmetics and cooking. For example, it is the essential oil of bergamot (in the citrus family) that gives Earl Grey tea its distinctive scent and flavor. Most of us are familiar with the uses of mint oil or lemon oil in the flavoring of foods, and few have escaped the ubiquitous lavender scented soaps, unguents, and moisturizers. Until synthetic scents were invented, all perfumes were made with essential oils. What makes the application of essential oils therapeutic, is the informed use of the highly concentrated essence of a plant for the purposes of healing.

Essential oils can be absorbed by the body through the skin, via the olfactory system, or by the digestive system. Aromatherapy oils are rarely ingested, however, because many of the oils are quite toxic if taken internally. Essential oils are most commonly applied to the skin in a massage oil or in a steam bath. Alternately, the oils can be put in a diffuser which allows the oil to evaporate into the air and enter the body through the nose.

Aromatherapy is used for a wide range of conditions: everything from athlete's foot (tea tree oil) to depression (bergamot, lavender, basil jasmine). Many essential oils have antiseptic properties (e.g., thyme, cedar, pine, bergamot, tea tree oils) and can be applied topically to prevent or treat infection. Others stimulate digestion (basil, rosemary, peppermint), act as analgesics (chamomile, lavender) or serve to reduce inflammation (eucalyptus, patchouli, bay). A wide variety of essential oils are said to be useful for treating mood disturbances, such as anxiety, depression, nervousness, agitation, insomnia, and irritability.

One of the reasons aromatherapy has rapidly become popular is that the essential oils are readily available in health food stores and are easily applied. However, *caveat emptor:* not all essential oils are created equal; some are mixed with synthetics or extracted using harsh chemicals and these are not suitable for aromatherapy. Pure essential oils are available from reputable vendors, but the buyer must know what to look for. Avoid vendors that sell inexpensive rose oil, for example, since pure rose oil is notoriously difficult to extract and tiny bottles of pure rose essential oil are very expensive. Most reputable health food stores screen out ersatz essential oils; purchasing oils that are certified organic will guarantee a certain level of quality.

Most of the clinical research conducted on aromatherapy for older adults has focused on the calming, uplifting, and soothing qualities of certain essential oils for patients suffering from chronic pain, agitation, and anxiety, often in hospice or long-term care settings (Lewis & Kowalski, 2002). One study found that the topical application of lemon balm *(Melissa officinalis)* decreased agitation among a group of nursing home residents with severe dementia (Ballard et al., 2002). Several studies have been conducted to explore aromatherapy as an adjunctive therapy with other invasive conventional treatments (e.g., dialysis, radiation). Generally, any essential oil known to have calming properties can be safely administered by putting a few drops into a base oil (i.e., safflower, sesame, sunflower) and massaging this gently into the skin. Precautions should be taken with some oils, such as citrus oils, known to irritate the skin; these can be used in a diffuser.

By Elizabeth Mackenzie

CONCLUSION

The use of phytomedicine in the United States is widespread and likely to increase over the coming decades. Many herbs and supplements show promise in the treatment of conditions and illnesses associated with aging, and phytomedicines and phytotherapies will no doubt be a major component of integrated medicine as it evolves. Understanding the benefits and drawbacks of using herbs and supplements for health promotion and the treatment of disease is crucial for those who provide care to aging patients.

RESOURCES

American Botanical Council, 6200 Manor Road, Austin, TX 78723; telephone: (512) 926–4900; fax: (512) 926–2345; Web site: http://www.herbalgram.org

American Herbal Pharmacopoeia, P.O. Box 66809, Scotts Valley, CA 95067; telephone: (831) 461–6318; fax: (831) 475–6219; Web site: http://www.herbal-ahp.org

American Herbalists Guild, 1931 Gaddis Rd., Canton, GA 30115; telephone: (770) 751-6021; fax: (770) 751-7472; Web site: http://www.americanherbalistsguild.com

Blumenthal, M., et al. (Eds.). (1998). *The Complete German Commission E monographs: Therapeutic guide to herbal medicines.* Newton, MA: Integrative Medicine Communications.

Blumenthal, M., Goldberg, A., & Brinckmann, J. (Eds.). (2000). *Herbal medicine: Expanded Commission E monographs.* Newton, MA: Integrative Medicine Communications.

Gruenwald, J. (Ed.). (2000). *PDR for herbal medicines.* Montvale, NJ: Medical Economics.

Herb Research Foundation, 4140 15th St., Boulder, CO 80304; telephone: (303) 449-2265; fax: (303) 449-7849; Web site: http://www.herbs.org

NAPRALERT (Natural Products Alert), Program for Collaborative Research in the Pharmaceutical Sciences, 833 S. Wood St., M/C 877, Chicago, IL 60612; telephone: (312) 996-7253; fax: (312) 413-5894. Also available through Scientific and Technical Information International, Web site: http://stneasy.cas.org

National Association for Holistic Aromatherapy, 3327 W. Indian Trail Rd., PMB 144, Spokane, WA 99208; telephone: (509)325-3419; fax (509) 325-3479; e-mail: info@naha.org; Web site: www.naha.org

National Center for Complementary and Alternative Medicine, National Institutes of Health, Health Information on Dietary Supplements, Web site: http://nccam.nih.gov/health/supplements.htm

NOTES

1. Petkov VD, Yonkov D, Mosharoff A, et al. Effects of alchol aqueous extract from Rhodiola rosea L. roots on learning and memory. *Acta Physiol Pharmacol Bulg.* 1986; 12(1):3–16.
2. Lee MW, Lee YA, Park HM, et al. Antioxidative phenolic compounds from the roots of Rhodiola sachalinensis A Bor. *Arch Pharm Res.* 2000 Oct; 23(5):455–8.
3. Linh PT, Kim YH, Hong SP, et al. Quantitative determination of salidroside and tyrosol from the underground part of Rhodiola rosea by high performance liquid chromatography. *Arch Pharm Res.* 2000 Aug; 23(4):349–52.
4. Bonanome A, Pagnan A, Caruso D, et al. Evidence of postprandial absorption of olive oil phenols in humans. *Nutr Metab Cardiovasc Dis.* 2000 Jun; 10(3):111–20.
5. Stancheva SL, Mosharrof A. Effect of the extract of Rhodiola rosea L. on the content of brain biogenic monamines. *Med Physiol.* 1987; 40:85–87.
6. Maimeskulova LA, Maslov LN, Lishmanov IuB, et al. The participation of the mu-, delta-, and kappa-opioid receptors in the realization of the anti-arrhythmia effect of Rhodiola rosea. *Eksp Klin Farmakol.* 1997 Jan–Feb; 60(1):38–9. [Article in Russian].

7. Lishmanov IuB, Trifonova ZhV, Tsibin AN, et al. Plasma beta-endorphin and stress hormones in stress and adaptation. *Biull Eksp Biol Med.* 1987 Apr; 103(4):422–4. [Article in Russian].

8. Darbinyan V, Kteyan A, Panossian A, et al. Rhodiola rosea in stress induces fatigue—a double blind crossover study of a standardized extract SHR-5 with a repeated low-dose regimen on the mental performance of healthy physicians during night duty. *Phytomedicine.* 2000 Oct; 7(5):365–71.

9. Spasov AA, Wikman GK, Mandrikov VB, et al. A double-blind, placebo-controlled pilot study of the stimulating and adaptogenic effect of Rhodiola rosea SHR-5 extract on the fatigue of students caused by stress during an examination period with a repeated low-dose regimen. *Phytomedicine.* 2000 Apr; 7(2):85–9.

10. Udintsev SN, Shakhov VP. The role of humoral factors of regenerating liver in the development of experimental tumors and the effect of Rhodiola rosea extract on this process. *Neoplasma.* 1991; 38(3):323–31.

11. Udintsev SN, Schakhov VP. Decrease of cyclophosphamide haematotoxicity by Rhodiola rosea root extract in mice with Ehrlich and Lewis transplantable tumors. *Eur J Cancer.* 1991; 27(9):1182.

12. Udintsev SN, Krylova SG, Fomina TI. The enhancement of the efficacy of adriamycin by using hepatoprotectors of plant origin in metastases of Ehrlich's adenocarcinoma to the liver in mice. *Vopr Onkol.* 1992; 38(10):1217–22.

13. Cada DJ, exec. Ed. *The Review of Natural Products.* St. Louis, MO: Walters & Kluwer Co.; 1997

14. Gohil, K, Rothfuss L, Lang J, et al. Effect of exercise training on tissue vitamin E and ubiquinone content. *J Appl Physiol.* 1987 Oct; 63(4): 1638–41.

15. Lockwood K, Moesgaard S, Hanioka T, et al. Apparent partial remission of breast cancer in 'high risk' patients supplemented with nutritional antioxidants, essential fatty acids and coenzyme Q10. *Mol Aspects Med.* 1994; 15 Suppl: s231–40.

16. Lockwood K, Moesgaard S, Yamamoto T, et al. Progress on therapy of breast cancer with vitamin Q10 and the regression of tumors. *Biochem Biophys Res Commun.* 1995 Jul 6; 212(1): 172–7.

17. Domae N, Sawada H, Matsuyama E, et al. Cardiomyopathy and other chronic toxic effects induced in rabbits by doxorubicin and possible prevention by coenzyme Q10. *Cancer Ther Rep.* 1981 Jan–Feb; 65(1–2): 79–91.

18. Iarussi D, Auricchio U, Agretto A, et al. Protective effect of coenzyme Q10 on anthracyclines cardiotoxicity: control study in children with acute lymphoblastic leukemia and non-Hodgkin's lymphoma. *Mol Aspects Med.* 1994; 15 Suppl: s207–12.

19. Shults CW, Oakes D, Kieburtz K, et al. Effects of coenzyme Q10 in early Parkinson disease: evidence of slowing of the functional decline. *Arch Neurol.* 2002 Oct; 59(10): 1541–50.

20. Mortensen SA, Leth A, Agner E, et al. Dose-related decrease of serum coenzyme Q10 during treatment with HMG-CoA reductase inhibitors. *Mol Aspects Med.* 1997; 18 Suppl: S137–44.

21. Simopoulos AP. Essential fatty acids in health and chronic disease. *AJCN.* 1999; 70(suppl): 560S–9S.

22. Mantzioris E, Cleland LG, Gibson RA, et al. Biochemical effects of a diet containing foods enriched with n-3 fatty acids. *AJCN.* 2000; 72: 42–8.

23. Stark KD, Park EJ, Maines VA, et al. Effect of a fish-oil concentrate on serum lipids in postmenopausal women receiving and not receiving hormone replacement therapy in a placebo-controlled, double-blind trial. *AJCN.* 2000; 72: 389–94.

24. Deutch B. Menstrual pain in Danish women correlated with low n-3 polyunsaturated fatty acid intake. *Eur J Clin Nutr.* 1995; 49: 508–16.
25. Calviello G, Palozza P, Piccioni E, et al. Dietary supplementation with eicospentanoic and docosahexanoic acid inhibits growth of morris hepatocarcinoma 3924a in rats: effects on proliferation and apoptosis. *Int J Cancer.* 1998; 75: 699–705.
26. Peet M, Horrobin DF. A dose-ranging study of the effects of ethyl eicosapentanoate in patients with ongoing depression despite apparently adequate treatment with standard drugs. *Arch Gen Psychiatry.* 2002; 59: 913–19.
27. Storlien LH, Kraegen WE, Chisholm DJ, et al. Fish oil prevents insulin resistance induced by high fat feeding in rats. *Science.* 1987; 237: 885–88.
28. Ajiro K, Sawamura M, Ikeda K, et al. Beneficial effects of fish oil on glucose metabolism in spontaneously hypertensive rats. *Clin Exp Pharm Physiol.* 2000; 6: 77–84.
29. Burns CP, Halabi S, Clamon GH, et al. Phase I clinical study of fish oil fatty acid capsules for patients with cancer cachexia: cancer and leukemia group B Study 9473. *Clin Cancer Res.* 1999; 5: 3942–47.
30. Virtanen JK, Voutilainen S, Rissanen TH, et al. Mercury, fish oils, and risk of acute coronary events and cardiovascular disease, coronary heart disease, and all-cause mortality in men in eastern Finland. *Arterioscler Thromb Vasc Biol.* 2005; 25: 228–33.
31. Lopes Vaz A. Double-blind clinical evaluation of the relative efficacy of ibuprofen and glucosamine sulphate in the management of osteoarthrosis of the knee in outpatients. *Curr Med Res Opin.* 1982; 8: 145–49.
32. Poolsup N, Suthisisang C, Channark P, et al. Glucosamine long-term treatment and the progression of knee osteoarthritis: systematic review of randomized controlled trials. *Ann Pharmacother.* 2005 Jun; 39(6): 1080–7.
33. Hoffer LJ, Kaplan LN, Hamadeh MJ, et al. Sulfate could mediate the therapeutic effect of glucosamine sulfate. *Metabolism.* 2001; 50: 767–70.
34. Qiu GX, Gao SN, Giacovelli G, et al. Efficacy and safety of glucosamine sulfate versus ibuprofen in patients with knee osteoarthritis. *Arzneimittelfroschung.* 1998 May; 48(5): 469–74.
35. Tapadinhas MJ, Rivera IC, Bignamini AA. Oral glucosamine sulphate in the management of arthrosis: report on a multi-centre open investigation in Portugal. *Pharmacotherapeutica.* 1982; 3: 157–68.
36. Thie NM, Prasad NG, Major PW. Evaluation of glucosamine sulfate compared to ibuprofen for the treatment of temporomandibular joint osteoarthritis: a randomized double blind controlled 3 month clinical trial. *J Rheumatol.* 2001 Jun; 28(6): 1347–55.
37. Anderson JW, Nicolisi RJ, Borzelleca JF. Glucosamine effects in humans: a review on glucose metabolism, side effects, safety considerations and efficacy. *Food Chem Toxicol.* 2005 Feb; 43(2): 187–201.
38. Virkamaki A, Daniels MC, Hamalainen S, et al. Activation of the hexosamine pathway by glucosamine in vivo induces insulin resistance in multiple insulin sensitive tissues. *Endocrinology.* 1997; 138: 2501–7.
39. Patti ME, Virkamaki A, Landaker EJ, et al. Activation of the hexosamine pathway by glucosamine in vivo induces insulin resistance of early postreceptor insulin signaling events in skeletal muscle. *Diabetes.* 1999; 48: 1562–71.

40. Kowalak JP, senior ed. *Professional Guide to Complementary & Alternative Therapies.* Springhouse, PA: Springhouse publishing; 2001. 338.
41. Garfinkel D, Laudon M, Nof D, et al. Improvement of sleep quality in elderly people by controlled-release melatonin. *Lancet.* 1995 Aug 26; 346(8974): 541–4.
42. Kayumov L, Brown G, Jindal R, et al. A randomized, double-blind, placebo-controlled crossover study of the effect of exogenous melatonin on delayed sleep phase syndrome. *Psychosom Med.* 2001; 63: 40–8.
43. Aldhous M, Franey C, Wright J, et al. Plasma concentrations of melatonin in man following oral absorption of different preparations. *Br J Clin Pharmacol.* 1985 Apr; 19: 517–21.
44. Haimov I, Lavie P, Laudon M, et al. Melatonin replacement therapy of elderly insomniacs. *Sleep.* 1995 Sep; 18(7): 598–603.
45. Andrade C, Srihari BS, Reddy KP, et al. Melatonin in medically ill patients with insomnia: a double-blind, placebo-controlled study. *J Clin Psychiatry.* 2001 Jan; 62(1): 41–5.
46. Petrie K, Dawson AG, Thompson L, et al. A double-blind trial of melatonin as a treatment for jet lag in international cabin crew. *Biol Psychiatry.* 1993 Apr 1; 33(7): 526–30.
47. Sauer LA, Dauchy RT, Blask DE. Polyunsaturated fatty acids, melatonin, and cancer prevention. *Biochem Pharmacol.* 2001 Jun 15; 61(12): 1455–62.
48. Lusardi P, Piazza E, Fogari R. Cardiovascular effects of melatonin in hypertensive patients well controlled by nifedipine: a 24-hour study. *Br J Clin Pharmacol.* 2000; 49: 423–27.
49. Seabra ML, Bignotto M, Pinto LR, et al. Randomized, double-blind clinical trial, controlled with placebo, of the toxicology of chronic melatonin treatment. *J Pineal Res.* 2000 Nov; 29(4): 193–200.
50. Agnusdei D, Bufalino L. Efficacy of ipriflavone in established osteoporosis and long-term safety. *Calcif Tissue Int.* 1997; 61 Suppl 1: S23–7.
51. Benevenuti S, Tanini A, Frediani U, et al. Effects of ipriflavone and its metabolites on a clonal osteoblastic cell line. *J Bone Miner Res.* 1991 Sep; 6(9): 987–96.
52. Tsutsumi N, Kawashima K, Nagata H, et al. Effects of KCA-098 on bone metabolism: comparison with those of ipriflavone. *Jpn J Pharmacol.* 1994 Aug; 65(4): 343–9.
53. Petilli M, Fiorelli G, Benevenuti S, et al. Interactions between ipriflavone and the estrogen receptor. *Calcif Tissue Int.* 1995 Feb; 56(2): 160–5.
54. Yamazaki I, Kinoshita M. Calcitonin secreting property of ipriflavone in the presence of estrogen. *Life Sci.* 1986 Apr 28; 38(17): 1535–41.
55. Melis GB, Paoletti AM, Cagnacci A, et al. Lack of any estrogenic effect of ipriflavone in postmenopausal women. *J Endocrinol Invest.* 1992 Nov; 15(10): 755–61.
56. Adami S, Bufalino L, Cervetti R, et al. Ipriflavone prevents radial bone loss in postmenopausal women with low bone mass over 2 years. *Osteoporosis Int.* 1997; 7(2): 119–25.
57. Gennari C, Adami S, Agnusdei D, et al. Effect of a chronic treatment with ipriflavone in postmenopausal women with low bone mass. *Calcif Tissue Int.* 1997; 61 Suppl 1: S19–22.
58. Passeri M, Biondi M, Costi D, et al. Effect of ipriflavone on bone mass in elderly osteoporotic women. *Bone Miner.* 1992 Oct; 19 Suppl 1: S57–62.

59. Alexandersen P, Toussaint A, Christiansen C, et al. Ipriflavone in the treatment of postmenopausal osteoporosis: a randomized controlled trial. *JAMA.* 2001 Mar 21; 285(11): 1482–8.
60. Cecchetin M, Bellometti S, Cremonesi G, et al. Metabolic and bone effects after administration of ipriflavone and salmon calcitonin in postmenopausal osteoporosis. *Biomed Pharmacother.* 1995; 49(10): 465–8.
61. Monostory K, Vereczkey L. The effect of ipriflavone and its main metabolites on theophylline biotransformation. *Eur J Drug Metab Pharmacokinet.* 1996 Jan–Mar; 21(1): 61–6.
62. Monostory K, Vereczkey L. Interaction of theophylline and ipriflavone at the cytochrome P450 level. *Eur J Drug Metab Pharmacokinet.* 1995 Jan–Mar; 20(1): 43–7.

REFERENCES

Andreatini, R., & Leite, J. R. (1994). Effect of valepotriates on the behavior of rats in the elevated plus-maze during diazepam withdrawal. *European Journal of Pharmacology, 260*(2–3), 233–235.

Bach, D., & Ebeling, L. (1996). Long-term drug treatment of benign prostatic hyperplasia—results of a prospective 3-year multicenter studey using sabal extract IDS 89. *Phytomedicine, 3*(2), 105–111.

Bahrke, M. S., & Morgan, W. R. (2000). Evaluation of the ergogenic properties of ginseng: An update. *Sports Medicine, 29*(2), 113–133.

Baillie, N., & Rasmussen, P. (1997). Black and blue cohosh in labour. *New Zealand Medical Journal, 110*(1036), 20–21.

Balderer, G., & Borbely, A. (1985). Effect of valerian on human sleep. *Psychopharmacology (Berlin), 87*(4), 406–409.

Ballard C. G., et al. (2002). Aromatherapy as a safe and effective treatment for the management of agitation in severe dementia: The results of a double-blind, placebo-controlled trial with Melissa. *Journal of Clinical Psychiatry, 63*(7), 553–558.

Barnes, J., et al. (1999). Articles on complementary medicine in the mainstream medical literature. *Archives of Internal Medicine, 159,* 1721–1725.

Bastianetto S., et al. (2000). The ginkgo biloba extract (EGb 761) protects and rescues hippocampal cells against nitric oxide-induced toxicity: Involvement of its flavonoid constituents and protein kinase C. *Journal of Neurochemistry, 74*(6), 2268–2277.

Bauer, B. A. (2000). Herbal therapy: What a clinician needs to know to counsel patients effectively. *Mayo Clinic Proceedings, 75*(8), 835–841.

Binns, S. E., et al. (2000). Light-mediated antifungal activity of echinacea extracts. *Planta Medica, 66*(3), 241–244.

Bisset, N. G. (1994). *Herbal drugs and phyopharmaceuticals.* Boca Raton, FL: CRC Press.

Blumenthal, M. (1995). Herb sales up 35 percent in mass market. *Herbal Gram,* 34–66.

Blumenthal, M., et al. (1998). *The ABC complete German Commission E monographs.* Austin, TX: American Botanical Council.

Blumenthal, M., Goldberg, A., & Brinckmann, J. (Eds). (2000). *Herbal medicine: Expanded Commission E monographs*. Newton, MA: Integrated Medicine Communications.

Boccafoschi, S., & Annoscia, S. (1983). Comparison of *Serenoa repens* extract with placebo by controlled clinical trial in patients with prostatic adenomatosis. *Urologia, 50*(6), 1257–1268.

Bombardelli, E., & Morrazzoni, P. (1997). *Serenoa repens* (Bartram) J K Small. *Fitoterapia, 68*(2), 99–114.

Boullata, J. I., & Nace, A. M. (2000). Safety issues with herbal medicine. *Pharmacotherapy, 20*(3), 257–269.

Braquet, P. (1987). The ginkgolides—potent platelet-activating factor antagonists isolated from ginkgo biloba L.: Chemistry, pharmacology and clinical applications. *Drugs of the Future, 12*, 643–699.

Braquet, P. (Ed.). (1989). *Ginkgolides—chemistry, biology, pharmacology and clinical perspectives* (Vol. 2). Barcelona: J. R. Prous.

Brevoort, P. (1996). The US botanical market—an overview. *Herbal Gram, 36*, 49–57.

Brinker, F. (1998). *Herb contraindications and drug interactions*. Sandy, OR: Eclectic Medical Publications.

Byers, T. (1999). What can randomized controlled trials tell us about nutrition and cancer prevention? *CA: A Cancer Journal for Clinicians, 49*, 353–361.

Cassileth, B. R. (1999). Evaluating complementary and alternative therapies for cancer patients. *CA: A Cancer Journal for Clinicians, 49*, 362–375.

Cauffield, J. S., & Forbes, H. J. (1999). Dietary supplements used in the treatment of depression, anxiety, and sleep disorders. *Lippincott's Primary Care Practice, 3*(3), 290–304.

Champault, G., Patel, J. C., & Bonnard, A. M. (1984). A double-blind trial of an extract of the plant *Serenoa repens* in benign prostatic hyperplasia [Letter]. *British Journal of Clinical Pharmacology, 18*(3), 461, 462.

Chatterjee, S., et al. (1998a). Antidepressant activity of Hypericum perforatum and hyperforin: The neglected possibility. *Pharmacopsychiatry, 31*(Suppl.), 7–15.

Chatterjee, S. S., et al. (1998b). Hyperforin as a possible antidepressant component of hypericum extracts. *Life Sciences, 63*, 499–510.

Croon, E., & Walker, L. (1995, November 6). Botanicals in the pharmacy: New life for old remedies. *Drug Topics*, 84–93.

Cui, J., Eneroth, P., & Bjoerkhem, I. (1994). What do commercial ginseng preparations contain? *Lancet, 344*, 134.

DeFeudis, F. G. (1991). *Ginkgo biloba extract (Egb 761): Pharmacological activities and clinical applications* (pp. 68–73). Paris: Editions Scientifiques Elsevier.

DerMarderosian, A. (1996). Milestones of pharmaceutical botany. *Pharmacy in History, 38*(1), 15–19.

DerMarderosian, A. (1998). Promising practices in the use of medicinal plants in the United States. In T. Tomlinson & O. Akerele (Eds.), *Medicinal plants: Their role in health and biodiversity* (pp. 177–190). Philadelphia: University of Pennsylvania Press.

Diamond, B. J., et al. (2000). Ginkgo biloba extract: Mechanisms and clinical indications. *Archives of Physical Medicine and Rehabilitation, 81*(5), 668–678.

Donath, F., et al. (2000). Critical evaluation of the effect of valerian extract on sleep structure and sleep quality. *Pharmacopsychiatry, 33*(2), 47–53.

Duker, E. M., et al. (1991). Effects of extracts from *Cimicifuga racemosa* on gonadotropin release in menopausal women and ovariectomized rats. *Planta Medica, 57*(5), 420–424.

Duran, N., & Song, P. S. (1986). Hypericin and its photodynamic action. *Photochemistry and Photobiology, 43*(6), 677–680.

Edzard, E. (2002). The risk-benefit profile of commonly used herbal therapies: Ginkgo, St. John's wort, ginseng, echinacea, saw palmetto, and kava. *Annals of Internal Medicine, 135,* 42–53.

Eisenberg, D. M., et al. (2001). Perceptions about complementary therapies relative to conventional therapies among adults who use both: Results from a national survey. *Annals of Internal Medicine, 135,* 344–351.

Ernst E. (1998). Harmless herbs? A review of the recent literature. *American Journal of Medicine, 104*(2), 170–178.

Filaretov, A. A., et al. (1988). Role of pituitary-adrenocortical system in body adaptation abilities. *Experimental and Clinical Endocrinology, 92,* 129–136.

Food and Drug Administration, Center for Food Safety and Nutrition. (1994). *Food label use and nutritional education survey.* Washington, DC: Author.

Forstl, H. (2000). Clinical issues in current drug therapy for dementia. *Alzheimer Disease and Associated Disorders, 14*(Suppl. 1), S103–108.

Garges, H. P., et al. (1998). Cardiac complications and delirium associated with valerian root withdrawal. *Journal of the American Medical Association, 280*(18), 1566–1577.

Geumei, A., et al. (1975). Evaluation of a new oral B2-adrenoceptor stimulant bronchodilator, terbutaline. *Pharmacology, 13,* 201–211.

Gillespie, S. (1997, December). Herbal drugs and phytomedicinal agents. *Pharmacy Times,* 53–62.

Goldman, P. (2001). Herbal medicines today and the roots of modern pharmacology. *Annals of Internal Medicine, 135*(8, Pt. 1), 594–600.

Gruber, J., & DerMarderosian, A. (1996a). Back to the future: Traditional medicinals revisited, the use of plants in medicine. *Laboratory Medicine, 27*(2), 100–108.

Gruber, J., & DerMarderosian, A. (1996b). An emerging green pharmacy, modern plant medicines and health. *Laboratory Medicine, 27*(3), 170–176.

Gunn, T. R., & Wright, I. M. (1996). The use of black and blue cohosh in labour [Letter]. *New Zealand Medical Journal, 109*(1032), 410–411.

Gurley, B. J., et al. (1998). Ephedrine pharmacokinetics after the ingestion of nutritional supplements containing *Ephedra sinica* (Ma Huang). *Therapeutic Drug Monitoring, 20,* 439–445.

Hardman, J., et al. (Eds). (1996). *Goodman and Gilman's The pharmacological basis of therapeutics* (9th ed.). New York: McGraw-Hill.

Hardy, M. L. (2000). Herbs of special interest to women. *Journal of the American Pharmaceutical Association, 40*(2), 234–242.

Harrer, G., et al. (1999). Comparison of equivalence between the St John's wort extract LoHyp-57 and fluoxetine. *Arzneimittel-Forschung, 49,* 289–96.

Hathcock, J. (2001). Dietary supplements: How are they used and regulated. *Journal of Nutrition, 131,* 1114S–1117S.

Henneicke-von Zepelin, H., et al. (1999). Efficacy and safety of a fixed combination pytomedicine in the treatment of the common cold (acute viral respiratory tract infection): Results of a randomised, double blind, placebo controlled, multicentre study. *Current Medical Research and Opinion, 15*(3), 214–227.

Heptinstall, S. (1988). Feverfew—an ancient remedy for modern times? *Journal of the Royal Society of Medicine, 81*(7), 373–374.

Heptinstall, S., et al. (1992). Parthenolide content and bioactivity of feverfew (Tanacetum parthenium (L) Schultz Bip): Estimation of commercial and authenticated feverfew products. *Journal of Pharmacy and Pharmacology, 44*(5), 391–395.

Houghton, P. J. (1988). The biological activity of valerian and related plants. *Journal of Ethnopharmacology, 22*(2), 121–142.

Houghton, P. J. (1999). The scientific basis for the ruputed activity of valerian. *Journal of Pharmacy and Pharmacology, 51*(5), 502–512.

Jacobs, B., & Browner, W. (2000). Ginkgo biloba: A living fossil. *American Journal of Medicine, 108,* 341, 342.

Jacobson, J. S., et al. (2001). Randomized trial of black cohosh for the treatment of hot flashes among women with a history of breast cancer. *Journal of Clinical Oncology, 19*(10), 2739–2745.

Johnson, E. S., et al. (1985). Efficacy of feverfew as prophylactic treatment of migraine. *British Medical Journal (Clinical Research Education), 291*(6495), 569–573.

Kagan, J. (Ed.). (2000, May). The mainstreaming of alternative medicine. *Consumer Reports,* 17–25.

Kanowski, S., et al. (1997). Proof of efficacy of the ginkgo biloba special extract EGb 761 in outpatients suffering from mild to moderate primary degenerative dementia of the Alzheimer type or multi-infarct dementia. *Phytomedicine, 4*(1), 3–13.

Kessler, R. C., et al. (2001). Long-term trends in the use of complementary and alternative medical therapies in the United States. *Annals of Internal Medicine, 135,* 262–268.

Kim, H. L., et al. (1999). St John's wort for depression: A meta-analysis of well defined clinical trials. *Journal of Nervous and Mental Disease, 187,* 532–539.

Klepser, T. B., & Klepser, M. E. (1999). Unsafe and potentially safe herbal therapies. *American Journal of Health-System Pharmacy, 56*(2), 125–138, 139–141.

Laakmann, G., et al. (1998). St John's wort in mild to moderate depression: The relevance of hyperforin for the clinical efficacy. *Pharmacopsychiatry, 31*(Suppl.), 54–59.

Lambrecht, J. E., et al. (2000, August). A review of herb-drug interactions: Documented and theoretical. *Pharmacist,* 42–53.

LeBars, P. L., et al. (1997). A placebo-controlled, double blind randomized trial of an extract of ginkgo biloba for dementia: North American EGb study group. *Journal of the American Medical Association, 278*(16), 1327–1332.

LeBars, P. L., Kieser, M., & Itil, K. Z. (2000). A 26-week analysis of a double-blind placebo-controlled trial of the ginkgo biloba extract Egb 761(R) in dementia. *Dementia and Geriatric Cognitive Disorders, 11*(4), 1230–1237.

Leathwood, P. D., et al. (1982). Aqueous extract of valerian root (*Valeriana officinalis* L) improves sleep quality in man. *Pharmacology, Biochemistry, and Behavior, 17*(1), 65–71.

Leathwood, P. D., & Chauffard, F. (1985, April). Aqueous extract of valerian reduces latency to fall asleep in man. *Planta Medica, 2,* 144–148.

Lewis, M., & Kowalski, S. D. (2002). Use of aromatherapy with hospice patients to decrease pain, anxiety, and depression and to promote an increased sense of well-being. *American Journal of Hospice and Palliative Care, 19*(6), 381–386.

Lieberman, S. (1998). A review of the effectiveness of Cimicifuga racemosa (black cohosh) for the symptoms of menopause. *Journal of Women's Health, 7*(5), 525–529.

Linde, K., et al. (1996). St. John's wort for depression—an overview and meta-analysis of randomized clinical trials. *British Medical Journal, 313*(7052), 253–258.

Linde, K., & Berner, M. (1999). Commentary: Has hypericum found its place in antidepressant treatment? *British Medical Journal, 319*, 1539.

Liske, E. (1998). Therapeutic efficacy and safety of Cimicifuga racemosa for gynecological disorders. *Advances in Therapy, 15*(1), 45–53.

Liu, C. X., & Xiao, P. G. (1992). Recent advances on ginseng research in China. *Journal of Ethopharmacology, 26*, 27–38.

Liu, Y. M., et al. (1993). A comparative study on commercial samples of *Ephedrae herba*. *Planta Medica, 59*, 376–378.

Logani, S., et al. (2000). Actions of ginkgo biloba related to potential utility for the treatment of conditions involving cerebral hypoxia. *Life Sciences, 67*(12), 1389–1396.

Lust, J. (1974). *The herb book* (pp. 199–200). New York: Bantam Books.

Marks, L., & Tyler, V. (1999). Saw palmetto extract: Newest (and oldest) treatment alternative for men with symptomatic benign prostatic hyperplasia. *Urology, 53*, 457–461.

Mathews, J. D., et al. (1988). Effects of the heavy usage of kava on physical health: Summary of a pilot survey in an Aboriginal community. *Medical Journal of Australia, 148*(11), 548–555.

McDermott, J., et al. (1998, February). Herbal chart for health care professionals. *Pharmacy Today,* center fold-out.

Miller, L. G. (1998). Herbal medicinals: Selected clinical considerations focusing on known or potential drug-herb interactions. *Archives of Internal Medicine, 158*(20), 2200–2211.

Moore, L. B., et al. (2000, June). St. John's wort induces hepatic drug metabolism through activation of the pregnane X receptor. *Proceedings of the National Academy of Sciences USA,* 13.

Muller, W., et al. (1998). Hyperforin represents the neurotransmitter reuptake-inhibiting constituent of hypericum extract. *Pharmacopsychiatry, 31*, 16–21.

Murray, M. (1995). *The healing power of herbs.* Rocklin, CA: Prima Publishing.

National Institutes of Health, Practice and Policy Guidelines Panel. (1997). Clinical practice guidelines in complementary and alternative medicine: An analysis of opportunities and obstacles. *Archives of Family Medicine, 6*(2), 155–156.

Newall, C., Anderson, L., & Phillipson, J. (1996). Ginseng, panax. In *Herbal Medicines: A Guide for Health Care Professionals* (pp. 145–150). London: Pharmaceutical Press.

Obach, R. S. (2000). Inhibition of human cytochrome P450 enzymes by constituents of St. John's wort, an herbal preparation used in the treatment of depression. *Journal of Pharmacology and Experimental Therapeutics, 294*(1), 88–95.

Ong, Y. C., & Yong, E. L. (2000). Panax (ginseng)—panacea or placebo? Molecular and cellular basis of its pharmacological activity. *Annals of the Academy of Medicine (Singapore), 29*(1), 42–46.

Parnham, M. J. (1996). Benefit-risk assessment of squeezed sap of the purple coneflower *(Echinaea purpurea)* for long-term oral immunostimulation. *Phytomed, 3*(1), 95–102.

Percival, S. S. (2000). Use of echinacea in medicine. *Biochemical Pharmacology, 60*(2), 155–158.

Philipp, M., et al. (1999). Hypericum extract versus imipramine or placebo in patients with moderate depression: Randomised multicentre study of treatment for eight weeks. *British Medical Journal, 319,* 1534–1539.

Pittler, M. H., & Ernst, E. (2000). Efficacy of kava extract for treating anxiety: Systematic review and meta-analysis. *Journal of Clinical Psychopharmacology, 20*(1), 84–89.

Price, S. (1983). *Practical aromatherapy.* London: Thorsons/HarperCollins.

The review of natural products. (2002). St. Louis, MO: Facts and Comparisons.

Roby, C. A., et al. (2000). St John's wort: Effect on CYP3A4 activity. *Clinical Pharmacology and Therapeutics, 67*(5), 451–457.

Roots, T. (1996). Evaluation of photosensitization of the skin and multiple dose intake of hypericum extract. Paper presented at the Second International Congress on Phytomedicine, Munich.

Rosenblatt, M., & Mindel, J. (1997). Spontaneous hyphema associated with ingestion of ginkgo biloba extract [Letter]. *New England Journal of Medicine, 336*(15), 1108.

Ruze, P. (1990). Kava-induced dermopathy: A niacin deficiency? *Lancet, 335*(8703), 1442–1445.

Ryu, S., & Chien, Y. (1995). Ginseng-associated cerebral arteritis. *Neurology, 45,* 829–830.

Scaglione, F., et al. (1990). Immunomodulatory effects of two extracts of panax ginseng C.A. Meyer. *Drugs Under Experimental and Clinical Research, 16,* 537–542.

Scaglione, F., et al. (1996). Efficacy and safety of the standardized ginseng extract G 115 for potentiating vaccination against common cold and/or influenza syndrome. *Drugs Under Experimental and Clinical Research, 22,* 65–72.

Schempp, C. M., et al. (2001). Single-dose and steady-state administration of *Hypericum perforatum* extract (St. John's wort) does not influence skin sensitivity to UV radiation, visible light, and solar-stimulated radiation. *Archives of Dermatology, 137*(4), 512, 513.

Scherer, J. (1998). Kava-kava extract in anxiety disorders: An outpatient observational study. *Advances in Therapy, 15*(4), 261–269.

Schmid, R., et al. (1994). Comparison of seven commonly used agents for prophylaxis of seasickness. *Journal of Travel Medicine, 1*(4), 203–206.

Schuckit, M. A. (1996). Ma-huang (ephedrine) abuse and dependence. *Drug Abuse and Alcohol Newsletter, 25,* 1–4.

Schulz, V., Hansel, R., & Tyler, V. (1998). *Rational phytotherapy: A physician's guide to herbal medicine* (3rd ed.). Berlin: Springer Verlag.

Schulz, V., Huebner, W. I., & Ploch, M. (1997). Clinical trials with phyto-psychopharmacological agents. *Phytomedicine, 4*(4), 379–387.

Schweizer, J., & Hautmann, C. (1999). Comparison of two dosages of ginkgo biloba extract Egb 761 in patients with peripheral arterial occlusive disease Fontaine's stage IIb. *Arzneimittel-Forschung (Drug Research), 49*(2), 900–904.

Shelton, R. C., et al. (2001). Effectiveness of St. John's wort in major depression: A randomized controlled trial. *Journal of the American Medical Association, 285*(15), 1978–1986.

Shin, K. S., et al. (1997). Rhamnogalacturonan II from the leaves of panax ginseng C.A. Meyer as a macrophage Fc receptor expression-enhancing polysaccharide. *Carbohydrate Research,* 239–249.

Shuster, J. (1997). Adverse drug reaction: Herbal remedies and seizures. *Nursing, 27*(4), 75.

Singh, Y. N. (1992). Kava: An overview. *Journal of Ethnopharmacology*, 37(1), 13–45.

Smith, R. M. (1983). Kava lactones in *Piper methysticum* from Fiji. *Phytochemistry*, 22(4), 1055–1056.

Sotaniemi, E., Haapakoski, E., & Rautio, A. (1995). Ginseng therapy in non-insulin dependent diabetic patients. *Diabetes Care, 18*, 1373–1375.

Sun, L. Z., et al. (1999). The American coneflower: A prophylactic role involving nonspecific immunity. *Journal of Alternative and Complementary Medicine*, 5(5), 437–446.

Talalay, P., & Talalay, P. (2001). The importance of using scientific principles in the development of medicinal agents from plants. *Academic Medicine, 76*(3), 238–246.

Tinkelman, D. G., & Avner, S. E. (1977). Ephedrine therapy in asthmatic children: Clinical tolerance and absence of side effects. *Journal of the American Medical Association*, 237–553.

Tyler, V. (1994). The therapeutic use of phytomedicinals. In *Herbs of choice* (pp. 28–35). Binghamton, NY: Haworth Press.

van Beek, T. A., & Lelyveld, G. P. (1992). Concentration of ginkgolides and bilobalide in ginkgo biloba leaves in relation to the time of year. *Planta Medica, 58*, 413–416.

Vandenbogaerde, A., et al. (2000). Evidence that total extract of Hypericum perforatum affects exploratory behavior and exerts anxiolytic effects in rats. *Pharmacology, Biochemistry, and Behavior, 65*(4), 627–633.

Vickers, A., & Zollman, C. (1999). ABCs of complementary medicine: Herbal medicine. *British Medical Journal, 319*, 1050–1053.

Victoire, C., et al. (1988). Isolation of flavonoid glycosides from ginkgo biloba leaves. *Planta Medica, 54*, 245–247.

Volz, H. P. (1997). Controlled clinical trials of hypericum extracts in depressed patients—an overview. *Pharmacopsychiatry, 30*(Suppl.), 72–76.

Volz, H. P., & Kieser, M. (1997). Kava-kava extract WS 1490 versus placebo in anxiety disorders—a randomized placebo-controlled 25 week outpatient trial. *Pharmacopsychiatry, 30*(l), 1–5.

Vorberg, G. (1985). Ginkgo biloba extract (GBE): A long term study on chronic cerebral insufficiency in geriatric patients. *Clinical Trials Journal, 22*, 149–157.

Wada, K., et al. (1988). Studies on the constitution of edible medicinal plants. 1. Isolation and identification of 4-O-methylpyridoxine, toxic principle from the seed of ginkgo biloba L. *Chemical and Pharmaceutical Bulletin, 36*, 1779–1782.

Wheatley, D. (1998). Hypericum extract: Potential in the treatment of depression. *CNS Drugs, 9*(6), 431–440.

Winslow, L. C., Kroll, D. J. (1998). Herbs as medicines. *Archives of Internal Medicine, 158*(20), 2192–2199.

Wustenberg, P., et al. (1999). Efficacy and mode of action of an immunomodulator herbal preparation containing echinacea, wild indigo, and white cedar. *Advances in Therapy, 16*(1), 51–70.

CHAPTER FOUR

Homeopathy as an Aid to Healthy Aging

Joyce Frye

One hundred years ago, the topic of homeopathy would not have been entertained in a book such as this. Homeopathy was mainstream medicine. Washington, D.C.'s only monument to a physician had been erected at Scott Circle honoring the founder of homeopathy, German physician Samuel Hahnemann (1755–1843), with President William McKinley and the U.S. Marine Band participating in the dedication.

Harris Coulter provided extensive documentation of the early history of homeopathy in the United States in his book *Divided Legacy: The Conflict Between Homeopathy and the American Medical Association* (Coulter, 1982). He provides exhaustive evidence documenting that in the late 19th and early 20th centuries homeopathic treatment was far superior to that offered by "regular" doctors, whom Hahnemann referred to as *allopaths*. Homeopathic practice was favored by the clergy, the press, and community leaders. Free dispensaries for the poor were more affordable, owing to the minimal cost of homeopathic medications. Homeopathic insane asylums were recognized as achieving more successful treatment. Some life insurance companies sought homeopathic patients as clientele and charged them lower premiums. The Homoeopathic Mutual Life Office of New York reported in 1879 that, in the previous 10 years, there had been 84 deaths among 7,929 policyholders who were followers of homeopathy, while there had been 66 deaths among the 2,258 others.

Subsequently, a variety of internal and external factors contributed to the near disappearance of homeopathic practice in the United States.

Pharmaceutical companies began to financially support medical journals. Allopathic treatment became more successful, with increasing understanding of the physiologic and biochemical mechanisms of human function, while the homeopathic paradigm became more difficult to comprehend. Among homeopathic physicians themselves, there were disagreements about the best form of practice. However, homeopathy remained popular in Europe and even gained popularity in South America and India, where there are currently more than 100 homeopathic medical colleges.

Hahnemann predicted that it would take at least 200 years to understand homeopathy. We are now at a time when chronic disease is prevalent, and conventional medicine provides symptomatic relief and delay of sequelae but seldom cures, a time when the cost of reparative procedures and pharmaceuticals threatens to bankrupt the national economy. A large sample size pharmaceutical study may need only a 5% to 7% difference in outcome between the treated and the placebo groups in order to demonstrate statistical significance, which tells us nothing about how to treat the 50% or so who do not respond. Furthermore, the new genomics demonstrate that individuals respond to medications differently.

The need for effective, affordable, individualized medical care has never been greater. With increasing appreciation for the many potential forms of biological information and energy transfer, the potential for better defining the potential value of homeotherapeutics and understanding the mechanism of action of homeopathy now seems bright. The convergence of factors necessary for the further investigation and application of homeopathy may finally be in place.

THE PARADIGM

Similia Similibus Curentur

The paradigm of homeopathy begins with two precepts that go against conventional wisdom in scientific culture. First is the principle of similars, meaning that medicines are chosen based on their ability to elicit symptoms similar to those suffered by the patient. In contrast, allopathy would have medicines do the work of "curing" by suppressing symptoms, as is common in the prevalent array of "anti-" medications (e.g., antibiotics, antihistamines, antispasmodics, antitussives, and antidepressants), which Hahnemann referred to as *antipathic* treatment. The principle of treatment with substances causing similar symptoms is actually first known to have been proposed by Hippocrates. Paracelsus (1493–1541) was also a proponent, stating that, "if given in small doses, what makes a man ill also cures him" (1990). Hahnemann was the first to test this hypothesis empirically and formalize it into a system of medicine.

Although he had already written a popular medical text, Hahnemann was disillusioned with the toxicity of current therapies and had stopped practice. In addition to medicine, he had been trained as a linguist (fluent in at least 11 languages), chemist, and medical historian and was making his living by doing translations. When he came upon William Cullen's theory (a Scottish physician and author of *Materia Medica*) that Peruvian bark (*Cinchona*, the source of quinine) was useful for malaria because it was bitter, he was skeptical that this was a sufficient explanation. Hahnemann experimented by ingesting some himself, whereupon he developed symptoms resembling malaria, which resolved when he stopped taking it and recurred when he rechallenged with the Peruvian bark. He began a series of experiments ingesting and, later, giving to willing colleagues medicinal doses of cinchona. In each case, symptoms like malaria resulted and spontaneously resolved when the dosing was stopped—a reasonable approximation of a phase 1 trial.

This observation led Hahnemann to further experimentation and the elucidation of the similia principle "Let likes be cured by likes." The development and refinement of this theory, with all of its ramifications, consumed the remaining 60 years of his life. Hahnemann set out his theories in the *Organon of the Medical Art,* first published in 1810. Further editions followed with the evolution of his work, ending with the sixth, published the year before his death in 1842 (Hahnemann, 1842).

To discover the potential medicinal value of substances, Hahnemann conducted *provings*—experiments in which a substance is given to a group of healthy people in order to observe the symptoms produced and thereby learn what symptoms might, according to the principle of similars, be treated by that substance. He named the new science *homeopathy,* from the Greek, meaning "similar suffering." Hahnemann cited Sir William Jenner's use of cowpox innoculum to vaccinate against smallpox as an example of his principle.

Hahnemann "proved" over 100 substances in his lifetime. This represents the first time that the effects of medicines were tested in healthy rather than in sick individuals. Hundreds of other provings have been conducted by later homeopaths. In the 1880s, homeopaths conducting provings also recognized that reported symptoms might come from factors other than the experimental substance. They were the first to introduce the concept of *placebo* and incorporate inert substances, blinded to the subject, into the proving trials.

The principle of similars seems quite reasonable when we consider the concept of homeostasis and recall that symptom formation occurs as the body's attempt at ridding itself of foreign invaders whether the source is infectious, allergenic, or toxic. Assuming a *vital force* (in other traditions *anima* or *qi*), the addition of a substance capable of producing similar symptoms pushes the organism to strain further—increasing the energy of the homeostatic effort without adding to the original pathogenic load. Hahnemann saw symptoms as the organism's signals about how the body was attempting to achieve homeostasis and which catalyst might augment and stimulate the organism to further its own healing process. He called this substance the *similimum*.

The Minimum Dose

Needless to say, creating further symptomatology is undesirable. Thus, the second precept is to give the *minimum dose*. In order to minimize the possibility of worsening symptoms, Hahnemann diluted his medicinal substances—either in 10-fold or 100-fold sequences—keeping track of the final strength. He agitated the dilutions at each level, known as *succussion*. The complete process of dilution and succussion is referred to as *potentization*. The final potency of a medicine is simply the number of 1:910 *(X)* or 1:99 *(C)* dilutions; for example, 6C represents six 1:99 dilutions.

At potencies higher than 12C or 24X, the dilutions exceed Avogadro's number, leading to the problem that there may be no molecule of original substance remaining and no chemical explanation for how the medicinal effect is obtained. Thus, at first glance, homeopathy seems implausible. Additionally, the medicines are counterintuitively observed to be more clinically effective with increasing dilution. Physicians have dismissed homeopathy because they are unable to conceive of information transfer in biological systems at a submolecular level. Clearly, the high dilution factor leads one to abandon theories at the molecular level and search in the areas of energy transfer.

Although the actual mechanism of action of homeopathic medicines has yet to be determined, one long-held theory is that the polarity of the molecular structure of the water used as diluent plays an important role. Recently reported research demonstrated that dissolved molecules, instead of moving farther apart with increasing dilution, actually did the opposite and clumped together (Samal & Geckeler, 2001). Furthermore, the importance of succussion in the potentization process has been demonstrated in the laboratory, where basophil degranulation was triggered by a dilute antiserum against immunoglobulin E (IgE) that had been created with 10-second vortexing, whereas use of an equal concentration created by repeated pipetting had no effect (Davenas et al., 1988). The successive action might help to distribute clumps of molecules more systematically.

This field of research has not been palatable to many conventional scientists. However, the BELLE (Biological Effects of Low Level Exposures) Group at the University of Massachusetts led by Dr. Edward Calabrese has more actively explored nonlinear and hormetic effects in toxicology, biology, and medicine. *Stedman's Medical Dictionary* defines *hormesis* as "the stimulating effect of subinhibitory concentrations of any toxic substance on any organism" (1996). Thus, normally toxic substances or effects may be beneficial when used in low doses. Calabrese states:

> The fundamental nature of the dose response is neither linear nor threshold, but rather U-shaped. When studies are properly designed to evaluate biological activity below the traditional toxicological threshold, low-dose stimulatory responses are observed with high frequency and display specific quantitative features. (Calabrese & Baldwin, 2001)

This action of potentized substance in accord with the similia principle is illustrated in a series of studies led by Doutremepuich at Bordeaux. In one of these (Doutremepuich et al., 1990), a 5C dilution of aspirin in distilled water, or distilled water alone, was given intravenously to 20 healthy male volunteers in a double-blind, randomized, controlled trial. The subjects receiving the aspirin were observed to have significantly shorter bleeding times ($p < .05$ at 2 hours) than those receiving the distilled water. This is in direct contrast to the common understanding that aspirin prolongs bleeding time. Subsequent studies attempting to elicit a mechanism of action isolated a specific effect on vessel wall activity (Lalanne et al., 1990, 1991, 1992). Clinically, a potentized dose of aspirin presumably could be used to treat delayed clotting. Some readers may recall that it was popular to give heparin in the treatment of disseminated intravascular coagulation (DIC) in the not so distant past. This line of treatment may deserve revisiting according to homeopathic principles with the use of smaller doses of heparin or aspirin.

THE MEDICINES

A homeopathic medicine can be made from any substance that creates symptoms (or side effects) for the healthy person in its natural state. While nearly half come from plants, they may also come from animal, mineral, or chemical sources. Additionally, there are *nosodes,* defined as "homeopathic attenuations of: pathological organs or tissues; causative agents such as bacteria, fungi, ova, parasites, virus particles, and yeast; disease products; excretions or secretions." Many standard drugs (e.g., nitroglycerin) were initially introduced through homeopathic use.

Current Status

Homeopathic medicines were included in the 1938 federal Food, Drug, and Cosmetic Act (FDCA). The Homoeopathic Pharmacopoeia Convention of the United States (HPCUS, www.hpcus.com) is charged by the Food and Drug Administration (FDA) with determining which medicines have undergone sufficient testing to be considered official homeopathic drugs within the meaning of the act. Homeopathic medicine was also included in the Medicare enabling legislation, and is a covered service except in those areas where the regional administration has opted out (e.g., the New York region does not cover any alternative medicine).[1]

Homeopathic drugs are delivered in numerous oral and topical dosage forms, including but not limited to liquids, tablets, medicated pellets, ointments, and suppositories. One of the most common forms is sublingual lactose tablets or pellets impregnated with the final potentized dilution of the substance. Medicines are prepared according to Good Manufacturing Practices, and the FDA regulates the manufacture, marketing, and sale of these drugs. With the exception of nosodes and dilutions of restricted substances, which require a prescription, the preparations are available over the counter (OTC) for treatment of self-limited conditions.

USING HOMEOPATHIC MEDICINE

In Hahnemann's initial provings, a variety of symptoms were observed—often as many as 150 different collected effects among the provers. These included general physical changes, such as lethargy and fever; specific physical symptoms, such as headache and diarrhea; mental symptoms, such as clouded sensorium or rush of thoughts; and emotional symptoms, such as irritability, tearfulness, and even excess laughter. These provings, as well as other symptoms not seen in original provings but subsequently demonstrated to resolve in a patient treated with the medicine, along with known effects from toxicology, became the core of the materia media for each medicine (also known as *remedy*).

---

[1]Title 42. The Public Health and Welfare, Chapter 7. Social Security Act Part C. Miscellaneous Provisions (t) Drugs and Biologicals (1) The term "drugs" and the term "biologicals," except for purposes of subsection (m)(5) and paragraph (2) of this section, include only such drugs and biologicals, respectively, as are included (or approved for inclusion) in the United States Pharmacopoeia, the National Formulary, or the United States Homeopathic Pharmacopoeia, or in New Drugs or Accepted Dental Remedies (except for any drugs and biologicals unfavorably evaluated therein), or as are approved by the pharmacy and drugs therapeutics committee (or equivalent committee) of the medical staff of the hospital furnishing such drugs and biologicals for use in such hospital.

Along with the symptoms experienced, homeopathy also considers *modalities,* the events or behaviors that aggravate or ameliorate symptoms (designated in the nomenclature by < or >, respectively). For example, one individual with difficult respiration secondary to influenza may feel the need to breathe deeply (> motion), whereas another splints the chest because of pain with every respiration (< motion). This symptom would indicate the need for different remedies for these individuals despite the common diagnosis of influenza. Other factors noted in provings included sensations and emotional symptoms (e.g., anger and grief) and the location and progression of symptoms (e.g., a sore throat starting on the right side and moving to the left).

A key feature of classical homeopathy is the goal of matching the entire spectrum, the totality of symptoms, between the medicine and the patient in order to treat the whole person—not merely the superficial disease. Consideration of the totality of symptoms is the aspect of homeopathic practice that is both most appealing and most challenging. It is the aspect that allows for the individualization of treatment of the person who has the disease rather than focusing on the disease itself. It emphasizes that the illness signifies an imbalance within the organism that expresses itself in the development of symptoms, not simply a failure of the organism to ward off more potent external forces.

As an example, in a group of individuals exposed to a virus, some will become ill and some will not. Individuals who do become ill may be in the midst of an emotional turmoil, or they may become ill after too little sleep or after exposure to the elements. Of those who become ill, some may have sore throats on the left and some on the right. Some sore throats will improve after swallowing cold beverages, some after swallowing warm beverages. Some may be made worse by swallowing. Some sore throats may progress to sinus congestion and some to a cough. Some coughs may be barking and some hacking, some dry and some productive. Some ill persons may be chilly; some may be feverish. Some may desire caretaking and attention; some will prefer to be left alone. All of the symptoms (and any others that are prominent) may be taken into consideration in choosing a remedy for an individual who is ill. What is clear is that, although all were exposed to the same virus, not all became ill, and not all are ill in the same way.

Taking the Case

The homeopathic interview attempts to elicit the symptoms most characteristic of the disease. Symptoms that are strange, rare, and peculiar are often especially helpful in choosing a remedy. Hahnemann states:

In the search for a homeopathically specific remedy, that is, in the comparison of the complex of the natural disease's signs with the symptom sets of the available medicines (in order to find among them an artificial disease potency that corresponds in similarity to the malady to be cured) the more *striking, exceptional, unusual, and odd* (characteristic) signs and symptoms of the disease care are to be especially and almost solely kept in view. *Those above all, must correspond to very similar ones in the symptom set of the medicine sought* if it is to be the most fitting one for cure. The more common and indeterminate symptoms (lack of appetite, headache, lassitude, restless sleep, discomfort, etc.) are to be seen with almost every disease and medicine and thus deserve little attention unless they are more closely characterized.(Hahnemann, 1842)

Unique symptoms specifically associated with a particular remedy are known as *keynotes;* for example, burning pain made better from hot applications is a keynote of the remedy *Arsenicum album* and also a peculiarity in that one would expect a burning pain to feel better with a cold rather than a hot application.

Repertorization to Find the Single Remedy

Lists of symptoms know as *rubrics,* along with the remedies known from provings to be associated with them, are collected in volumes referred to as *repertories.* Rubrics are classified according to general body part or system and in increasing order of specificity. In using the old repertories, the language of the time also must be understood. Thus, in J. T. Kent's *Repertory of the Homeopathic Materia Medica,* one that is still widely used, motion sickness is classified under "Stomach, Nausea," from riding in a carriage (Kent, 1897). Yasgur's dictionary of the old terminology can be a useful tool in finding a particular symptom in the repertory (Yasgur, 1990).

The process of *repertorization* (finding the remedy from the group of symptoms and signs elicited from the patient) traditionally involves searching a repertory for the symptoms most characteristic of the case, followed by cross-matching the associated remedies to find the one with the best fit. This is generally more time-consuming than the average patient–physician encounter, but the required time will vary considerably depending on the acuity of the illness. In trauma and in exposure to particularly potent environmental conditions or virulent organisms, individual responses become more uniform, making it possible to select one or a very few remedies that will work for most people under those conditions. The process has also been made considerably easier with the advent of computer software that accomplishes what is essentially a database search (2003a,b).

Combination Remedies

For occasions when such aids are not available or the choice of medicine is not obvious, homeopathic pharmaceutical companies have created *combination* or *complex* remedies. These combine, in a single formulation, several of the remedies most commonly indicated for a disease or condition, thus sidestepping the need for any repertorization. While combination remedies are not individualized, they are frequently effective for symptom relief and less costly than conventional medicines for self-limited conditions.

Although extensive modern studies of combination remedies are limited (as is all homeopathic research), evidence suggests that they are effective. One study comparing Vertigoheel (Heel Inc., Albuquerque, NM) with standard therapy betahistine hydrochloride demonstrated equal efficacy (Weiser, Strosser, & Klein, 1998). Another combination remedy, Calms Forte (Hylands Inc., Los Angeles, CA), is the third best selling sleep aid in the United States according to the manufacturer To the extent that repeat sales (i.e., sales to those who are satisfied enough to repurchase) demonstrate satisfaction with a product, this one would seem to be efficacious. Numerous other combination products address such maladies as headache, allergies, diarrhea, joint pain, leg cramps, and many other symptoms.

It is unclear whether combination remedies work through the combined activity of individual components or whether an entirely new substrate is formed. In any case, they are usually very low potency and unlikely to get at deep underlying issues. Thus, even when effective, if the condition persists or recurs frequently (e.g., ongoing insomnia), an individualized prescription (often referred to as *constitutional care*) is more likely to provide long-term relief and restore overall general health.

Following the administration of a successful remedy, the expected direction of cure follows Hering's law. Constantine Hering was the father of homeopathy in the United States and the founder of the first homeopathic medical colleges that became Hahnemann University, Philadelphia. Hering observed that *cure proceeds from above downward, from within outward, from the most important organs to least important organs, and in the reverse order of appearance of symptoms* (Vithoulkas, 1980, p. 231) As a practical matter, this means that a patient may have a rapid improved sense of wellness prior to any objective improvement in physical symptoms, and that superficial symptoms such as rashes and discharges may initially appear worse while healing occurs at a deeper level. Once improvement is under way, the medicine should only be repeated if there is a relapse.

Hering also introduced the first "self-help" homeopathic book in the United States, which was distributed with a kit of 42 remedies. Numerous books are currently available to assist the first-time user in selecting a medication that fits the symptoms. A more recent classic is *Homeopathic Medicine at Home,* which has been translated into several languages and contains useful charts for distinguishing the characteristics among the 28 most frequently needed medicines for minor ailments (Panos & Heimlich, 1980).

When uncertain about which homeopathic medicine to use, practitioners and individuals can fairly safely "experiment" by prescribing or taking one. Because of the high dilution factor, toxicity and side effects are not a concern. If the remedy is not correct for the situation, there will simply be no response. After a reasonable interval—usually only a few minutes in an acute situation—if there is no response, another one can be tried. However, numerous repeated doses of a medicine that does not seem to be working should be avoided. This can lead to a proving, that is, a creation of the symptoms of the medicine.

CONDITIONS

Injuries and First Aid

While constitutional care is the gold standard in homeopathy, in acute trauma there is little individual variation in patient response. Pain, swelling, and bruising or hemorrhages are common responses, and the appropriate remedy given at the earliest opportunity may relieve pain as well as limit the sequelae of injury. A number of remedies are commonly considered among people familiar with homeopathy. *Arnica* is used as the first-line treatment for head injury and for trauma where there is hemorrhage or the potential for bruising. This would suggest that it might also be useful for hemorrhagic stroke. On the emotional level, the traumatized patient needing arnica may think he or she is all right even when objectively injured.

Arnica has become especially popular in recent years with plastic surgeons. Significantly decreased postoperative bruising and swelling have been demonstrated in two recent randomized controlled trials using an arnica dose pack (SinEcch, Alpine Pharmaceuticals, San Rafael, CA) containing specific potencies for pre- and postoperative use (Quinn, 2003). *Hypericum perforatum* is used for injuries to nerves and nerve-rich areas such as digits. For burns, *Cantharis vesicatoria* is used internally and *Calendula officinalis* topically. Calendula is also generally used for any superficial skin wounds or ulcers. However, if the wound is deep, calendula is discouraged because the deep layers may heal less rapidly, leaving the potential for complications from dead space.

For strains and sprains, *Bryonia alba* is commonly used where the modality "pain worse from movement" is prominent. Traumeel (Heel Inc., Albuquerque, NM) is a combination remedy available in both oral and topical form that is widely used for soft tissue injury, and according to the manufacturer, it is used by the German Olympic teams. A similar combination, Traumeel S (Heel Inc., Albuquerque, NM), also worked significantly better than placebo in a randomized trial for prophylaxis against stomatitis in children undergoing chemotherapy prior to stem cell transplantation (Oberbaum et al., 2001). A larger study funded by the National Institutes of Health (NIH) is currently under way to corroborate these results.

Fracture union has been expedited experimentally using homeopathic treatment in a guinea pig model. At a meeting of the Homeopathic Research Network in 1995, Oberbaum (Oberbaum et al., 2001) reported a study in which uniform fractures were created with a dental instrument in anesthetized guinea pigs. The animals were randomized to receive daily 7C *Symphytum* and *Calcarea phosphoricum* or placebo. Radiographs demonstrated significantly more rapid fracture healing in the verum group.

Epidemic Infections

In epidemic disease, homeopathy historically worked equally well for both viral and bacterial vectors. Homeopathy was used in the influenza pandemic of 1918. The illness struck with such force that people often died within 24 hours. Twenty percent of the entire world population was infected, and 20 million to 40 million people died (Perko, 1999). Dr. T. A. McCann, of Dayton, Ohio. reported in the *Journal of the American Institute of Homeopathy* in May 1921 that 24,000 cases of flu treated allopathically had a mortality rate of 28.2%, while 26,000 cases of flu treated homeopathically had a mortality rate of 1.05%. Another homeopathic physician working on a troop ship during World War I reported treating 81 cases during one crossing with 100% survival, while another ship suffered 31 deaths en route (JAIH).

Those few homeopathic drugs that are specific to the epidemic are known as the *Genus epidemicus* (GE). In the 1918 flu pandemic, only three remedies were needed to treat almost all cases. Just as the flu vaccine changes from year to year, the GE will vary from one epidemic to another due to such factors as season, weather conditions, and the strain of infectious agent—even when the name of the infectious agent remains the same. Thus, the GE must be learned with the first few cases of an infectious epidemic, making it important for expert homeopathic practitioners to be involved in the early stages of an outbreak.

The GE can also be used for prophylaxis. Homeopathic medicine was first used for prevention in a wide-scale epidemic in 1801when Hahnemann observed that a child who was being treated with a homeopathic preparation of belladonna resisted scarlet fever even though all three siblings were affected. Wondering whether the *Atropa belladonna* had acted prophylacticly, Hahnemann began giving it to children in other families when the first ones fell ill. He found it to be protective despite a 90% attack rate among the untreated. The method was so successful that regular physicians adopted it, and by 1838 the Prussian government made its use mandatory (Hoover, 2001).

Disease nosodes are also used for prophylaxis and in the first stage of infectious disease treatment when the GE has not yet been discovered. *Variolinum* (created from smallpox pustules) and *Vaccinium* (created from the pustule formed after smallpox vaccination from scarification) given orally were both found to be at least as effective as scarification for smallpox prevention by the Iowa courts in 1905 (Winston, 2001). A variety of remedies have been used for the successful prevention and treatment of smallpox as well as for treatment of the sequelae of smallpox vaccination. Arthur Grimmer, MD, practicing in Chicago for over 40 years in the first half of the 20th century, had great success using *Thuja occidentalis* (1996).

Some physicians theorized that nosodes were more effective in the prophylaxis and early stages of disease, but that the GE was more likely to be effective as the disease progressed and the patient's preceding chronic illness played more of a role in the peculiar disease manifestation. The role of nosode prophylaxis was demonstrated in more modern times during a meningococcus outbreak in Brazil in 1974. In a group of 18,640 patients given the nosode *Meningococcinum* as prophylaxis, there were 4 reported cases, while a cohort of 6,430 receiving no treatment had 32 cases. The nosode prophylaxis was 23 times more effective than no treatment.

Jonas (1999) has demonstrated the potential value of creating nosodes experimentally using a mouse model. Protection from tularemia was achieved in a significant number of mice given *Tularemia* nosode prior to exposure to the *Tularemia* bacterium (Jonas, 1999). Although nosode prophylaxis was less effective than known vaccine in this study, the disease was 100% fatal in the mice that received no prophylaxis. This would seem to be a worthwhile line of investigation for emerging infections, such as West Nile virus and severe acute respiratory syndrome (SARS), when no standard prophylaxis or treatment is available—particularly for the elderly, who have the highest fatality rate when only supportive care is available. A nosode can be quickly made from disease secretions such as sputum using standard methodology available from the *Homeopathic Pharmacopoeia of the United States (HPUS)*.

Acute Infections

Individualized homeopathic treatment offers prompt relief from minor infections and may be lifesaving in serious infections when antibiotics are ineffective and supportive measures are insufficient. Individual acute infections (e.g., pneumonia unrelated to an epidemic) require individualized prescribing. It is best to take into consideration the patient's general constitution, the emotional and environmental factors surrounding the onset of illness, and the specific symptoms and modalities that are unusual for the patient or unusual for the customary course of the disease. However, some generalizations are still possible. For example, pyrogen, a medicine potentized from rotting meat, can be invaluable in septicemia.

Chronic Disease

In general, the need for an individualized homeopathic prescription is equally important when seeking relief in chronic disease. The total complex arises from those symptoms caused by the disease, along with predispositions, preexisting conditions, environmental factors, and emotional state. Thus, persons with the same conventional diagnosis are frequently treated with one of a variety of different medicines due to the unique symptom picture of each individual. With long-standing pathology, complete resolution may not be possible even with homeopathy. However, palliation can almost always be offered with decreased dependence on conventional drugs, usually at much less cost and with fewer side effects.

The need for individualization of therapy has made research in homeopathy particularly challenging. One strategy is preselection of the study population on the basis of symptomatology matching a particular homeopathic medicine. This method was used by Peter Fisher, a rheumatologist at the Royal London Homeopathic Hospital (where homeopathy is provided through the National Health Service) in a study of fibrositis (fibromyalgia). In a randomized controlled trial (RCT), a group of 30 patients were selected for symptoms matching *Rhus toxicodendron*. Those receiving the study medication had a significant 25% reduction in tender spots compared to those receiving placebo (Fisher et al., 1989).

Heart Disease

Heart disease represents a situation where chronic disease (previously known or unknown) may have acute manifestation in the form of myocardial infarction. While the usual risk factors of smoking, lipid levels, inactivity, and overweight are well established, it has been more recently recognized that emotional factors such as depression are also associated (Frasure-Smith & Lesperance, 2003). These are particularly amenable to homeopathic intervention. Ideally, if the constitutional state is recognized early, an acute cardiac event might be deterred.

Paul Herscu, ND, who has been practicing homeopathy for over 20 years, states that no one in his practice has had a myocardial infarction. He distinguishes among the personality traits of individuals who have both chronic heart disease and work issues. For example, the person needing aurum metallicum (potentized gold) wants to achieve perfection and works to the point of alienation, then feels himself or herself a failure and is embarrassed by it. The person needing nux vomica (from *Strychnos nux-vomica*, the poison nut tree) works hard because there's a job that needs to be done. He worries when things are incomplete and uses more stimulants to keep going. Digitalis (from *Digitalis lanata*, foxglove) types are moral people who work a lot and feel responsible. They feel tremendously guilty when something goes bad because they've made the wrong decision, whereas those needing naja (from the venom of Naja naja, the Asian cobra) feel more generally unsuccessful in their work.

Many physical signs, sensations, and modalities also differentiate the cardiac indications for various homeopathic medicines. Kreuzel (1992) lists the specific qualities of 23 of them in the "Cardiac Pain" section of his *Homeopathic Emergency Guide* and notes that "[t]reatment with homeopathic medicines while in transit to an emergency facility has been credited with saving more than one life."

Cancer

Choosing the correct medicine in cancer is the most challenging aspect of using homeopathy. Although treating the whole person with the medicine that matches the totality of symptoms as well as the tumor type is ideal, as the stage of disease advances, the symptoms often become more characteristic of the tumor than of the patient, and the homeopath and patient need to extensively explore the patient's memory of the time before cancer to recall the contributing factors and identifying symptoms in order to choose the constitutional remedy. Additionally, the preceding or concurrent use of radiation and/or chemotherapy alters the symptom picture, making the homeopathic prescription more difficult to discern.

Most homeopathic physicians advocate primary surgical removal of the tumor followed by homeopathy, as homeopathy alone is unlikely to be successful where significant pathological change has occurred and the tumor burden is too great for the vital force (Ernst, 1998; Jonas & Jacobs, 1996). However, Arthur Grimmer is said to have treated several thousand cases of cancer in his 57-year career. Specific data between 1925 and 1929 revealed 150 cured cases of biopsy-diagnosed cancers and prolonged palliation (7–15 years), with excellent quality of life in another 75 cases. The greatest successes occurred where there was little preceding allopathic treatment.

With the paucity of modern case series, few practitioners or patients choose to forgo conventional treatment. Thus, homeopathy currently is most often used in an adjunctive role. Most homeopaths would agree that systemic chemotherapy is more disruptive to the organism's ability to heal and, given the choice, would opt for local radiation alone alongside constitutional homeopathy. Obviously, some patients will succumb to their disease. In these cases, the goal is to keep the patient as alert, functional, and comfortable as possible until the very end, when death may come quickly and easily. With homeopathy, this is often possible.

PRACTICE PATTERNS

Homeopathy is included in the scope of practice for physicians in all 50 states. Arizona, Connecticut, and Nevada require separate homeopathic licensure. Naturopathic physicians trained in 4-year colleges may also elect to specialize in homeopathy. In addition, dentists, advanced practice nurses, licensed physician's assistants, and veterinarians may all use homeopathic medicines within the scope of practice defined by the state of licensure.

At this time there are no specific CPT codes for homeopathic care, and practitioners typically bill the patient or third-party insurer using standard International Classification of Diseases (ICD-9) and Evaluation and Management codes. An additional lay class of homeopathic practitioners has arisen among individuals who have devoted significant study to homeopathy but have no license to practice medicine. Some have passed a certification examination and use the initials CCH after their names. In the United Kingdom, an analogous group has gained official recognition for legal practice.

The absence of CPT codes has made it difficult to track economic data in the United States. However, in France, where homeopathy is used more frequently, Social Security data compiled in 1991 showed significantly reduced cost from homeopathic care versus conventional medical care. The totality of costs associated with homeopathic care per physician was approximately one half of the totality of care provided by conventional primary care physicians. It also appeared that these savings increased the longer a physician had been using homeopathy. A subsequent analysis also revealed that the number of paid sick leave days by patients under the care of homeopathic physicians was 3.5 times less (598 days/year) than patients under the care of general practitioners (2,017 days/year). CNAM (National Inter-Regulations System) 61, 1991).

CONCLUSION

Homeopathic medicine has stood the test of time with millions of case histories to document its efficacy. Much research is needed to bring it into the modern realm of evidence-based medicine. This has been particularly challenging due to scientific and paradigmatic issues that are in direct contrast with popular beliefs about the nature of illness and information transfer in biological systems. But, historically, the greatest proponents of homeopathy have been those who set out to disprove it and found that they could not. Hopefully, more funding will become available to find new strategies for research that focuses on hormesis and on patient-centered therapies.

In the meantime, the concerns of toxicity and drug interactions common to herbs and dietary supplements are absent in homeopathic medicines due to standard regulated manufacturing practices and miniscule dosages. Aging patients may find much relief and lower costs with use of homeopathic medicines at home. And geriatricians and hospitalists may find gentler and more satisfying tools if they include homeopathic medicines in their armamentarium.

RESOURCES

American Institute of Homeopathy, 801 N. Fairfax Street, Suite 306, Alexandria, VA 22314; telephone: (888) 445-9988; Web site: www. homeopathyusa.org

The oldest national medical organization in the United States, founded in 1844. A professional organization for MDs, DOs, dentists, advanced practice nurses, and physician's assistants. Publishes the *American Journal of Homeopathic Medicine*. Sponsors an annual conference and 36-hour primary care courses for licensed medical professionals in various locations. A listing of practitioner members is available on the Web site.

Homeopathic Association of Naturopathic Physicians, 1412 W. Washington St., Boise, ID 83702; telephone: (208) 336-3390; Web site: www.hanp.net

Professional organization for naturopathic physicians (NDs) who specialize in homeopathic practice. Publishes *Simillimum* and sponsors an annual conference.

National Center for Homeopathy, 801 N. Fairfax St., Suite 306, Alexandria, VA 22314; telephone: (877) 624-0613; Web site: www.homeopathic.org

Membership organization advocating for more widespread use and availability of homeopathic medicine. Publishes *Homeopathy Today*, the most complete source of homeopathic courses and resources. Sponsors an annual conference open to the public, Affiliated Study Groups for learning home use, and a 2-week summer school with a variety of class offerings including specialized classes in pharmacy and animal care. Offers books to members at 10% discount.

BOOKS

A number of books, too numerous to list completely, are available to learn more about homeopathy and specific indications for remedies. Along with the usual book dealers, see:

Homeopathic Educational Services, 2124B Kittredge St., Berkeley, CA 94704; telephone: (510) 649-0294; Web site: www.homeopathic.com

Minimum Price Homeopathic Books, Inc., P.O. Box 2187, Blaine, WA 98231; telephone: (800) 663-8272; Web site: www.minimum.com

REFERENCES

Calabrese, E. J., & Baldwin, L. A. (2001). Hormesis: U-shaped dose responses and their centrality in toxicology. *Trends in Pharmacological Sciences, 22*(6), 285–291.

CNAM (National Inter-Regulations System) 61. (1991). French Social Security Data. Retrieved from http://homeopathic.org/cost.htm.

Coulter, H. (1982). *Divided legacy: The conflict between homeopathy and the American Medical Association*. Berkeley, CA: North Atlantic Books.

Currim, A. (Ed.) (1996). *The collected works of Arthur Hill Grimmer, M.D.* Norwalk, CT: Hahnemann International Institute for Homeopathic.

Davenas, E., Beauvais, F., Amara, J., Oberbaum, M., Robinzon, B., Miadonna, A., et al. (1988). Human basophil de-granulation triggered by very dilute antiserum against IgE. *Nature, 333*(6176), 816–818.

Doutremepuich, D., deSeze, O, LeRoy, D., et al. (1990). Aspirin at very low dosage in healthy volunteers: Effects on bleeding time, platelet aggregation and coagulation. *Haemostasis, 20*, 99-105.

Ernst, E. (1998). Are highly dilute homoeopathic remedies placebos? *Perfusion, 11*(7), 291, 292.

Fisher, P., Greenwood, A., Huskisson, E. C., Turner, P., & Belon, P. (1989). Effect of homoeopathic treatment on fibrositis (primary fibromyalgia). *British Medical Journal, 199*, 365–366.

Frasure-Smith, N., & Lesperance, F. (2003). Depression—a cardiac risk factor in search of a treatment [Editorial]. *Journal of the American Medical Association, 289*(23), 3171–3173.

Hahnemann, S. (1842). *Organon of the medical art* (W. B. Reilly, Ed.). Redmond, WA: Birdcage Books.

Hoover, T. A. (2001). Homeopathic prophylaxis. *Journal of the American Institute of Homeopathy, 3,* 168–175.

Jonas, W. B. (1999). Do homeopathic nosodes protect against infection? An experimental test. *Alternative Therapies in Health and Medicine, 5*(5), 36–40.

Jonas, W. B., & Jacobs, J. (1996). *Healing with homeopathy.* New York: Warner Books.

Kent, J. T. (2003). *Kent's comparative repertory of the homeopathic materia medica.* New Delhi: B. Jain.

Kreuzel, T. (1992). *The homeopathic emergency guide.* Berkeley, CA: North Atlantic Books.

Lalanne, M. C., deSeze, O., Doutremepuich, D., & Belon, P. (1991). Could proteolytic enzyme modulate the interaction platelets/vessel wall in presence of ASA at ultra low doses? *Thrombosis Research, 63,* 419–426.

Lalanne, M. C., Doutremepuich, D., deSeze, O., & Belon, P. (1990). What is the effect of acetylsalicylic acid at ultra low dose on the interaction platelets/vessel wall? *Thrombosis Research, 60,* 231–236.

Lalanne, M. C., Ramboer, I., deSeze, O., & Deutremepuich, C. (1992). In vitro platelets/endothelial cells interactions in presence of acetylsalicylic acid at various dosages. *Thrombosis Research, 65,* 33–43.

MacRepertory. San Rafael, CA: Kent Homeopathic Associates.

Oberbaum, M., Yaniv, I., Ben-Gal, Y., Stein, J., Ben-Zvi, N., Freedman, L. S., et al. (2001). A randomized, controlled clinical trial of the homeopathic medication TRAUMEEL S (R) in the treatment of chemotherapy-induced stomatitis in children undergoing stem cell transplantation. *Cancer, 92*(3), 684–690.

Panos, M., & Heimlich, J. (1980). *Homeopathic medicine at home.* Los Angeles: Jeremy P. Tarcher.

Paracelsus. (1990). *Micropædia* (Vol. 9, pp. 134–135). Chicago: Encyclopædia Britannica.

Perko, S. (1999). *The homeopathic treatment of influenza.* San Antonio, TX: Benchmark Homeopathic Publications.

Quinn, M. (2003). SinEcch(tm) in plastic surgery. Retrieved from http://www.alpinepharm.com/sinresreswri.html.

Radar™. Archibel software. Retrieved from http://archibel.com/homeopathy/radar.

Samal, S., & Geckeler, K. E. (2001). Unexpected solute aggregation in water on dilution. *Chemical Commununications, 21,* 2224–2225.

Stedman's medical dictionary. (1996). Baltimore: Williams & Wilkins.

Vithoulkas, G. (1980). *The science of homeopathy.* New York: Grove Press.

Weiser, M., Strosser, W., & Klein, P. (1998). Homeopathic vs conventional treatment of vertigo—a randomized double-blind controlled clinical study. *Archives of Otolaryngology—Head and Neck Surgery, 124*(8), 879–885.

Winston, J. (2001). Some history of the treatment of epidemics with homeopathy.

Yasgur, J. (1990). *A dictionary of homeopathic medical terminology.* Greenville, PA: VanHoy Publishers.

CHAPTER FIVE

Music, Health, and Well-Being

Elaine Abbott and Kathleen Avins

For many people, the connection between music and health is a natural one. Most of us have some sort of relationship with music, and many of us have intuitively used music to help ourselves feel better in some way—perhaps by playing a favorite recording to lift our spirits, perhaps simply by singing in the shower. As human beings, we possess an innate musicality, whether or not we think of ourselves as musicians per se. What may not be readily apparent, however, is the fact that music itself can be viewed as a valuable metaphor for health. As Western society begins to expand its concepts of health and wellness, with the traditional view of body-as-machine seeming increasingly limited, there is a need for new metaphors.

CHANGING VIEWS OF HEALTH

In *Merriam-Webster's New Collegiate Dictionary* (2005, italics added), health is defined as "a condition of being *sound* in body, mind, and spirit." It is not at all uncommon, when discussing the pursuit of health, to speak in terms of restoring harmony within a person. Indeed, the very etymology of the word *person* is *per son,* or *through sound* (Updike, 1994).

Within the traditional Western medical model, health has been viewed as *pathogenic,* that is, as a dichotomy in which one is either healthy or ill. In this framework, humans are perceived as having an ideal homeostasis, the balance of which must be protected, either through preventive measures that focus on maintaining wellness or through interventive measures that focus on removing illness. This homeostasis is viewed as the "normal" human condition; hence, illness is seen as an aberration. There is, however, an increasing emphasis on health as heterostasis rather than homeostasis, particularly within more holistic approaches to medicine. In this *salutogenic* perspective, health is viewed not as a dichotomy but as a continuum, with all points along the continuum being viewed as part of the "normal" human condition. Experiences of illness are therefore no more abnormal than experiences of wellness; health is viewed not as an either-or state, but as an ongoing process (Antonovsky, 1987).

There are some subtle but powerful implications in the salutogenic model. If health is a continuum, with all points along the continuum being "normal," then much will depend on how the individual perceives his or her experience of wherever he or she is along the continuum. What one individual might consider intolerable, another might thrive upon. Hence, concepts of health are intrinsically subjective rather than objective; health is largely self-defined (Aldridge, 1996). As such, this broader view of health contains a number of qualities, such as meaningfulness, free action, process, and interrelationship of self to a larger whole. All of these qualities can also be found within music.

A MUSICAL PERSPECTIVE ON HEALTH

Music consists of artfully ordered sound. Health includes a sense of the natural order, which music can restore (Kenny, 1989). In experiencing music, one directly perceives an implicate order and wholeness that may be seen as analogous to the ordered universe (Bruscia, 2000; Eagle, 1991), or indeed the ordered self. Our perception of music can heighten our sense of ourselves as part of a higher order, with profound meaning encoded within the beauty of the music: "[I]n experiencing the intricate, ordered and beautiful patterns of music, we are attuned, spiritually and acoustically, to our universe" (Salas, 1990, p. 5).

Music is also an invitation to participate; whether though actively making music or actively listening to it, music promotes action. This is implicit within the very term playing music; the ability to play may be seen as very much akin to the capacity for choice and free action in the world (Kenny, 1989). Creating a work of art, such as music, can be seen as analogous to creating a life (Salas, 1990). Good music has an unencumbered flow of energy among its constituent parts; so too does good health: "[T]o embrace creation, and hence creative activity, is to embrace life" (Aigen, 1991, p. 94).

Music can also promote social and cultural health. It accesses a means of nonverbal communication (Pavlicevic, 1997; Stige, 2002) that may have originated with the interactions of mother and infant. Music is also a part of our individual and collective identities (Ruud, 1998), and as such can strengthen the sense of belonging among group members. It can also provide powerful shared experience (Aigen, 1991) and serve as a field in which to co-construct meaning and beauty (Bruscia, 2000; Kenny, 1989).

Rhythm is a particularly basic, essential quality that is commonly shared by musical structure and human health. Our bodies are made of rhythms: pulse, respiration, movement. Rhythm has been described as the key to the integrative process that underlies both musical perception and physiological coherence. Our ability to grow, change, and work within our environment is "dependent on a global rhythmic strategy . . . [D]isruption in this overall global strategy will influence a person's ability to detect new or changed non-temporal information. We may not be aware of certain changes and become either out of tune or out of time" (Aldridge, 1996, p. 31). At all stages of life, the rhythm of our movement is a reliable measure of health; there exists a natural connection between the extent of our health and the musicality of how we move (Pavlicevic, 1997). Thus, the human body and its musical workings—its harmony, rhythm, tempo, and dynamics—are the traces of our health activity (Aldridge, 1996).

The ways in which we order ourselves can be compared to the ways in which we order our music, and vice versa. It could be said that to increase our health, we need to be more like music, more able to flow from one position to another (Bruscia, 2000). Music, like health, has a natural ebb and flow in which highs and lows are equally meaningful as parts of the overall process (Kenny, 1989).

Music also contains, within its balance of rhythm and harmony, a natural wholeness. Appreciation for this wholeness, in the eyes of some music therapists, can be very helpful in countering the old Cartesian concept of a mind–body split (Aldridge, 1996; Kenny, 1989; Pavlicevic, 1997; Ruud, 1998), which has recently been called into question. The experience of music is not only an experience of wholeness, it *requires* wholeness and integration on the part of the one who experiences it. We enter into music with our whole selves—body, mind, spirit, and culture.

TYPES OF MUSIC EXPERIENCES

One may enter into and benefit from music through different types of experiences. Bruscia (1998) has identified four general categories of therapeutic music experiences: compositional, improvisational, receptive, and re-creative. These categories describe typical music experiences, but exact definitions may allow for clarification.

A *compositional* music experience is one in which the participant writes new musical material (songs, instrumental pieces, lyrics) or creates a musical product (video or audiotape). An *improvisational* music experience is one in which the participant is able to freely express himself or herself in the moment on chosen rhythmic (tambourine, drum, etc.) and/or melodic (xylophone, piano, etc.) instruments. *Receptive* music experiences are ones during which the participant engages in listening and responding to music, either live or recorded. The participant may respond to the music in any of several different ways, some of which include drawing, moving his or her body, and reporting imagery. *Re-creative* music experiences involve learning or performing precomposed music. In a re-creative music experience, the participant might learn a piece of music in much the same way he or she might for a piano or voice lesson, or perform an existing piece of music in such a way that it allows for personal interpretation (Bruscia, 1998).

SELF-GUIDED VERSUS EXPERT-DESIGNED THERAPEUTIC MUSIC EXPERIENCES

Therapeutic experiences in music can be either self-guided or expert-designed. The self-guiding of music experiences simply entails choosing for oneself music experiences that promote personal health and well-being. Examples include joining a community choir in order to spend more time interacting socially, taking piano lessons to ease arthritic hand pain, and listening to self-selected, recorded music for 15 minutes a day to induce relaxation.

Expert-designed therapeutic music experiences are those designed and implemented by experts for participants. There are a growing number of experts in this area, and several different groups of practitioners have organized. Some of these groups are music therapists, fellows of the Association of Guided Imagery and Music, music practitioners, and sound healers. Examples of expert-designed music experiences include sessions with a music therapist who will work with a participant to develop specific piano exercises to ease the participant's arthritis pain, sessions with a sound healer or music practitioner who will play live music to influence the mood or the physical state of the participant, and sessions with a music therapist who will improvise with the participant to work with his or her feelings regarding pertinent life issues.

This chapter was written by music therapists, and as a result, is largely informed by the profession of music therapy. A music therapist designs and implements different types of therapeutic music experiences within the context of a therapist–participant relationship in order to address health issues. Members of the music therapy profession must complete a degree program approved by the American Music Therapy Association (AMTA) in order to be eligible to sit for the Certification Board for Music Therapists certification exam (AMTA, 2003). Music therapy was established as a profession in the United States during the 1940s (Davis, Gfeller, & Thaut, 1999) and currently has a growing body of literature that is published not only in music therapy journals, but also in medical and psychological publications (see References and Resources).

HEALTH ISSUES AND THERAPEUTIC MUSIC EXPERIENCES

For the purposes of this chapter, health issues have been divided into three primary areas: physical, psychological, and social. This division is somewhat simplistic and artificial, as current literature is indicating that these areas are interrelated. Health professionals are finding that when a therapeutic intervention is designed and implemented to address one health area (working from a primary goal), it can lead to positive outcomes in another health area (creating a secondary outcome) (Dileo, 1999).

Although music is typically used in therapeutic settings with the intention of addressing the individual as a "whole" person whose health issues are interrelated, when planning treatment music therapists do target primary health goals. Following this form of therapeutic practice, the ensuing examples of different types of therapeutic music experiences are organized according to the above three health areas. Further clarification of these areas is as follows: Physical health issues pertain to the individual's physical body, psychological health issues relate to the individual's inner world or psyche, and social health issues concern the individual's roles and relationships with other people.

Physical Health Issues

Some physical health issues related to aging that have been addressed with therapeutic music experiences include exercise (Bernard, 1992), pain (Kelley, 1996), recovery from surgery (Reilly, 2000), physical rehabilitation (Johnson, Otto, & Clair, 2001), cognition (O' Callaghan, 1999), and speech (Cohen, 1992). Examples of how three of these issues can be addressed with a specific type of music experience are given below.

Exercise

Listening to recorded music is a receptive music experience that can aid with exercise. Different research studies have shown that recorded music listening can increase motivation to exercise (Bernard, 1992), can increase repetition frequencies during physical therapy rehabilitation exercises (Johnson et al., 2001), and can increase distances walked (Becker, Chambliss, Marsh, & Montemayor, 1995). These music listening experiences can be self-guided, or a music therapist can assist a participant in selecting music and music listening equipment. When choosing music to aid with motor functioning, it is important to choose preferred music with appropriate rhythms and tempos.

Pain

Pain perception can be altered through a music therapy technique called entrainment. Entrainment can combine both compositional and receptive music experiences, and requires specific training to implement. The concept of entrainment is based on several different principles, which draw from theories of music therapy and physics. One specific entrainment technique, developed by Cheryl Dileo (1999), involves a process during which both the therapist and the participant work to assess the participant's pain, set appropriate goals for the entrainment session, compose pain music, compose healing music, and then allow the participant's reception of the music as it is played by the therapist (Dileo & Bradt, 1999).

Recovery From Surgery

Recovery from surgery can be assisted by physioacoustic therapy. Physioacoustic therapy is a receptive therapeutic music experience during which the participant is exposed to "pure tone sounds (without music) using frequencies which stimulate resonant vibration in human muscle fibers and nervous system" (Butler & Butler, 1997, p. 198). Initial case study research (Butler & Butler, 1997) has shown evidence of increased cardiac output as a result of treatment. This was a positive patient response to physioacoustic therapy in recovery from heart surgery. Physioacoustic therapy should be expert-designed and implemented; literature in this area implies that its use is currently limited to medical institutions and other types of therapeutic centers (Wigram & Dileo, 1997).

Psychological Health Issues

Aging brings about changes not only of a physical nature, but also of a psychological nature. These changes may affect the aging adult's sense of identity and mental well-being. Aging adults may find themselves adjusting to new societal roles (Mullins & McNicholas, 1986), as well as to other significant life changes. As these changes occur, feelings of depression, grief, and loss may arise (Eckford & Lambert, 2002). Aging adults may also begin to look back on their lives in search of meaning and purpose (Butler, 1971), and find them selves desiring greater connections to spirituality (Hughes & Peake, 2002), family, and friends (Troll, 1994) as they seek satisfaction in life. Therapeutic music experiences can successfully address these psychological health issues. Examples are given below.

Life Review

When an aging adult begins to look back on his or her life in search of meaning and purpose, participation in compositional therapeutic music experiences can be helpful. Compositions do not have to entail full symphonic scores, nor do they even have to include writing music. A therapeutic compositional music experience can involve writing lyrics to fit precomposed music, or using recording technology to compile a personal musical memoir on tape or CD. When used in the context of life review, compositional music experiences can stimulate memories (McCloskey, 1990), allow the participant to reminisce as he or she works (Tomaino, 1994), and allow the participant to share his or her life history with others through the finished product, or even as he or she works on the composition. These types of experiences can be self-guided or expert-designed. A music therapist might inform the process by providing supportive physical and relational environments from within which the participant could work during the compositional process, and by assisting with compositional logistics such as locating recordings, operating recording equipment, and tutoring in music theory and notation.

Loss and Grief

An aging adult's loss and grief might be addressed through a receptive music experience commonly referred to as guided imagery and music (GIM). GIM can be used in numerous different ways but generally involves listening to music in order "to evoke and support imaginal processes or inner experiences" (Bruscia, 1998, p. 125). The Bonny Method of Guided Imagery and Music (BMGIM) is a specific method of GIM that requires institute training to implement and can address issues of loss and grief (Bonny, 2002a; Schulberg, 1999; Smith, 1996–1997). A typical BMGIM session begins with an opening conversation between the therapist and the participant, then moves to the music listening section of the session. As this section of the session begins, the therapist chooses one of several specially designed classical music programs for the participant to listen to, and after engaging the participant in a short directed imagery exercise to induce relaxation, begins the music. At this point the therapist and the participant begin what could be called a BMGIM conversation. During this verbal conversation, the participant reports his or her experiences in the music and the imagery to the therapist, and the therapist responds to the participant with interventions intended to help the participant to stay actively engaged in the music and in his or her imagery. After the music listening section of the session concludes, the therapist and participant work together to help the participant understand the meaning and import of the imagery in his or her life. BMGIM is, for the most part, based in theories of humanistic psychology, and supports a process of deep, participant-directed self-exploration (Bonny, 2002a).

Life Satisfaction

As aging creates change in an adult's life, he or she may be required to travel down new roads in search of life satisfaction. Re-creative music experiences, such as participation in a community or church-affiliated musical ensemble, can provide opportunities to satisfy this search. Performing in, or helping to organize musical ensembles, can be self-affirming contributions to society that engender learning, self-exploration, and a sense of accomplishment (Palmer, 1980). One may self-guide participation in a re-creative therapeutic music experience by making a personal choice to offer one's musical or organizational services to an ensemble, or seek out a music therapist who directs an intergenerational choir or a community choir specifically developed for the needs and interests of aging adults.

Social and Interpersonal Health

The elderly face a number of social challenges in our society. McCloskey (1985) observed that "music is effective therapeutically because it is the most social of all the arts and it is precisely the social aspects of life that are affected through . . . old age" (p. 73). Although many older adults maintain active lifestyles in their later years, others may find themselves disengaging from former levels of social interaction (Davis, 1986). Certainly, aging members of our society are often faced with the need to cope with changing roles and relationships.

Societal Perceptions of Aging

Adjusting to life as an older adult can be particularly challenging when one is confronted with attitudes of ageism in younger members of the community. Reuer and Crowe (1995) have identified several of these misconceptions, which include that senility is an inevitable part of the aging process (actually, only 20% to 25% of older adults ever experience organic brain disorders), that all elderly people are much the same (in fact, older adults have had more time to develop individual differences, and thus are more heterogeneous than other age groups), and that older adults are relatively unproductive and no longer have very much to offer (they actually tend to remain concerned community members who wish to pass on their ideas to future generations).

One possible means of altering these negative attitudes may be to engage older and younger adults in shared music-making experiences. Music is widely believed to have the potential to bring different kinds of people closer together, and indeed a number of recent studies have borne this out. Darrow and Johnson (1994) studied the attitudes of teenagers and elderly persons toward each other before and after participation in an intergenerational choir. Analysis of pre- and post-test scores demonstrated that both teens and elders developed more positive attitudes toward one another during the course of their time singing together. An additional benefit was that the elderly participants' attitudes toward themselves became more positive as well. In a similar study, Bowers (1998) used an intergenerational choir to examine the attitudes of college students and seniors toward each other. Pre- to post-test scores in this study also indicated a positive shift in these two groups' perceptions of each other.

Discovering New Roles, Learning New Skills

Often, older adults have begun to move beyond the roles and responsibilities that may have defined them for many years. They may have retired from full-time work; their children have grown and moved on. As these life changes occur, there is a need to find new creative outlets and ways of feeling valuable within the community.

Participation in music making can be a rewarding and effective means of supporting older adults in assuming leadership roles within a group. Reuer and Crowe (1995) have developed a program in which elderly volunteers are trained by music therapists in the use of carefully selected, rhythm-based music activities. The purpose of this program is not to train these volunteers to function as music therapists, but rather to encourage them to serve as recreational music group leaders and/or activity assistants to professional music therapists. The end result, then, is very positive in that it not only provides these elderly volunteers with a sense of purpose, self-growth, and the many benefits of participation in rhythmic activities, but also allows these volunteers to pass on many of these benefits to less functional members of the elderly community, in situations in which a music therapist may not be readily accessible.

Considerations for Caregivers

One particularly poignant interpersonal challenge that older adults may face is the impact of age-related illness upon their relationships with spouses, children, and other significant persons. From either side of this equation, there are often difficult adjustments to face and feelings of loss or grief to endure.

In treating elderly persons, a number of music therapists have expanded their practice to include working with their clients' family members, especially those who must face the stresses of caring for their frail or cognitively impaired loved ones. Korb (1997) used instructional tapes containing specially composed songs whose lyrics reminded elderly clients of specific improvements they wished to make in their daily living. Caregivers were encouraged to play these tapes for their elderly family members on a regular basis. Results were somewhat mixed, but generally clients exhibited better short-term memory and more positive affect, and caregivers reported experiencing relief from stress. Clair and Ebberts (1997) found that caregivers who participated in music therapy sessions with their care receivers reported a significant increase in feelings of satisfaction with the time they spent together. Hanser and Clair (1995) have developed clinical practice protocols specifically for use with dementia patients and their family caregivers, with differing approaches depending upon the severity of cognitive impairment. Both of these authors see music therapy as a means of retrieving some of the many losses in interpersonal relationships that can occur as the older adult declines.

At times, it may become necessary for caregivers to enlist the support of professional care settings such as adult day centers or nursing homes. When making such decisions, it may well be valuable for caregivers to inquire about opportunities for participation in music experiences, as there is strong support in the research literature for the benefits of music with the frail or cognitively impaired elderly. One simple gift that a caregiver can provide for his or her loved one is a recording of favorite music; familiar and preferred music has been found to reduce levels of agitation (Gerdner & Swanson, 1993). It is worth bearing in mind, however, that impaired older adults need not be limited to receptive experiences; with the right kind of support, they are often able to engage in meaningful music making. Smith (1992), the director of an adult day program, spearheaded a highly successful and high-profile performing arts program for her participants. She began with group singing, later hired a music therapist to enhance the program and lead a handbell choir, and ultimately took the participants on tour. Benefits of this ambitious program included increased self-esteem, a more positive profile within the community, and pure aesthetic pleasure.

CONCLUSION

This chapter provides a brief overview of some of the many possible uses of therapeutic music experiences in the lives of older people. The examples provided are not intended to be prescriptive, nor can they be, as each individual's relationship with music is unique.

As it was beyond the scope of this book to fully address the depth and breadth of this area of practice and research, the hope of the author has been to stimulate interest in the many benefits music can offer adults as they age. For those interested in more specific information on this topic, or in contacting practitioners, further resources are provided below.

RESOURCES

The Bonny Method of Guided Imagery and Music: Association for Music and Imagery, P. O. Box 4286, Blaine, WA 98231-4286; Web site: www.bonnymethod.com/ami

Clair, A. A. (1996). *Therapeutic uses of music with older adults*. Baltimore: Health Professions Press.

Jacobi, E. M., & Eisenberg, G. M. (2001). The efficacy of guided imagery and music (GIM in the treatment of rheumatoid arthritis. *Journal of the Association for Music and Imagery, 8,* 57–74.

Katsh, S., & Merle-Fishman, C. (1998). *The music within you* (2nd ed.). Gilsum, NH: Barcelona.

Music practitioners: The Music for Healing and Transitions Program Inc., 22 West End Rd., Hillsdale, NY 12529; Web site: www.mhtp.org

Music therapists: American Music Therapy Association, Inc., 8455 Colesville Rd., Suite 1000, Silver Spring, MD 20910; telephone: (301) 589-3300; fax: (301) 589-5175; e-mail: info@musictherapy.org

Short, A. E. (1991). The role of guided imagery and music in diagnosing physical illness or trauma. *Music Therapy, 10*(1), 22–45.

Sound healers: Sound Healers Association, P.O. Box 2240, Boulder, CO 80306; telephone: (800) 246-9764; fax: (303) 443-6023; Web site: www.healingsounds.com

REFERENCES

Aigen, K. (1991). The voice of the forest: A conception of music for music therapy. *Music Therapy, 10*(1), 77–98.

Aldridge, D. (1996). *Music therapy research and practice in medicine.* London: Jessica Kingsley.

American Music Therapy Association. (2003). *AMTA member sourcebook.* Silver Spring, MD: Author.

Antonovsky, A. (1987). *Unraveling the mystery of health: How people manage stress and stay well.* San Francisco: Jossey-Bass.

Becker, N., Chambliss, C., Marsh, C., & Montemayor, R. (1995). Effects of mellow and frenetic music and stimulating and relaxing scents on walking by seniors. *Perceptual and Motor Skills, 80,* 411–415.

Bernard, A. (1992). The use of music as purposeful activity: A preliminary investigation. *Physical and Occupational Therapy in Geriatrics, 10*(3), 35–45.

Bonny, H. (2002a). Guided imagery and music (GIM): Mirror of consciousness. In L. Summer (Ed.), *Music and consciousness: The evolution of guided imagery and music* (pp. 93–102). Gilsum, NH: Barcelona.

Bonny, H. (2002b). Sounds as symbol: Guided imagery and music in clinical practice. In L. Summer (Ed.), *Music and consciousness: The evolution of guided imagery and music* (pp. 133–140). Gilsum, NH: Barcelona.

Bowers, J. (1998). Effects of an intergenerational choir for community-based seniors and college students on age-related attitudes. *Journal of Music Therapy, 35*(1), 2–18.

Bruscia, K. E. (1998). *Defining music therapy* (2nd ed.). Gilsum, NH: Barcelona.

Bruscia, K. (2000). The nature of meaning in music therapy: Kenneth Bruscia interviewed by Brynjulf Stige. *Nordic Journal of Music Therapy, 9*(2), 84–96.

Butler, R. N. (1971). Age: The life review. *Psychology Today, 5*(7), 49–51, 89.

Butler, C., & Butler P. J. (1997). Physioacoustic therapy with cardiac surgery patients. In T. Wigram & C. Dileo (Eds.), *Music vibration* (pp. 197–204). Cherry Hill, NJ: Jeffrey Books.

Clair, A. A., & Ebberts, A. G. (1997). The effects of music therapy on interactions between family caregivers and their care receivers with late stage dementia. *Journal of Music Therapy, 34*(3), 148–164.

Cohen, N. (1992). The effect of singing instruction of the speech production of neurologically impaired persons. *Journal of Music Therapy, 29*(2), 87–102.

Darrow, A. A., & Johnson, C. M. (1994). Junior and senior high school music students' attitudes toward individuals with disabilities. *Journal of Music Therapy, 31,* 266–279.

Davis, L. J. (1986). Gerontology in theory and practice. In L.J. Davis & M. Kirkland (Eds.), *The role of occupational therapy with the elderly* (pp. 29–39). Rockville, MD: American Occupational Therapy Association.

Davis, W. B., Gfeller, K. E., & Thaut, M. H. (1999). *An introduction to music therapy: Theory and practice* (2nd ed.). New York: McGraw-Hill.

Dileo, C. (1999). Introduction to music therapy and medicine: Definitions, theoretical orientations and levels of practice. In C. Dileo (Ed.), *Music therapy and medicine: Theoretical and clinical applications* (pp. 1–10). Silver Spring, MD: American Music Therapy Association.

Dileo, C., & Bradt, J. (1999). Entrainment, resonance, and pain-related suffering. In C. Dileo (Ed.), *Music therapy and medicine: Theoretical and clinical applications* (pp. 1–10). Silver Spring, MD: American Music Therapy Association.

Eagle, C. (1991). Steps to a theory of quantum therapy. *Music Therapy Perspectives, 9,* 56–60.

Eckford, L., & Lambert, A. (2002). *Beating the senior blues: How to feel better and enjoy life again.* Oakland, CA: New Harbinger Publications.

Gerdner, L. A., & Swanson, E. A. (1993). Effects of individualized music on confused and agitated elderly patients. *Archives of Psychiatric Nursing, 7*(5), 284–291.

Hanser, S. B., & Clair, A. A. (1995). Retrieving the losses of Alzheimer's disease for patients and caregivers with the aid of music. In T. Wigram & B. Saperston (Eds.), *The art and science of music therapy: A handbook* (pp. 342–360). Philadelphia: Harwood Academic Publishers/Gordon and Breach Science Publishers.

Hughes, D. E., & Peake, T. H. (2002). Investigating the value of spiritual well-being and psychosocial development in mitigating senior adulthood depression. *Activities, Adaptation and Aging, 26*(3), 15–35.

Johnson, G., Otto, D., & Clair, A. (2001). The effect of instrumental and vocal music on adherence to a physical rehabilitation exercise program with persons who are elderly. *Journal of Music Therapy, 38*(2), 82–96.

Kelley, B. J. (1996). Music and music vibration plus relaxation/imagery for pain relief with independent elderly. Unpublished master's thesis, Texas Woman's University, Denton, Texas.

Kenny, C. (1989). *The field of play: A guide for theory and practice in music therapy.* St. Louis: MMB Music.

Korb, C. (1997). The influence of music therapy on patients with a diagnosed dementia. *Canadian Journal of Music Therapy, 5*(1), 26–54.

McCloskey, L. (1985). Music and the frail elderly. *Activities, Adaptation and Aging, 7*(2), 73–75.

McCloskey, L. (1990, Winter). The silent heart sings. *Generations Counseling and Therapy,* 63–65.

Merriam-Webster's New Collegiate Dictionary. (2005). Springfield, MA: G. & C. Merriam Company.

Mullins, L. C., & McNicholas, N. (1986). Loneliness among the elderly: Issues and considerations for professionals in aging. *Gerontology and Geriatrics Education, 7*(1), 55–65.

O' Callaghan. (1999). Recent findings about neural correlates of music pertinent to music therapy across the lifespan. *Music Therapy Perspectives, 17*(1), 32–36.

Palmer, M. (1980). Music therapy and gerontology. *Activities, Adaptation and Aging, 1*(1), 37–40.

Pavlicevic, M. (1997). *Music therapy in context.* London: Jessica Kingsley.

Reilly, N. P. (2000). Music, a cognitive behavioral intervention for anxiety and acute pain control in elderly cataract patient (UMI No. AAI9938255). *Dissertation Abstracts International, 60*(7), 3195B.

Reuer, B., & Crowe, B. (1995). *Best practice in music therapy: Utilizing group percussion volunteerism in the well older adult.* San Diego, CA: University Center on Aging.

Ruud, E. (1998). *Music therapy: Improvisation, communication, and culture.* Gilsum, NH: Barcelona.

Salas, J. (1990). Aesthetic experiences in music therapy. *Music Therapy, 9,* 1–15.

Schulberg, C. (1999). Out of the ashes: Transforming despair into hope with music and imagery. In J. Hibben (Ed.), *Inside music therapy: Client experiences* (pp. 7–12). Gilsum, NH: Barcelona.

Schwoebel J., Coslett, H., Bradt, J., Friedman, R., & Dileo, C. (2002). Pain and the body schema: Effects of pain severity on mental representations of movement. *Neurology, 59*(5), 775–777.

Smith, B. B. (1992). Treatment of dementia: Healing through cultural arts. *Pride Institute Journal of Long-Term Health Care, 11*(3), 37–45.

Smith, B. (1996–1997). Uncovering and healing hidden wounds: Using GIM to resolve complicated and disenfranchised grief. *Journal of the Association for Music and Imagery, 5*(1), 1–23.

Stige, B. (2002). *Culture-centered music therapy.* Gilsum, NH: Barcelona.

Tomaino, C. M. (1994). Music and music therapy for frail non-institutionalized elderly persons. *Journal of Long-Term Home Health Care, 13*(2), 24–27.

Troll, L. E. (1994). Family connectedness of old women: Attachments in later life. In B. F. Turner & L. E. Troll (Eds.), *Women growing older: Psychological perspectives* (pp. 169–201). Thousand Oaks, CA: Sage Publications.

Updike, P. A. (1994). Aesthetic, spiritual, and healing discussions in music. In P. L. Chinn & J. Watson (Eds.), *Art and aesthetics in nursing* (pp. 291–300). New York: National League for Nursing Press.

Wigram, T., & Dileo, C. (1997). *Music vibration.* Cherry Hill, NJ: Jeffery Books.

CHAPTER SIX

Art Therapy

Caroline Peterson

Art therapy encourages health-related quality of life through creative expression in the context of a supportive relationship. Expression through art making and dialogue around visual imagery fosters improvement in emotional well-being, cognitive orientation, the integration of life change and loss, recollective experience, physical engagement, and social role. As an interventional modality in complementary and alternative medicine (CAM), art therapy offers a range of assessments and treatments to support the diverse needs of the wide spectrum of aging adults.

As described by the American Art Therapy Association (AATA), art therapy is based on the tenet that the "creative process involved in the making of art is healing and life enhancing. Art therapists are professionals trained in both art and therapy. They are knowledgeable about human development, psychological theories, clinical practice, spiritual, multicultural, and artistic traditions, and the healing potential of art (2004)." Art therapists use art in treatment, assessment, and research, and provide consultations to allied professionals. They are among other clinically trained colleagues in the creative arts, including dance, music, drama, and expressive therapists. "Art therapy is the therapeutic use of art making, within a professional relationship, by people who experience illness, trauma, or challenges in living, and by people who seek personal development. Through creating art and reflecting on the art products and processes, people can increase awareness of self and others; cope with symptoms, stress, and traumatic experiences; enhance cognitive abilities; and enjoy the life-affirming pleasures of making art (AATA, 2004)."

Creative arts therapists are not the sole proprietors of the arts in health care, though they constitute a large contingent of the multidimensional and growing movement that is nominally defined as arts in health care or arts medicine. Contributors to this larger field are those who work to enhance the health care environment through art, architecture, and environmental design, and professional artists who volunteer or work as hospital staff offering performances and arts-expressive opportunities within their respective fields to patients and often their caregivers. Additionally, nurses have often used art making and arts-based interventions in a variety of health care settings and contribute significantly to the health literature on this use. All persons in the arts medicine field share a deep belief in the power of creativity as a wellspring for healing for each person receiving health care regardless of diagnosis or prognosis. In 1994, the National Institutes of Health defined art therapy, as well as other creative arts therapies, in the domain of complementary and alternative medicine. In subsequent years, the emergence of patient-centered integrated approaches to health care, inclusive of arts approaches, has grown significantly (Malchiodi, 1999a).

ART AS PSYCHOTHERAPY, ART AS THERAPY

According to *A History of Art Therapy in the United States* (Junge, 1994), the evolving field of psychoanalysis, developmental theories such as Jean Piaget's, and the ideas of the late 19th-century progressive education movement influenced the establishment of art therapy as a profession. Maxine Junge (1994) reports that the emphasis Sigmund Freud and Carl Jung placed on dreams and symbolic images, as the means to understand the unconscious mind, influenced Margaret Naumberg, the founder of the Walden School in New York and one of the founders of the art therapy profession. Naumberg (1966) was greatly influenced by psychoanalytic theory in developing what she called "dynamically oriented art therapy," which evolved from her work with children and adults at the New York Psychiatric Institute beginning in 1941. Naumberg, who also studied with John Dewey and Maria Montessori, advanced the view that spontaneous art making provided the ground for the psychotherapeutic process to unfold and for the development of insight.

Edith Kramer, another influential theorist in the development of art therapy, emphasized that the process of art making by itself provided the primary healing benefit of art therapy as an intervention. Challenging Naumberg's emphasis on art as psychotherapy, and based on her early work with emotionally disturbed boys, Kramer (1971) theorized that the value of the process of art making and the problem solving around producing an aesthetically satisfying picture or sculpture supported the development of a healthy ego; the picture thus contained internal conflicts that were sublimated through the art-making process. Naumberg's and Kramer's theories were expanded by Rhyne (1973), Ulman (1975), Kwiatkowska (1978), Rubin (1978), Wadeson (1980), Landgarten

(1981), Levick (1983), and others, providing art therapists with a rich theoretical ground from which to develop their work with children, adults and families.

Art therapy is reported to have developed along a somewhat parallel course in Great Britain, with the use of art therapy expanding in psychiatric settings in both countries during and after World War II, most notably in the United States at the Menninger Clinic. In Germany and other parts of Europe, art therapy developed as part of the anthroposophical medicine tradition based on the theories of Rudolph Steiner (1998). The British artist Adrian Hill coined the term *art therapy* in 1942. Hill shared the healing properties of painting with fellow patients who had tuberculosis, later receiving permission to work with soldiers returning from the war (Junge, 1994).

WHO RECEIVES ART THERAPY SERVICES?

Art therapists view their work as grounded across cultures, beginning with the earliest use of art making in collective rituals and the ongoing production of art by nonartists from the earliest times. As a precursor and adjunct to the use and cultivation of spoken language, from cave paintings to subway graffiti, humans have made meaning of their lives through image and symbol. Today, art therapists work with people of all ages: individuals, couples, families, groups, and communities. The American Art Therapy Association reports that art therapists "provide services, individually and as part of clinical teams, in settings that include mental health, rehabilitation, medical, and forensic institutions; community outreach programs; wellness centers, schools, and nursing homes; corporate structures; and open studios and independent practices" (2004). Advances and theoretical developments in general medicine and psychiatry have influenced art therapy over time. Art therapists approach their work from a variety of theoretical perspectives across what Lusebrink (1990) describes as a continuum from psychodynamic to psychoanalytic to humanistic to structuralist. This continuum includes Jungian, cognitive, phenomenological, Gestalt, psychocybernetic, transpersonal, visual expressive, shamanistic, anthroposophical, and mindfulness-based approaches.

ART THERAPY IN GENERAL:
SETTINGS, SESSIONS, SERVICES, AND ASSESSMENT

Art therapists like other health care professionals may have general or specialty practices or work in health care institutions or other community settings. Such services are found in diverse institutional settings, including schools, community mental health clinics, psychiatric day and inpatient programs, cancer centers, skilled nursing and rehabilitation settings, integrative medicine programs, geriatric day and residential centers, and forensic institutions. Art therapists may work as consultants or as part of clinical teams where they play an integral role in treatment planning and implementation. Depending on the population being served, their team of colleagues may include physicians, psychologists, nurses, social workers, substance abuse counselors, occupational and physical therapists, other creative arts or expressive therapists, school counselors, forensics professionals, and research scientists.

Planning Treatment

Whatever the clinical setting or practice, treatment planning is developed on a case-by-case basis. An interview and evaluative assessment by the art therapist or team members are part of this process in which the client's goals are the basis for planning. Therapist or team recommendations are reviewed in this context with the client, and a contract for treatment is agreed upon. In cases where the client is in the care of a custodian, the same process as described above would occur, with the client and his or her custodian or family members. In institutional settings, adjunctive therapists such as art therapists provide psychological/behavioral services that are complementary to treatment with medications, medical interventions, and/or physical therapy. In such group treatment milieus, art therapists may have daily contact hours with a client/patient/resident. Art therapists see individuals, children, and/or adults, conduct family sessions, or offer groups for special populations. Art therapy sessions may be held in offices, hospital rooms, schoolrooms, or open studios, with nonambulatory or ambulatory persons, with individuals or groups. Session times vary depending on the purpose of the session and the client's capacity for session duration and usually generally vary from 30 minutes to 90 minutes in length.

Evaluating Needs and Progress

In the field of art therapy numerous evaluative approaches have been developed, some consisting of a single drawing and others of a series of drawings. These assessment tools support the art therapist's clinical decision making and enable the therapist to meet the client through verbal and nonverbal interaction. Some evaluative approaches have been under development for decades and include the cataloguing of pictures, the development of rating scales based on graphic indicators or picture elements, and the validation of those scales relative to diagnostic categories.

Two such evaluative tools are the Diagnostic Drawing Series (Cohen, Hammer, & Singer, 1988; Cohen, Mills, & Kijak, 1994) and the Formal Elements Art Therapy Scale (Gantt, 2001). As Wadeson (1980) suggested, the concrete and permanent record the art productions afford is valuable to practitioners and clients alike for identifying problems and clarifying strengths, charting progress, recalling what has been learned, observing state change toward improvement or illness progression, and providing a review of the art therapy journey for closure when treatment concludes. The development of valid and reliable measures for diagnostic purposes using art productions is an ongoing challenge in the fields of art therapy, psychology, and psychiatry (American Art Therapy Association, 1998; Hacking, 2000).

ART THERAPY IN PRACTICE: FOSTERING CREATIVITY THROUGHOUT THE LIFE CYCLE

To reiterate, art therapy is based on the belief that the creative process involved in the making of art is healing and life-enhancing. Art making is not the only way to be creative; however, it is one of the first or primary ways we come to know ourselves as distinct individuals. Whether we have drawn a sun in the dirt with a stick, made an impression of our bodies in the snow, or had the fortune of the pleasurable use of a box of crayons, creating meaning in relation to ourselves and the world through the external expression of internal images is natural to our earliest activities of being. The interplay of creativity and image plays a role in our development as individuals whether we think of ourselves as particularly creative or not.

As a quality of being, creativity is a complex topic and was addressed in early philosophical writings. Plato conceived of creativity as derived from mysterious external forces; Aristotle disagreed and wrote of creativity as obedient to natural laws. Possibly they were both correct. Abraham Maslow (1968), the humanistic psychologist, is best known for describing a hierarchy of needs for self-actualization. In *Towards a Psychology of Being,* Maslow states that he once believed that creativity was related to special talent; however, after years of observing human beings, he found there was "self-actualizing creativeness (p. 137)" in ordinary individuals that was related to personality rather than achievement. He concluded that self-actualizing creativity "seems to be sometimes synonymous with health itself . . . a defining characteristic of essential humanness (p. 145)." Maslow's colleague Carl Rogers (1961), in his influential article "Towards a Theory of Creativity," suggested that the directed tendency to self-actualize is at the heart of our creativity. Creativity supports our endeavors to be more in relation to others, the environment, and ourselves. Thus, creativity is constructive to our being. Rogers suggested that the conditions within the individual for creativity include an openness to experience, an internal capacity for self-evaluation, and an ability to play spontaneously. Play is not the sole domain of the young, and creativity is not an age-based function. Simonton (1990), with over a dozen years studying age and creativity, suggests that in the later years of life creativity can even be resurgent. Whether an older individual is aware or unaware of their creative-expressive energies or not, what distinguishes art therapy is that it is relational, and the relationship between therapist and client revolves around the creativity of both persons.

It is the art therapist's task to provide a milieu that will foster the conditions Rogers describes within each person with whom they work. Rogers' constructs for accomplishing this are standard to general therapeutic practice and include empathy, unconditional positive regard, nonjudging, and facilitation of free symbolic expression.

In this context, treatment goals will vary according to the needs of the individual receiving art therapy services. The types of art materials provided and whether the image making is structured as a therapist-directed art therapy task or a free drawing by the client or both are a function of the goals of treatment as well as the context of time and place in which the treatment is received. A highly delusional senior with schizophrenia, an executive facing retirement, an individual grieving over the loss of a spouse of many years, a grandparent with a cancer diagnosis, or a person with midstage Alzheimer's dementia differ in their age-related adaptive challenges. In each case, the mobilization and use of creative energy offer the opportunity for healing and life enhancement and provides the opportunity to give shape and meaning to one's lived experience within a therapeutic relationship.

ART THERAPY IN PRACTICE: FOSTERING SUCCESSFUL LIFE SPAN DEVELOPMENT FOR EACH PERSON

Art therapists work with people of all ages and are clinically trained in life span development theory. Given that older adults may be as young as 60 and as old as the growing number of persons reaching 100, gerontologists now view "old people" as young-old, old-old, and oldest-old. Aging adults are a very large and diverse group of persons. Standard to complementary and alternative medicine practices, from a biopsychosocial-spiritual or holistic perspective, art therapists approach each person receiving services as an individual. In a call for an integrated biopsy-chosocial approach to research on successful aging in the *Annals of Internal Medicine,* "successful aging is defined not by longevity alone but by sufficient well-being (in multiple domains) to sustain a capacity for functioning adequately in changing circumstances" (Inui, 2003, p.391).

When we consider the psychosocial aspects of aging, one theory that describes age-related developmental tasks and needs is Erik Erikson's (1963) psychosocial model of the stages of development. This theory has served as a springboard for much of life span development theory. Erikson's theories have influenced many art therapists in conceptualizing treatment approaches for adults from a developmental perspective.

Erikson describes sets of experiences that define the developmental tasks for each stage of life from infancy to late age. Unresolved developmental tasks from one stage to the next are viewed as making later stages more challenging. Successful resolution of developmental tasks, at each stage of life, is therefore, the building block of successful aging and personal wisdom. In the Eriksonian developmental sequence, cultivating trust as an infant, purposefulness as a preschooler, competency as a student, an identity as an adolescent, to be in-relation to others as a young adult, and to have the capacity for caring in the middle years are all precursors to sustain integrity with and engagement in the world in older adulthood. The alternative to integrity is isolating despair resulting from unresolved loss and hopelessness. Healthy aging, then, in this perspective, includes understanding interdependence and having humor and resilience, self-acceptance, and an equal acceptance of others (Erikson, Erikson, & Kivnick, 1986).

Even for the older person who has gracefully accomplished all these developmental tasks, the stresses of aging and the onset of acute and/or chronic changes in functional status can undermine one's confidence. Individuals can find themselves despairing and even stuck in a pattern of struggle reflective of struggle earlier in life. Shore (1997) emphasizes the utility of Erickson's model for art therapists working with older adults, suggesting that the natural tensions that arise as we struggle with change can be worked through with two- and three-dimensional art materials. "(A)rt therapy can be used to promote the struggle for successful aging. Even severely impaired individuals may use the creative process to tap into their capacity for wisdom (p. 177)."

The psychosocial despair Erikson describes in late adulthood may often be undiagnosed clinical depression, a common mental health disorder in the aging population. The value of adjunctive therapies, such as art therapy, as a nonpharmacological intervention for the treatment of depression is recommended as efficacious in care guidelines for geriatric nurses (Gerstenlauer, Maguire, & Wooldridge, 2003).

CONCEPTUALIZING TREATMENT FOR OLDER ADULTS: KEY COMPONENTS OF HEALTHY AGING

A search of current health literature offers a view of how healthy aging is conceptualized, and the specific elements deemed sufficient to the maintenance of well-being in multiple domains for older adults are identified. When themes that emerge from this review are considered as a constellation, a more holistic view of the mind–body connection in healthy aging and the utility of art therapy become apparent.

Physical activity, cognitive stimulation, mental outlook, and finding meaning in life (Hartman-Stein & Potkanowicz, 2003) are key components of healthy aging that need to be supported by improved outcomes and the management of chronic illness for all generations of the aging population (Kane, 2003; Rigaud, Hanon, Seux, & Forette, 2001). Emotional well-being, the maintenance of social identity, and engagement in generative activities as well as those that foster integrating one's inner life with external experience are all reported as factors in the maintenance of physical well-being. These play an important compensatory role as well in the capacity to adapt to reductions in functional health status (Bailis & Chipperfield, 2002; Carlson, Seeman, & Fried, 2000; Meeks & Murrell, 2001).

Creativity and Successful Aging

This adaptive being in old age is often linked in the geriatric literature to creativity. In a review of key components of successful aging reported by the Menninger Clinic (Aronson, 1999), the necessity of adaptive skills to support coping in late life is reviewed, and the role of creativity is highlighted. In assessing the meanings of successful aging and creativity, as reported in the *Journal of Aging Studies,* outcomes suggest that creative activity fosters a sense of competence, purpose, and growth and transferable problem-solving skills for daily life (Fisher & Specht, 1999). Healthy or successful aging is therefore not solely predicated on physical health, the undoing of which is common to later life span development, but rather to adaptive skills sets, an integrated self-relation, and a connectedness to an identified meaningful social role. In this light, art therapy, as a beneficial mind–body intervention, is easily conceptualized and made practical. Key to treatment planning in art therapy interventions with older persons are the cultivation of competency, an ongoing sense of purposefulness, developmental persistence, and transferable skills in the face of inevitable life changes. In this way art therapy fosters improvement in cognitive orientation, affective well-being, the integration of life change and loss, recollective experience, physical engagement/motor skills maintenance, and social role.

Configuring Health Through Imagery

The art therapist engages persons in expression, in the concretization of images using art materials. Expression therefore includes both the process of making the image and the image itself. Understanding is derived from the process, the image, and how we interact with both. Art media vary from more structured (pencil, marker) to less structured (pastel, water-color) and are often utilized based on their facilitative function and thus their influence on the quality of the image creation experience. Whether expressed two dimensionally on paper or three dimensionally in sculp-tural material like clay, the resulting art images are derived from internal representations of both internal and external experience.

Creative expression through art media may be appreciated for the fullness of the direct experience it affords and the mind–body relationship that it enlivens. The experience of images and image making is as multi-dimensional as our ways of knowing: kinesthetic, sensory, perceptual, af-fective, cognitive, symbolic, and creative, according to Kagin and Lusebrink (1978), who formulated a model of an expressive therapies continuum (ETC). The kinesthetic is then related to active movement as images are drawn, painted, and given shape. The sensory field engaged re-lated to how the art materials feel in hand, and their smell, sound, and vi-sual impact; perceptual knowing follows related to form, structure, organizing within the materials' fluidity, or constraints. Active engage-ment in forming and structuring gives rise to the affective (emotion); felt emotion gives itself back to form; image making and reflection ensue.

In this expressive continuum, a range of cognitive processes unfold, including how to utilize the art materials and organize steps in the process of the art making. Unconscious and conscious dialogue, with the emer-gent image, support conceptual thinking and movement toward symbolic expression. Kagin and Lusebrink (1978) posit that creative actualization may occur at any stage within this process and may reflect interaction with the art materials, the created image, and the in-relation verbal pro-cessing between the client and the art therapist. Within this model, mak-ing art as a way of knowing has both depth and utility. A full and technical exploration of ETC and its practical applications can be found in Vija Lusebrink's (1990) book *Imagery and Visual Expression in Therapy.*

WORKING WITH IMAGES:
A NEUROSCIENCES PERSPECTIVE

Lusebrink's attention to the mind–body process in imagery and visual ex-pression is consistent with the heightened mind–body focus of research in the neurosciences in the 21st century. This research focuses broadly on neural interactions that influence biology and behavior. Research at the Department of Psychology and Laboratory for Affective Neuroscience at the University of Wisconsin-Madison, for example, has recently focused on the relationship between emotion and immune functioning (Davidson, Kabat-Zinn, Schumacher, Rosenkranz, Muller, Santorelli, et al., 2003). Exposure to images has served as the basis for a number of research protocols conducted there relative to emotional expression and brain physiology (Davidson, Ekman, Saron, Senulis, & Friesenm, 1990). Essentially, Davidson (2000) proposes that in the circuitry of the prefrontal cortex of the human brain there are "both behavioral and biological variables related to affective style and emotion regulation,"(p. 1196) as well as plasticity that may serve the transformation and cultivation of positive affective states and impact personal resilience. Outcomes in neuroscience research thus suggest that we have the potential to change our minds, our bodies, and therefore our health and well-being.

The potential for these evidence-based outcomes and the role of images in this process were extensively explored by Jeanne Achterberg in her book *Imagery in healing: Shamanism and modern medicine* (1985). Within this model, images in the prefrontal cortex link conscious levels of information processing with physiological shifts in the body. In discussing images as a bridge between the mind and body, Achterberg places emphasis on the right hemisphere having predominant domain over image and the right hemisphere's strong link both to affect (emotion) and to the autonomic nervous system that regulates our internal environment, including our fight/flight response and capacity to evoke calm. Formative, stored, and recalled images in the prefrontal cortex serve as a gateway between emotion and direct experience in our physical bodies whether automatic (reactive) or self-regulated (chosen/directed).

Therefore, if we think of the mind as a dimensional library of images, in relaxed conscious awareness (a condition that supports plasticity in the brain), we can work with and develop images that support our capacity for self-organizing well-being. Conversely, we can release or alter images that bind us to confusion and dis-ease. This can be done with guided imagery as well as art making; many art therapists use both approaches and often integrate the two.

Building on Achterberg's and Lusebrink's work, the neurodevelopmental approach in art therapy has been further advanced by the work of Linda Chapman and colleagues (Chapman, Morabito, Ladakaos, Schreier, & Knusdon, 2001), who developed and researched the Chapman Art Therapy Treatment Intervention (CATTI) for hospitalized injured children diagnosed with incident-based post-traumatic stress disorder. Chapman et al.'s intervention is intended to repair communication across the right (image) and left (language) hemispheres in the brain, which can become disregulated in trauma. The CATTI process supports the development of a visual narrative as a method to access bound affect/emotion. The release of affect supports a physiological relaxation in the body leading to the unfolding of verbal narrative, greater understanding around the experience, and restoration of equilibrium. Outcomes with the CATTI, as reported by Chapman et al. (2001), confirm that the recollection of a blocked pattern of memory (perceived experience stored as images) due to stress trauma can be (1) restored from partial data, (2) tolerated affectively, and (3) integrated into consciousness when the pathway for recovery follows a neurodevelopmental course, as described by Lusebrink (1990), from kinesthetic to sensory to perceptual/affective to cognitive/symbolic. Developed as a trauma recovery model for acute care, the CATTI has theoretical applicability for art therapy as an effective intervention in illnesses common to older adults where there is often persistent stress and chronicity.

Working directly with an understanding of how we, neurally, know ourselves and the world through images, Achterberg, Lusebrink, and Chapman have forged a path in art therapy theory and practice relative to developments in neuroscience. Advances in the neurosciences represent advances in mind–body medicine and complementary and alternative practices. This progression invigorates interventions around health and aging such as mindfulness-based art therapy (MBAT), a multimodal intervention that combines meditation-based stress reduction, art therapy, and group support for adults with chronic illness. The 8-week MBAT program has been the subject of a recent clinical trial, conducted at Thomas Jefferson University in Philadelphia, for persons with cancer funded by the National Institutes of Health National Center for Complementary Medicine. In the MBAT randomized clinical trial, adult women with cancer, who received the MBAT program and usual oncologic care had significant reductions in psychological distress and improvements in health-related quality of life as compared to women receiving usual oncologic care alone. (Monti, Peterson, Shakin Kunkel, Hauck, Pequiqnot, et al., 2005). Funding for ongoing research into the MBAT intervention, at Thomas Jefferson, was awarded by the National Cancer Institute in the fall of 2005.

ART THERAPY IN PRACTICE:
ILLNESS WITH WELLNESS

In practice, art therapy supports health-related quality of life through the cultivation of competency, a sense of purpose, personal development and growth, and transferable skills in the face of inevitable life changes. In this way art therapy fosters improvement in emotional well-being, cognitive orientation, the integration of life change and loss, recollective experience, physical engagement, and social role.

Rehabilitation

Persons in geriatric rehabilitation settings are often older adults receiving services following a stroke or cerebrovascular accident (CVA), recovering from a fall, and/or joint replacement surgery. The physical activity involved in art making is a key component to the value of art therapy in rehabilitation. Art making engages non- and recovering ambulatory patients in movement as they are able. Art materials can be provided that support treatment goals relative to gross or fine motor skills reactivation. Art therapists, working closely with physical and occupational therapists, reinforce themes for recovery with alternative activities that cultivate adaptive functioning. Even as patients may be renewing fine and/or gross motor skills while making art, the art productions provide opportunities for expressions of grief, explorations of pain and fear, and the emergence of reality testing about what is possible and not relative to resuming one's life. For post-CVA patients who have expressive or receptive aphasia and/or impaired sensory functioning, the art media, such as precut collage pictures, torn tissue paper, and clay provide opportunities for a variety of modes of adaptive expressive opportunities.

Healing Without Words

There is enormous value to art therapy in rehabilitation settings because exchanges within the art therapy relationship are not verbally dependent. Persons with impaired language skills have immediate access to self-expression using the language of images that may be self-generated in drawing or coloring, or constructed from colored and textured shape forms, images from magazines, or even accumulated get well cards. Alternatively, the art therapist can initiate a visual art-based dialogue by choosing or making the first image that begins an art production. This action can support word processing, verbal conversation, and/or a nonverbal picture-building exchange between the therapist and the client. The client can be given support for autonomous functioning and direct the art therapist to paste picture elements based on the choice and placement by the client, thus constructing their own understanding and meaning.

Much of the research in art therapy has been conducted in geriatric settings. Specific to rehabilitation for stroke, Yaretsky, Levinson, and Kfar-Saba (1996) report on the benefits of group art therapy using clay with geriatric rehabilitation patients. Work with clay supported both "bilateral sensorimotor activities of the upper limbs with social interaction directed towards future leisure time activity (p. 75)." The focus of the clay constructions was "home." Outcomes included an increased level of shared communication among patients on the rehabilitation unit about their personal lives and a reported sense of pleasure with the creative activity. Individuals with severe aphasia are reported by Sacchett and colleagues (Sacchett, Byng, Marshall, & Pound, 1999) to have benefited from a communicative drawing intervention over 12 weeks, with caregivers reporting that the beneficial effects of the therapy were felt at home.

HOME: PICTURING AND INTEGRATING CHANGE

Landgarten (1981) describes the clinical art therapy approach in rehabilitation as one that supports (1) confronting reality; (2) expressing one's deepest emotions, such as feelings of rage regarding one's health status; (2) concretizing one's experience; (3) exploring fears, fantasies, and adaptation through symbolic expression; and (4) rehearsing for home. When return to home is planned, the independent maintenance of activities of daily life requires practice and creativity. Pictures can be made about expected changes in the home environment, problem solving homecare management, and general well-being issues such as exercise, compliance with medication schedules, and dietary regimens.

For many older adults, the severity of injury may signal permanent change, such as not returning home. In this case, the art productions may serve to process feelings of grief and separation as well as fears regarding a new environment. On the other hand, the real benefits the new environment may offer for safety and well-being may be explored. In both cases, the art productions serve as containers for the exploration of personal meanings. In that personal meaning affects motivation, creatively envisioning changes at home or in a new environment, imaging what may be uncomfortable, as well as the configuring of comfort through imagery, supports adaptation in the face of situational change.

MAXIMIZING COGNITIVE SKILLS, WORKING WITH EMOTIONS

For some time, researchers in aging have understood that, as individuals age and the structures that support their needs satisfaction change, they may operate below capacity unless presented with opportunities for success and increased environmental expectation. Older individuals retain a need for recognition, and this need is often overlooked in the general culture and institutional settings. Wigdor (1992) concludes that mental health, more so than physical health, is an important component of goal-directed behavior that facilitates recognition and reward for older persons. As external controls are diminished with age, internal locus of control becomes increasingly important as circumstantial change is negotiated.

Conversely, with age, external stimulus, in manageable doses appropriate to one's health, becomes more significant to invigorate active engagement in the world, to maintain our reason for being, as well as levels of wellness and connection. In this context, ability is less a factor than the meaningfulness of tasks. Activities that support creativity and productivity are noteworthy resources for successful aging. Works of art, art materials, and art making are well suited to this paradigm, particularly to maximize cognitive functioning and emotional well-being.

IMAGE-BASED COMMUNICATION

The value of visual art-based dialogues has been studied with functional elderly persons, and outcomes are believed by the researchers to suggest innovative models for nursing interventions using imagery. Wikstrom (2000) conducted a randomized clinical trial with 40 residents of a senior housing facility assessing the health effects of social interaction and aesthetics. Participants in the experimental group were engaged in communication with the added support of works of art as a stimulus and are reported to have had improved psychological and physical health over the controls who had equal time and attention of the experimenter without the hypothesized benefit of concrete art images as a variable. Using masterworks of art, Hodges, Keeley, and Grier (2001) suggest "the image bridges the limitations of language and experience" (p. 391). The elderly often integrate chronicity into a way of life without benefit of reflection from a caring other. "Masterworks of art have the potential for being the catalyst for generating this interpretive reflection and shared understanding, for co-creating a shared reality, and for getting patients unstuck" (p. 396).

Recollective processing as one ages is key to healthy aging, and art-based recollection activity has numerous therapeutic benefits, including facilitating social engagement, developing memory skills, and concretizing and making visible what may seem lost. Chaudhury (2003) used picture making to study recollection of home by patients with mild to moderate dementia in which their recollected home images shared features with actual pictures of their previous homes. Outcomes from this study led the author to endorse the value to health care providers of such interventions for their dynamic benefits in the treatment of cognitively impaired elders, the pictures a means to expand exchanges between patients and their health care providers.

IMPAIRED FUNCTIONING, RETAINED STRENGTHS

The strengths of older persons with dementing illness include access to distant memories, a connection to feeling states, retention of motor skills, and sensory pathway receptivity. For such older persons, art therapy interventions have been implemented in a variety of settings employing diverse approaches: painting as a clinical tool for geriatric patients (Rosin Matz, & Carmi, 1977); nonverbal dialogue with brain-damaged elderly (Fischer and Fischer, 1977); art therapy for patients with Alzheimer's disease and related disorders (Wald, 1989); multisensory art experience (Jensen, 1997); art therapy with geriatric dementia clients (Kahn-Denis, 1997); the role of art therapy to promote wisdom in geriatric settings (Shore, 1997); psychodynamic art therapy groups for the cognitively impaired elderly (Byers, 1998); a weekly art program, Memories in the Making (Rentz, 2002); and the potential of art therapy to slow deterioration in dementia and Alzheimer's patients (Madori, 2002).

In common, these interventions are designed so that the art-making tasks build success through sensory stimulation, physical activity, nonverbal communication, opportunities for self-organizing, self-reflection, and reminiscence. Consistent outcomes, across interventions, include the pleasure afforded through the use of the art materials, increased physical engagement, and improvements in patient-reported psychological well-being. In addition, art therapists Jensen (1997) and Madori (2002) both suggest that an outcome of their work, using art therapy in a multimodal context with dementia patients, is improved cognitive functioning. Jensen (1997) reported that participants in her structured weekly group began needing reminders for attendance, and closed with participants knowing that it was time for the group. Madori (2002) hypothesized that the stimulation of the right side of the brain through a multimodal intervention, which included music, discussion, and pictorial representation (art making) over a 2-day period, created opportunities for new memory retrieval and enhanced regeneration of brain cells in the brain's mapping area. Support for Madori's hypothesis comes from a recent neuropsychological study of cognitive skills in adults. Bunce (2003) concluded that bimodal presentation of words (words were spoken as well as presented in visual form on cards) in an episodic memory task improved recollection for adults over 67 years of age. As Madori hypothesizes and Bunce concludes, cognitive support, the additional inclusion of right brain–mediated image/visual information formatting, at the time information is encoded, appears to improve cognitive performance.

WORKING THROUGH DEPRESSION

Changes in cognitive performance and general health, along with economic and social status, contribute significantly to the onset of depression in aging persons. Rubenstein and Lawton (1997) describe a phenomenon of depression among residents in nursing homes and residential care. Depression is reported by Shmuely and colleagues (Shmuely, Baumgarten, Rovner, & Berlin, 2001) to be the predominant psychiatric syndrome of aging, and its affects of health-related quality of life may be significant. Goldberg (1993) reported that depression is often underdiagnosed in medically ill patients, of which a high proportion are older adults. The utility of individual and group art therapy as an intervention in the treatment of mood disorders including depression has been standard practice on inpatient psychiatric units, in outpatient day programs, and in geriatric settings. Art making supports the emergence of expressiveness that depression mutes and offers opportunities for satisfaction and goal fulfillment. Goal satisfaction improves self-esteem, a benefit of art therapy reported as an outcome in clinical studies such as Doric-Henry's (1997) use of art therapy (throwing clay pots on a wheel) with elderly nursing home residents. In this study, those most likely to benefit were residents with low self-esteem, depression, and anxiety as measured by pre- and post intervention testing. Malchiodi (1999b) reports increasing opportunities for art therapy in diverse medical settings, including cancer treatment centers and integrative medicine centers in traditional allopathic medical hospitals, where the introduction of CAM-centered practices has shifted the focus from biomedical treatment alone to integrative treatments across the biopsychosocial-spiritual domain. Art therapy as an adjunctive therapy supports this approach.

ART THERAPY IN PALLIATIVE CARE

Realistically, healthy aging may include dying well. For individuals whose illness is not responsive to cure, palliative approaches within the domain of complementary alternative medicine, such as spiritual support, meditation, massage, nonpharmaceutical pain remedies, and expressive arts therapies, have much to offer. Within this framework, the cultivation of wholeness regardless of expected illness trajectory is the primary focus, with art therapy facilitating the creative potential at the end of life.

Connell (1998) suggests that the psyche remains fully engaged even as the physical body weakens and declines in terminal illness and that creative action liberates individuals from the confines of the physical. The art therapy context is one of holding and facilitating a deeper understanding of self and existential meanings and to process and be present to experiences for which words may be inadequate.

Patients who participated in a phenomenological study of a creative arts program in a hospice day program in Great Britain are reported by Kennett (2000) to have experienced enjoyment, pride, surprise, a sense of achievement, acquisition of new skills, a sense of purpose, goal incentive, mutual support, satisfaction in the permanent nature of their art productions, and hope. Researchers concluded that these themes constituted successful treatment as conceptualized in palliative care with outcomes that fostered hope, self-esteem, autonomy, and social integration. Additionally, the literature in palliative care points to an outcome, also seen in geriatric settings, where the art productions of the clients serve to consolidate a connection between caregivers and those for whom they offer care.

The level of engagement in creative activity by persons with terminal illness reported by Connell and Kennett is consistent with earlier research. Zlantin and Nucho (1983) conducted a critical analysis of the art productions of nursing home residents who died during or soon after participation in a descriptive study examining drawings produced by the elderly. Based on nine cases, they observed three stages of involvement in the creative process prior to death. Initial participation reflected declining functional status; this was followed by a period of heightened expressiveness, an increase in physical vitality, alertness, and selectivity of focus. In this stage picture content is reported to be integrative and reconciling and produced verbal exchanges with the therapist that reflected new engagement. This stage was followed by a period of calm and serenity that the authors associated with acceptance. The cultivation of acceptance and the ability to be present to the range of emotional states life-threatening illness stimulates are at the heart of Luzzatto's (1998) approach to working with patients facing illness, pain, and death. In offering a "creative journey" for persons with cancer, openness to negative thoughts or stress in the mind and body is the source of personal imagery, which serves as well as for possible transformation.

CONCLUSION

Art therapy as an interventional modality in complementary and alternative medicine offers a range of assessments and treatments to support the diverse needs of the wide spectrum of aging adults. Essential to the practice of art therapy is meeting each client where he or she is and supporting the client's capacity for ongoing development throughout his or her life span. This includes maximizing autonomous functioning, coherence, and deepening relation to self, others, and the world. Art therapy offers opportunities for pleasure, insight, adaptive skills development, and transformation using tools and materials that invite physical engagement, play, and discovery. Directed art therapy tasks provide structured, supported opportunities for exploration, expansion of expression, problem solving, and dialogue within the therapeutic relationship. The art therapist provides a nonjudgmental holding environment and human connection that join with the client to invigorate self-acceptance and engagement. This creative environment supports the cultivation of internal harmony and the capacity to be in relation; these together are the meeting ground for healthy aging.

RESOURCES

American Art Therapy Association, 1202 Allanson Rd., Mundelein, IL 60060-3808; telephone: (888) 290-0878 or (847) 949-6064; fax: (847) 566-4580; e-mail: info@arttherapy.org

AATA, a national association founded in 1969, is a not-for-profit organization of approximately 4,750 professionals and students that has established standards for art therapy education, ethics, and practice. Its mission is to serve its members and the general public by providing standards of professional competence, and developing and promoting knowledge in, and of, the field of art therapy. Publishes *Art Therapy: Journal of the American Art Therapy Association*. AATA sets educational, professional, and ethical standards for its members. To locate a credentialed art therapist in your community, contact AATA or ATCB (see below).

Art Therapy Credentials Board, Inc. 3 Terrace Way, Suite B, Greensboro, NC 27403-3660; telephone: (877) 213-2822, fax: (336) 482-2852.Web site: http://www.atcb.org/public.htm

The ATCB, an independent organization, grants credentials. Some states regulate the practice of art therapy, and in many states art therapists can become licensed as counselors or mental health therapists.

Society for the Arts in Healthcare 1632 U St. N.W., Washington, DC 20009; telephone: (202) 299-9770; (202) 299-9887; e-mail: mail@TheSAH.org

SAH is a member-based, nonprofit organization advocating on a national and international level for the integration of the arts into health care settings.

The Literature, Arts, and Medicine Database, telephone: (212) 263-5401; Web site: http://endeavor.med.nyu.edu/lit-med/medhum.html

MedHum online database is an annotated bibliography of prose, poetry, film, video, and art that was developed to be a dynamic, accessible, comprehensive resource in medical humanities, for use in health/pre-health, and liberal arts settings. It is a multi-institutional project that was initiated at the New York University School of Medicine in the summer of 1993. This Web site is produced and maintained by the Hippocrates Project, the multidisciplinary development laboratory for application of information technologies to medical education at New York University School of Medicine.

International Arts-Medicine Association, 714 Old Lancaster Rd., Bryn Mawr, PA 19010; telephone (610) 525-3784; fax: (610) 525-3250, e-mail: IAMAorg@aol.com

IAMA is a nonprofit organization formed in Philadelphia in 1985 by Richard A. Lippin, MD, IAMA founding president and president through 1995. The organization has about 300 members in 20 countries. The IAMA's purpose is to provide a forum for interdisciplinary, international communication between arts and health professionals. Members include clinicians, educators, researchers, and artists who have an interest in one or more of the many aspects of the relationships between arts and health. International Journal of Arts Medicine, http://library.berklee.edu:8080/ipac20/periodicals/Inter_Journal_of_Arts_Med.php

Published 1991–2000. Contains peer-reviewed articles by educators in the creative arts as well as prominent physicians at a seminal period in the development of Arts Medicine.

REFERENCES

Achterberg, J. (1985). *Imagery in healing: Shamanism and modern medicine.* Boston: New Sciences Library.

American Art Therapy Association. (1998). Art therapy and research [Special Issue]. *Art Therapy: Journal of the American Art Therapy Association, 15*(1).

American Art Therapy Association. (2004). Information and Membership Brochure. Mundelein, IL. Retrieved from http://www.arttherapy.org/.

Aronson, S. M. (1999). Adaptational challenges and coping in late life. *Bulletin of the Menninger Clinic, 63*(2, Suppl. A), A4–15.

Bailis, D. S., & Chipperfield, J. G. (2002). Compensating for losses in perceived control over health: A role for collective self-esteem in healthy aging. *Journals of Gerontology Series B: Psychological Sciences and Social Sciences, 57*(6), 531–539.

Bunce, D. (2003). Cognitive support at encoding attenuates age differences in recollective experience among adults of lower frontal lobe function. *Neuropsychology, 17*(3), 353–361.

Byers, A. (1998), Candles slowing burning. In S. Skaife & V. Huet (Eds.), *Art psychotherapy groups: Between pictures and words* (pp. 109–132). London: Routledge.

Carlson, M. C., Seeman T., & Fried, L. P. (2000). Importance of generativity for healthy aging in older women. *Aging-Clinical and Experimental Research, 12*(2), 132–140.

Chaudhury, H. (2003). Remembering home through art. *Alzheimer's Care Quarterly, 4*(2), 119–124.

Chapman, L., Morabito, D., Ladakakos, C., Schreier, H., & Knudson, M. (2001). The effectiveness of an art therapy intervention in reducing posttraumatic stress disorder (PTSD) symptoms in pediatric trauma patients. *Art Therapy: Journal of the American Art Therapy Association, 18*(2), 100–104.

Cohen, B. M., Hammer, J., & Singer, S. (1988). The Diagnostic Drawing Series: A systematic approach to art therapy evaluation and research. *Arts in Psychotherapy, 15*(1), 11–21.

Cohen, B. M., Mills, A., & Kijak, A. K. (1994). An introduction to the Diagnostic Drawing Series: A standardized tool for diagnostic and clinical use. *Art Therapy: Journal of the American Art Therapy Association, 11*(2), 105–110.

Connell, C. (1998). The search for a model which opens: Open group at the Royal Marsden Hospital. In M. Pratt & M. J. M. Wood (Eds.), *Art therapy in palliative care: The creative response* (pp. 75–87). London: Routledge.

Davidson, R. J. (2000). Affective style, psychopathology, and resilience: Brain mechanisms and plasticity. *American Psychologist, 55*(11), 1196–1214.

Davidson, R. J., Ekman, P., Saron, C. D. Senulis, J. A. & Friesen, W. V. (1990). Approach-withdrawal and cerebral asymmetry: Emotional expression and brain physiology I. *Journal of Personality and Social Psychology, 58*(2), 330–341.

Davidson, R. J., Kabat-Zinn, J., Schumacher, J., Rosenkranz, M., Muller, D., Santorelli, S. F., Urbanowski, et al. (2003). Alterations in brain and immune function produced by mindfulness meditation. *Psychosomatic Medicine, 65*(4), 564–570.

Doric-Henry, L. (1997). Pottery as art therapy with elderly nursing home residents. *Art Therapy: Journal of the American Art Therapy Association, 14*(3), 163–171.

Erikson, E. (1963). *Childhood and society.* New York: W. W. Norton.

Erikson, E., Erikson, J., & Kivnick, H. (1986). *Vital involvement in old age.* New York: W. W. Norton.

Fischer, T., & Fischer, R. (1977). Non-verbal dialogue with brain damaged elderly. *Confinia Psychiatrica, 20*(2–3), 61–78.

Fisher, B. J., & Specht, D. K. (1999). Successful aging and creativity in later life. *Journal of Aging Studies, 13*(4), 457–472.

Gantt, L. M. (2001). The Formal Elements Art Therapy Scale: A measurement system for global variables in art. *Art Therapy: Journal of the American Art Therapy Association, 18*(1), 50–55.

Gerstenlauer, C. J., Maguire, S. R., & Wooldridge, L. (2003). Geriatric nurse practitioner care guidelines: Depression in older adults. *Geriatric Nursing, 24*(3), 185–187.

Goldberg, R. J. (1993). Depression in medical patients. *Rhode Island Medicine, 76*(8), 391–396.

Hacking, S. (2000). The descriptive assessment for psychiatric art (DAPA): Update and further research. *Journal of Nervous and Mental Diseases, 188*(8), 525–529.

Hartman-Stein, P. E., & Potkanowicz, E. S. (2003). Behavioral determinants of healthy aging: Good news for baby boomer generation. *Online Journal of Issues in Nursing, 8*(2), 6.

Hodges, H. F., Keeley, A. C., & Grier, E. C. (2001). Masterworks of art and chronic illness experiences in the elderly. *Journal of Advanced Nursing, 36*(3), 389–398.

Inui, T. S. (2003). The need for an integrated biopsychosocial approach to research on successful aging. *Annals of Internal Medicine, 139*(5, Suppl. 2), 391–394.

Jensen, S. M. (1997). Multiple pathways to self: A multisensory art experience. *Art Therapy: Journal of the American Art Therapy Association, 14*(3), 178–186.

Junge, M. (1994). *A history of art therapy in the United States.* Mudelein, IL: American Art Therapy Association.

Kagin, S. L., & Lusebrink, V. B. (1978). The expressive therapies continuum. *Art Psychotherapy, 5*(4), 171–179.

Kahn-Denis, K. B. (1997). Art therapy with geriatric dementia clients. *Art Therapy: Journal of the American Art Therapy Association, 14*(3), 194–199.

Kane, R. L. (2003). The contribution of geriatric health services research to successful aging. *Annals of Internal Medicine, 139*(5, Suppl. 2), 460–462.

Kennett, C. (2000). Participation in a creative arts project can foster hope in hospice day center. *Palliative Medicine, 14*(5), 419–425.

Kramer, E. (1971). *Art as therapy with children.* New York: Schocken.

Kwiatkowska, H. Y. (1978). *Family therapy and evaluation through art.* Springfield, IL: Charles C. Thomas.

Landgarten, H. (1981). *Clinical art therapy: A comprehensive guide.* New York: Brunner/Mazel.

Levick, M. F. (1983). *They could not talk and so they drew: Children's styles of coping and thinking.* Springfield, IL: Charles C. Thomas.

Lusebrink, V. B. (1990). *Imagery and visual expression in therapy.* New York: Plenum Press.

Luzzatto, P. (1998). From psychiatry to psycho-oncology: Personal reflections on the use of art therapy with cancer patients. In M. Pratt & M. J. M. Wood (Eds.), *Art therapy in palliative care: The creative response* (pp. 169–175). London: Routledge.

Madori, L. L. (2002, November). *Art therapy and the potential to slow deterioration process in dementia and Alzheimer's patients.* Paper presented at the meeting of the American Art Therapy Association, Washington, D.C.

Malchiodi, C. A. (1999a). Art therapy, arts medicine, arts in healthcare: A vision for collaboration in the next millennium. *International Journal of Arts Medicine, 6*(2), 13–16.

Malchiodi, C. A. (Ed.). (1999b). *Medical art therapy with adults.* Philadelphia: Jessica Kingsley Publishers.

Maslow, A. (1968). *Towards a psychology of being* (2nd ed.). Toronto: Van Nostrand.

Meeks, S., & Murrell, S. A. (2001). Contribution of education to health and life satisfaction in older adults mediated by negative affect. *Journal of Aging and Health, 13*(1), 92–119.

Naumberg, M. (1966). *Dynamically oriented art therapy.* New York: Grune & Stratton.

Monti, D., Peterson, C., Shakin-Kunkel, E., Hauck, W. W., Pequignot, E., Brainard, G. C., & Rhodes, L. (2005, November 15). A randomized, controlled trial of mindfulness-based art therapy (MBAT) for women with cancer. *Psycho-Oncology.*

Peterson, C. (2003, April). *Models of connection in care: Mindfulness-based art therapy for cancer patients.* Paper presented at the Center for Mind Body Medicine Comprehensive Cancer Care Conference, Washington, D.C.

Rentz, C. A. (2002). Memories in the making: Outcome-based evaluation of an art program for individuals with dementing illness. *American Journal of Alzheimer's Disease and Other Dementias, 17*(3), 175–181.

Rhyne, J. (1973). *The Gestalt art experience.* Monterey, CA: Brooks/Cole.

Rigaud, A. S., Hanon, O., Seux, M. L., & Forette, F. (2001). Hypertension and dementia. *Current Hypertension Reports, 3*(6), 454–457.

Rogers, C. (1961). Towards a theory of creativity. In *On becoming a person.* London: Constable.

Rosin, A. J., Matz, E., & Carmi, S. (1977). How painting can be used as a clinical tool. *Geriatrics, 32*(1), 41–46

Rubenstein, R. L., & Lawson, M. P. (Eds.). (1997). *Depression in residential and long term care: Advances in research and treatment.* New York: Springer.

Rubin, J. A. (1978). *Child art therapy.* New York: Van Nostrand Reinhold.

Sacchett, C., Byng, S., Marshall, J., & Pound, C. (1999). Drawing together: Evaluation of a therapy programme for severe aphasia. *International Journal of Language Disorders, 34*(3), 265–289.

Shmuely, Y., Baumgarten, M., Rovner, B., & Berlin, J. (2001). Predictors of improvement in health-related quality of life among elderly patients with depression. *International Psychogeriatrics, 13*(1), 63–73.

Shore, A. (1997). Promoting wisdom: The role of art therapy in geriatric settings. *Art Therapy: Journal of the American Art Therapy Association, 14*(3), 172–177.

Simonton, D. K. (1990). Creativity in the later years: Optimistic prospects for achievement. *The Gerontologist, 30*(5), 626–631.

Steiner, R. (1998). *Art as a spiritual activity: Selected lectures on the visual arts* (Michael Howard, Ed.). Hudson, NY: Anthroposophic Press.

Ulman, E. (1975). Art therapy: Problems of definition. In E. Ulman & P. Dachinger (Eds.), *Art therapy in theory and practice* (pp. 3–13). New York: Schocken.

Wadeson, H. (1980). *Art psychotherapy.* New York: John Wiley.

Wald, J. (1989). Art therapy for patients with Alzheimer's disease and related disorders. In H. Wadeson, J. Durkin, & D. Perach (Eds.), *Advances in art therapy* (pp. 181–204). New York: John Wiley.

Wigdor, B. T. (1992). Drives and motivation with aging. In J. E. Birren, R. B. Sloane, & G. D. Cohen (Eds.), *Handbook of mental health and aging* (2nd ed., pp. 245–261). San Diego, CA: Academic Press.

Wikstrom, B. M. (2000). Visual art dialogues with elderly persons: Effects on perceived life situation. *Journal of Nursing Management, 8*(1), 31–37.

Yaretsky, A., Levinson, M., & Kfar-Saba, I. (1996). Clay as a therapeutic tool in group processing with the elderly. *American Journal of Art Therapy, 34*(3), 750–782.

Zlatin, H., & Nucho, A. (1983). The final picture in art. *Journal of Geriatric Psychiatry, 16*(1), 113–147.

CHAPTER SEVEN

Massage Therapy and Older Adults

Eileen Kennedy and Cheryl Chapman

If any group of people is in need of touch, it is the aging population. Massage, in a light, modified style can have a profound effect on older adults in our touch-deprived society. According to Ashley Montague, world-renowned anthropologist and author of *Touching: The Human Significance of the Skin* (1986), "The impersonality of life in the Western world has become such that we have produced a race of untouchables." He went on:

> It is well known in professional circles that young nursing students tend to avoid touching elderly people. Touching as a therapeutic event is not as simple as a mechanical procedure or drug, because it is, above all, an act of communication, and the use of touch and physical closeness may be the most important way to communicate to persons that they are important as human beings.

With the accelerating advancements within the medical field, we may tend to forget that the simple act of touching can be so effective and beneficial. "Hands-on" techniques for healing have been around since the beginning of time. Ancient Chinese, Egyptian, Japanese, and Arab medical literature frequently refer to massage as a health treatment. Hippocrates prescribed massage for patients and athletes. An exploration of the aging process can put the benefits of massage into proper perspective and inform the reader who wishes to work with the elderly or may want to experience the benefits of touch.

THE AGING PROCESS

Every species ages, undergoing noticeable changes from birth to death. A number of theories have surfaced as to why this occurs. The "programmed senescence" theory suggests that the rate at which a species grows old is predetermined by genes. Yet another possible explanation is the "free-radical" theory that says cells age as a result of accumulated harm from continuous chemical reactions within cells. During the chemical reactions, toxins called free radicals are produced, and ultimately cause cells to die and the individual to age. The potential life span of a human being is finite, at around 115 years. Therefore, some kind of deterioration in body function seems inevitable. In the words of the French composer Daniel-François-Esprit Auber, "Aging seems to be the only available way to live a long time."

The body changes gradually, and this process is noticeable in a variety of ways. Impulses become slower, joints decline, and brain function slows by as much as 20%. The elderly my lose their sense of balance and become disoriented more easily. Calcium deposits may appear in the body, and the integrity of muscle and connective tissue changes on a cellular level. The human body consists of about 75% water. It is the main ingredient of blood, interstitial and intracellular fluid, lymph, and feces. Water is present in bone, muscle, connective tissue, and all cells. Most elderly experience water loss and dehydration. As one naturally loses 15% of that water, every organ and system are affected (Abrams & Berkow, 1999). The circulatory system slows down and exhibits a loss of elasticity and gauge of blood vessels. The heart works harder, and cardiac output decreases. Waste products and toxins are not processed and carried away as quickly and efficiently via the blood, lungs, kidneys, spleen, liver, and skin as they once were (Chapman, 1995). The lymphatic/immune system slows as well, leaving the elderly more susceptible to infection. By 70 years of age, the body's natural defenses against infection begin to fail. As a result, the recovery from illness is often prolonged (Chapman, 1995). In addition, the respiratory system decreases by age 75, often with a 30% loss of overall pulmonary function. Respiration becomes more shallow, and total respiratory volume is diminished. As more air remains in the lungs after exhalation, there is an increase in carbon dioxide retention. Decreased mobility and increased rigidity of chest muscles diminish the efficiency of the diaphragm and the expansion of the rib cage. Alveoli and capillary tissues become thicker and less elastic. Mucous membranes can dry out, and hair cilia lose their resilience. Smoking, air pollution, and other environmental factors contribute to the deterioration of this body system (Chapman, 1995), while health-promoting activities (e.g., yoga and exercise) can slow this process. The genitourinary system loses its tone, and the bladder is unable to retain the same volume of urine. This factor causes many elderly to drink less in order to lessen the need for urination. As a result, dehydration can occur. Dehydration can lead to edema as the body tries to retain the fluids it needs to flush and clean the interstitial spaces. Urinary incontinence is common. There can be a loss of kidney function, which can lead to kidney stones (Chapman, 1995). Skin tends to become drier and less resilient after the age of 50. Perspiration decreases, and skin and subcutaneous tissue become less elastic due to decreases in collagen. Fingernails and toenails become harder and thicker. Skin spots, moles, and changes in pigmentation occur more frequently, and there is a greater prevalence of malignant skin lesions (Chapman, 1995). The endocrine system also undergoes change. Many signs and symptoms of endocrine dysfunction are seen as "old age," as estrogen, progesterone, testosterone, adrenal, thyroid, and insulin levels diminish (Chapman, 1995). The gastrointestinal system can weaken due to years of poor eating habits. Nutritional absorption is often reduced, and the gastrointestinal tract can atrophy. A deterioration of the mucosal lining and a decrease in enzymes and hydrochloric acid can lead to poor digestion. Delayed stomach emptying may lead to constipation and gas (Chapman, 1995). The skeletal system weakens, and bone density loss can result in osteoporosis. Bones and vertebra compress and become brittle. Bone spurs are common on the spine and heels of the feet. Some elderly can shrink 2 to 4 inches in height. Fractures are more common at this stage of life (Chapman, 1995).

PSYCHOLOGICAL ASPECTS OF AGING

Massage therapists working with the elderly can attest that depression is common. Clearly, the reasons for depression are many and complex. Symptoms of depression include weight loss or gain, insomnia, abuse, despair, loneliness, fatigue, irritability, seclusion, and decreased interest in participating in activities or socializing with family or friends. Changes in social status or relationships with family may become strained, and patience on the part of caregivers may be tested. Anxiety and fear (the major psychological factor in depression) may be exacerbated by dependency on caregivers, financial insecurity, loss of self-esteem and self-control, body degradation, and loss of home and friends, spouse, or family. There may also be a fear of the future, fear of dying a painful death, or fear of dying alone. As the aging process progresses, there may be increased physical limitations such as sensory impairment or immobility, and the psychological toll of these conditions can be devastating to the elderly. The social and behavioral status of life for older Americans can make the difference between good health and disease and disorder. Many older adults no longer have spouses, children, or other family members available to participate in their lives. Not only do these people lack a sense of community, they also crave the need for touch, even though they may not be aware of it. If the elderly experience a temporary or permanent loss of independence, feelings of vulnerability arise. For these reasons, geriatricians often recommend multidisciplinary holistic care. In this model, a team of medical personnel, social workers, occupational/physical therapists, and massage therapists all participate in an enhanced level of care.

BENEFITS OF MASSAGE

The benefits of massage and bodywork are numerous. Though aging is unavoidable, individuals can take the steps necessary to prolong quality of life, while improving strength, flexibility, coordination, and energy. Regardless of why elderly people may consider massage, they will only benefit by being touched. Unfortunately, many clients view massage as an "extravagance" or "luxury" and do not consider it a form of therapy.

Specific training in massage for the older person is necessary to successfully access this population. The appropriate touch or modality is based on the therapist taking a good medical history, as well as a physical and emotional assessment. Caring touch can have a profound, positive effect on one's physical, mental, and emotional status. Daily living can be stressful, lonely, and depressing. A person may feel isolated from community and society at large. Skilled touch by a massage therapist may enable the client to be more physically active and mentally alert, or may help reconnect the person with those around him or her. Nurturing touch can calm anxious or agitated clients who feel frightened, worried, or depressed. Knowing that someone cares can make all the difference. Some elderly seek massage therapy simply for relaxation, whereas others come for relief from medical conditions. Massage can:

1. Ease pain and discomfort brought on by sore or tight muscles or years of pain from arthritic joints or structural misalignments. By softening hardened musculature and releasing areas of holding and knots, blood is brought to the area, the accumulation of lactic acid is released, cells are cleansed and nourished, and toxins are excreted. Several massage sessions may be required to provide relief.

2. Promote restful sleep and relieve insomnia, releasing endorphins, natural hormones that reduce pain as well as provide a greater sense of well-being.

3. Speed recovery from surgery and increase mobility and range of motion once the musculature is softened. Massage enhances the effectiveness of physical therapy, and many clients report incredible rates of recovery from hip replacement surgeries.

4. Improve all body systems affected by the aging process as discussed previously.

Most importantly, massage feels good and can reconnect clients to their bodies, minds, and emotions during a time when they may be at risk for being overwhelmed by physical pain and/or psychological loss.

CONTRAINDICATIONS FOR MASSAGE

Knowing the contraindications for performing or recommending massage is an important factor within the aging population. Before defining specific contraindications, it is prudent to make some generalizations that may add to the confidence level of both client and therapist. If there are any doubts as to the appropriateness of massage for an elderly individual, a physician or other health care practitioner should be consulted. Sometimes, written medical authorization is desirable. Keep in mind that even if massage therapy is contraindicated, engaging in simple, respectful touching and holding can be a great source of comfort. Simple hand massage, for example, can be of benefit. Light stroking can be as effective as a deeper massage for many people. All health professionals should ask their clients and patients for permission to touch them, of course. Energy work such as Reiki, therapeutic touch, or polarity therapy can complement physical touch and provide a feeling of balance and alignment.

Some situations that contraindicate massage therapy are listed below.

Do not:
1. Massage any area that looks inflamed, blistered, or has a rash
2. Attempt to move any joint beyond resistance
3. Massage an open sore or wound
4. Massage a client with a fever
5. Massage areas that feel "hot" (possibly indicating an inflammation or an acute arthritic condition)
6. Massage deeply on calves of elderly clients, as these areas can be the sites of thrombosis or blood clots
7. Massage varicose veins (areas surrounding veins can be touched gently through "holding")

8. Provide deep massage on the cervical area, as there may be compromised circulation in the carotid artery or the presence of osteoarthritis
9. Use strong traction or "rocking" motions without assessing a client's physical condition. Gentle traction may be appropriate, and gentle rocking movements from the side often feel good. Strong rocking from the feet is not advised. These movements can increase strain on the knees, hips, and vertebral joints already damaged or unstable.
10. Massage any individual who appears to be acutely ill, displaying such signs as profuse perspiration, confusion, labored breathing, or unfocused eyes.

PAIN

Pain is another consideration in working with the elderly, and chances are this population will exhibit the greatest amount of discomfort. Pain is a subjective sensation and is experienced in different ways by different people. It can be localized to one area or generalized throughout the body. It is important for the massage therapist to document the nature of the pain that is expressed, either verbally or nonverbally. Questions the therapist may ask include

1. Where do you feel the pain?
2. How often does the pain occur?
3. What is the "quality" of the pain (e.g., dull, sharp, spasmodic, throbbing, radiating, or diffuse)?
4. How long have you lived with the pain?
5. When did it start?
6. Has it gotten progressively worse?
7. Does medication, movement, or time release it?

Pain can be acute where the sensation is short and/or severe. Chronic pain persists over a long period; sensations may run from mild, to moderate, to severe. Pain is hard to quantify or "prove." In most cases where the client feels the pain is not the origin. Searching for the origin can be a challenge. Pain can also indicate a need for attention, gives a client permission to "feel," and may fill an emotional need. Experience has proven that the elderly can experience a remarkable release from pain, not by the application of specific therapeutic techniques, but simply through the power of being touched. Many elderly on pain medications report needing less pain medication or can better tolerate pain as a result of nurturing touch.

MASSAGE SETTINGS

Touch can be administered anywhere. A table may not always be appropriate, depending on the physical setting and the physical status of the individual. Whatever the space, it should be quiet, softly lit, and warm and create a mood of comfort and relaxation. Music plays a large part in enhancing the setting. If an individual is able to come into a fully equipped office setting, music, soft lighting, candles, and so on, are usually provided. The massage table should be low enough to allow the client to get on and off the table easily. Some clients may also need help dressing and undressing, as well. Assistance is sometimes necessary, depending on the client's physical condition. Elderly people can experience a drop in blood pressure after the session, making them light-headed, so be ready to help. Always provide a drink of water and encourage the client to drink water frequently to remove toxins from the system released during the massage. Using a massage table in a nursing home or hospice setting is generally not appropriate. The client's bed will work fine when properly adjusted. Asking a nursing assistant to help reposition the client is suggested. Massage in a chair or wheelchair is appropriate. The client may even be fully clothed. Some clients carry a personal history that makes disrobing anxiety-producing. The anxiety of being exposed will defeat the purpose of massage and discourage the client. Massage and touch the areas that can be reached easily. Always create a setting that is conducive to relaxation. Bring music, candles, and a lovely scented cream. Music is especially soothing for Alzheimer's patients.

No matter where touch is administered, it is important for the practitioner to stay focused on his or her "intent." Movement must be purposeful and slower in speed. It is the quality, not the quantity, of the work that truly matters. For some clients, less is more—15 minutes of massage may be just as effective as an hour. The length of the session will depend on the physical and mental condition of the client. Massage with some depth effectively stimulates the sensory nervous system and heart. A 50-minute massage increases blood flow throughout the body. In the elderly or ill, too much massage may overload the entire body, especially the heart, kidneys, and nervous system. In some cases energy work such as Reiki or polarity therapy may be all that is needed. Energy work can be subtle, yet powerful. Talking on the part of the therapist or client during a massage may prevent the client from focusing on the sensation of touch and detract from the concentration and intent of the therapist. Massage and touch create an unconscious transfer of energy between the client and the therapist. One might say that both parties are "touched." Similarly, for an effective session, sometimes quiet time is required to allow the parasympathetic nervous system (relaxation response) to take over.

Closure is important after the session, whether it is done on a table, chair, or bed. A proper ending to the massage provides an opportunity for the elderly client to regain a sense of stability and to remain in the relaxation mode. Feedback about the session usually takes place at this time.

MASSAGE MODALITIES

Modalities will vary according to the physical status of the person. Swedish massage must be modified with the elderly, as osteoporosis, which can begin as early as 40 years of age in both men and women, may be present. Techniques such as compression and hacking are not advised. Deep tissue massage should be modified, as bruising may occur. Avoid using elbows and thumbs—it is not necessary to do invasive techniques on aging people. Neuromuscular therapy (NMT), another invasive technique, should be reserved for such conditions as sciatica. Causing bruising, pain, or discomfort to a client will discourage him or her from returning, and the person may develop a negative attitude toward massage.

Effective Techniques

1. Fluffing—movement of fingers on the muscles without squeezing
2. Rocking—gentle movement of a limb in a back-and-forth motion
3. Effleurage—gliding stroke that is light and long stroking with the hands
4. Holding—placing hands on a specific part of the body and just "being" with that area
5. Petrissage—light kneading of the muscles

Positioning

The rule "Massage what is available" usually works well. As previously mentioned, it is the quality rather than the quantity of touch that matters, not how much skin has been covered or the number of strokes or techniques performed that will ensure a successful massage. It is not necessary to move a person to any position other than supine (face up). The massage school training that describes two or three positions will not always apply with the elderly. Always elevate the head and support the neck of older clients. Few people are able to lie totally flat. The mature "hale and hearty" client will usually tolerate multiple positions, including prone (face down) and side lying. The aged person may have structural limitations, such as a dowager's hump of the cervical spine, lordosis (an increase in the concave curve of the lumbar region), or kyphosis (an exaggerated convex curve in the dorsal region). For these conditions, the upper body placement is important to accommodate the spinal malfunctions. Shortened leg muscles will require the proper support of a bolster or pillow under the knees. Arthritic joints should not be touched if inflamed. Stretching, pulling, or rigorous range of motion is not indicated here.

Scientific Evidence of the Benefits of Massage Therapy

The Touch Research Institute (TRI) has conducted over 90 studies on the positive effects of massage therapy on many functions and medical conditions in varied age groups, including conditions that can affect the elderly. According to TRI, among the significant research findings are decreased autoimmune problems, reduction in pain, enhanced immune functioning, and improved alertness and performance. Specific studies documented by TRI include the following.

Back Pain

Massage lessened lower back pain, eased depression and anxiety, and improved sleep. The massage therapy group also showed improved range of motion, and participants' serotonin and dopamine levels were higher (Hernandez-Reif et al., 2001).

Breast Cancer

Massage therapy reduced anxiety and depression and improved immune function, including increased natural killer cell numbers (Hernandez-Reif et al., 2005).

Hypertension

Massage therapy decreased diastolic blood pressure, anxiety, and cortisol (stress hormone) levels (Hernandez-Reif et al., 2000).

Circulatory and Respiratory Conditions

Massage increases thoracic gas volume, peak flow, and forced vital capacity (Beeken et al., 1998).

Cardiovascular Health

Massage has been shown to reduce heart rate (Curtis, 1994) and blood pressure (Fakouri et al., 1987).

Psychological/Emotional/Neurological Conditions

Back massage, as an alternative or adjunct to pharmacological interventions, has been shown to be an effective intervention for the promotion of sleep (Meek, 1993).

Dementia

Dementia is a disorder that impairs the vascular (blood vessels) or neurological (nerve) structures of the brain. Patients suffering with dementia often express anxiety and dysfunctional behavior. A study by the Department of Nursing in South Korea explored the effect of using expressive physical touch with verbalization in dementia patients. The results of the study revealed that anxiety is considerably lowered immediately following touch and verbalization (Kim et al., 1999).

Alzheimer's Disease

Alzheimer's disease is a neurological disorder characterized by loss, speechlessness, agitation, and, sometimes, paralysis. The lack of effective treatments for this debilitating disease prompted researchers at the University of Texas to carry out a slow-stroke massage on outpatients. The researchers found that patients' agitated behavior increased from dawn to dusk. The study revealed that the more physical aspects of agitation, such as pacing, wandering, and resistance, significantly decreased after slow-stroke massage was administered (Rowe et al., 1999).

Delirium

Delirium is a combination of neurological conditions that include cognitive impairment, sleep deprivation, immobility, dehydration, and impaired vision or hearing. A study, conducted at Yale-New Haven Hospital in Connecticut and published in the *New England Journal of Medicine,* found that a combination of modalities including massage, relaxation tapes, and word games, had fewer episodes and a reduction in the number of days of delirium (Inouye et al., 1999).

CONCLUSION

The benefits of massage therapy for older adults are multifaceted. As a holistic therapy, massage works on several dimensions of health simultaneously. The health benefits of deep relaxation and appropriate touch are obvious. In addition, massage therapy can increase blood and lymphatic circulation, improve muscle tone, lower blood pressure, lessen pain, diminish insomnia, increase range of motion, and ameliorate agitation associated with dementia. As more research is conducted into this noninvasive, low-risk, low-cost nonpharmacological therapy, it is likely that even more scientific evidence of the health benefits of massage therapy will emerge.

RESOURCES

Specialized Training

Day-Break Geriatric Massage Project/Institute

Day-Break Geriatric Massage Project was founded by Dietrich Miesler in 1982. The project developed out of a need to teach the theoretical knowledge and technical skills necessary in working with the elderly. Over the decades, the project has culled pertinent facts from the fields of medicine, psychology, sociology, gerontology, and, of course, the various bodywork disciplines. The project is now known as the Day-Break Geriatric Massage Institute. Miesler has since retired, and Dr. Sharon Puszko is the owner and director of Day-Break (http://www.day-break-massage.com).

American Massage Therapy Association

The AMTA represents more than 46,000 massage therapists in 27 countries. The association works to establish massage therapy as integral to the maintenance of good health and complementary to other therapeutic processes. It currently has a link on its Web site that can be used for finding a massage therapist in your area (http://www.amta.org). The American Massage Therapy Association (AMTA) Foundation Research Database (http://www.amtafoundation.org) documents a growing body of research that confirms the efficacy of massage for a variety of illnesses and conditions. The AMTA Foundation advances the knowledge of massage therapy by supporting scientific research, education, and community service.

Government/Trade Association/Agencies Web Sites

There are a number of institutions exploring complementary modalities and issues for the aging population. The institutions and Web sites below are rich in information on the topic.

   1. The National Institutes of Health (NIH), National Institute on Aging (NIA) (http://www.nia.nih.gov)

2. Agency for Healthcare Research and Quality (AHRQ) (http://www.ahrq.gov)
3. Centers for Disease Control (CDC), National Center for Chronic Disease Prevention and Health Promotion (http://www.cdc.gov/aging)
4. National Institutes of Health, National Center for Complementary and Alternative Medicine (NCAM) (http://nccam.nih.gov)
5. American Massage Therapy Association (AMTA) (http://www.amta.org)
6. American Massage Therapy Association (Foundation Research and Grants) (http://amtafoundation.org)

REFERENCES

Abrams, W., & Berkow, R. (1988). *The Merck manual of geriatrics.* Rahway, NJ: Merck Sharp and Dome Research Laboratories.

Beck, M. (1999). *Milady's theory and practice of therapeutic massage* (3rd ed.). Clifton Park, NY: Thomson Delmar Learning.

Beeken, J., Parks, D., Cory, J., & Montopoli, G. (1998). Effectiveness of neuromuscular release massage therapy on chronic obstructive lung disease. *Clinical Nursing Research, 7*(3), 309–325.

Benjamin, P. (1994, September/October). A Massage Magazine interview with Dietrich Miesler: Founder of the Geriatric Massage Project. *Massage Magazine.*

Berkow, R., & Beers, M. (1997). *Merck manual home edition.* West Point, NJ: Merck Research Laboratories.

Burch, S. (1997). *Recognizing health and illness: Pathology for massage therapists and bodyworkers.* Health Positive! Publishing.

Chapman, C. (1995). Massage for the mature and aging client [Class Syllabus].

Colton, H. (1996). *The gift of touch.* New York: Kensington Books.

Curtis, M. (1994). The use of massage in restoring cardiac rhythm. *Nursing Times* (England), *90*(38), 36, 37.

Erickson, E., & Kivnick, H. (1988). *Vital involvement in old age.* New York: Norton & Co.

Fakouri, C., & Jones, P. (1987). Relaxation Rx: Slow-stroke back rub. *Journal of Gerontological Nursing, 13*(2).

Federal Interagency Forum on Aging-Related Statistics. (2000). *Older Americans 2000: Key indicators of well being.*

Hernandez-Reif, M., Field, T., Krasnegor, J., & Theakston, H. (2001). Low back pain is reduced and range-of-motion increased after massage therapy. *International Journal of Neuroscience, 106,* 131–145.

Hernandez-Reif, M., Field, T., Ironson, G., Beutler, J., Vera, Y., Hurley, J., et al. (2005). Natural killer cells and lymphocytes increase in women with breast cancer following massage therapy. *International Journal of Neuroscience, 115*(4), 495–510.

Hernandez-Reif, M., Field, T., et al. (2000). High blood pressure and associated symptoms were reduced by massage therapy. *Journal of Bodywork and Movement Therapies, 4,* 31–38.

Inouye, S. K., Bogardus, S. T., Charpentier, P. A., Leo-Summers, L., Acampora, D., et al. (1999, March 4). A multicomponent intervention to prevent delirium in hospitalized older patients. *New England Journal of Medicine,* 669–676.

Kim, E. J., & Buschmann, M. T. (1999). The effect of expressive physical touch on patients with dementia. *International Journal of Nursing Studies, 36*(3), 235–243.

King, R. (1986, Summer). Massage for seniors. *Massage Therapy Journal.*

Kreiger, D. (1986). *Therapeutic touch.* Englewood Cliffs, NJ: Prentice-Hall.

Kwei, C. (1992, May/June). Therapeutic massage for the elderly. *Massage Magazine.*

Lohman, J. S. (2001. Fall). Massage for elders. *Massage Therapy Journal.*

Martz, S. (Ed.). (2003). *When I am an old woman I shall wear purple* (4th ed.). Watsonville, CA: Papier Mache Press.

Maxwell Hudson, C. (1988). *The complete book of massage.* New York: Random House.

Meek, S. S. (1993). Effects of slow-stroke back massage on relaxation in hospice clients. *Image—The Journal of Nursing Scholarship, 25*(1), 17–21.

Miesler, D. (1991, September/October). Geriatric massage. *Massage Magazine.*

Miesler, D. (1993, Fall). Geriatric massage: The day-break way. *Massage and Bodywork Quarterly.*

Miesler, D. (1995, Spring). Chair massage in geriatric care? *Massage and Bodywork Quarterly.*

Miesler, D. (1996, Summer). Geriatric massage: Assessment and contraindications for the geriatric client, Part 1. *Massage and Bodywork.*

Miesler, D. (1998, Summer). Geriatric massage: Assessment and contraindications for the geriatric client, Part II. *Massage and Bodywork.*

Miesler, D. (1998b, Fall). Geriatric massage. *Massage and Bodywork.*

Montague, A. (1986). *Touching: The human significance of skin.* New York: Harper & Row.

Nelson, D. (1993a). *Compassionate touch: Hands-on caregiving for the elderly, the ill and the dying.* Station Press.

Nelson, D. (1993b, Fall). Therapeutic touch in long-term care. *Massage and Bodywork Quarterly.*

Nelson, D. (1996, Summer). The use of touch in Alzheimer's care. *Massage Therapy Journal.*

Nelson, D. (2001, February/March). The power of touch in facility care. *Massage and Bodywork.*

Physiological changes in sedentary adults. (1997, September/October). *American Fitness.*

Pomfret, S. (1999, March/April). Seniors and massage: The rewards for clients and therapists. *Massage Magazine.*

Rikkers, R. (1987, Spring). Physiology of aging. *Massage Therapy Journal.*

Rosenfeld, A. (1988, Spring). Massage for the elderly. *Massage Therapy Journal.*

Rowe, M., et al. (1999). The effectiveness of slow-stroke massage in diffusing agitated behaviours in individuals with Alzheimer's disease. *Journal of Gerontological Nursing, 25*(6), 22–34.

Saton, M. (1988). *After the stroke.* New York: Norton & Co.

Sharpe, P., et al. (2002, Fall). Methods for improving the range of motion for older clients. *Massage Therapy Journal.*

Signell, K. (1990). *Wisdom of the heart.* New York: Bantam Books.

Skeist, R. (1987, Winter). Aging—White Crane Senior Health Center spreads its wings. *Massage Therapy Journal.*

Sprott, R. L. (1993). *The biology of aging.* New York: Springer.

Tappan, F. M. *Healing massage techniques.* Norwalk, CT: Appleton & Lange.

Versagi, C. M. (2002, May/June). Expert advice. *Massage Magazine.*

CHAPTER EIGHT

Daoist Spirituality and Philosophy: Implications for Holistic Health, Aging, and Longevity

Amy L. Ai

Daoism, or Taoism, is an ancient legacy of the East Asian culture. Although Daoism is sometimes considered to be one of the world's religions, it may be the least organized, has few temples for worship, and attributes no human nature to its divinity. With respect to its spirituality, Daoism is more cosmological than psychological in comparison with other Eastern religions such as Buddhism, while it is perhaps more philosophical than religious in comparison with monotheistic Western religions. In *Dao Te Jing,* or the *Doctrine of the Way (Dao) and the Virtue (Te),* the founder of Daoism, Lao Zi or Lao Tze, mentioned neither a path to an afterlife nor the existence of heaven. Nor did he describe a benevolent divinity. Instead, he presented a portrait of an unintentional Nature. As he said:

> Nature acts without intent,
> so cannot be described
> as acting with benevolence,
> nor malevolence to any thing.
> In this respect, the Tao is just the same,
> though in reality it should be said
> that nature follows the rule of Tao. (Ch. 5)

149

Daoism, therefore, does not address the relationship between human beings and God as the Creator as does monotheistic theology. Nor does it teach an afterlife reward for present good deeds, such as through reincarnation to an upper hierarchical order, as does Buddhism. Rather, its primary interest lies in an intuitive and dialectical inquiry into universal law, into the nature of *Dao*, or *Tao*, especially patterns of ultimate changes driven by underlying energetic force (Ai, in press). In his *Dao Te Jing*, Lao Zi describes the infinite and indefinable nature of Dao:

> The Tao is abstract
> and therefore has no form.
> . . . without form or image, without existence,
> for form of the formless, is beyond defining,
> cannot be described,
> and is beyond our understanding.
> It cannot be called by any name. (Ch. 14)
> When the consistency of the Tao is known,
> The mind is receptive to its states of change. (Ch. 16)

It is difficult to portray the richness of Daoism in a short chapter, especially because Daoism presents a quite different worldview from most other spiritual traditions in the West, ontologically and epistemologically. This article will briefly address the basics of Daoism which are fourfold: the origin of Daoist spirituality, the basics of Daoist spirituality, the influence of Daoist spirituality in holistic health care and traditional medicine in East Asia, and impacts of Daoist spirituality on aging today.

THE ORIGIN OF DAOIST SPIRITUALITY

In ancient times, the emergence of major religions or spiritual belief systems tended to echo the impact of the historical environment of their founders. Lao Zi is believed to have lived between 571 and 471 BCE during the Spring and Autumn Period of the late Zhou dynasty, which extended for 242 years. He spent most of his life in cultivating the Dao and the Te. Yet, as a modest wise sage, he did not attempt to make his name in the world. During these two and a half centuries, the preunified China was divided by large and small feudal dukedoms, which engaged in 473 cycles of brutal wars with each other in the historical record. Countless political conflicts led to not only the misery of ordinary citizens but also the uncertainty and migration of Lao Zi during his life. In his earlier years, Lao Zi served as a librarian for the Zhou Royal Library. It was said that Lao Zi attempted to flee from Zhou Kingdom after experiencing its declination and turmoil. An officer at the gate stopped him and requested that he write a book. Lao Zi wrote the famous *Dao Te Jing* to explain the meaning of Dao and Te and then was allowed to leave.

THE BASICS OF DAOIST SPIRITUALITY

Daoism uses the word *Qi* as the description of or a metaphor for the unifying energy underlying all changing patterns. The Chinese character *Qi* means "air," which although invisible is perceivable by its moving pressure (Ai, 2003). Qi is further presented in a paradoxical pattern as two contradictory but intertwined forces, Yin and Yang, as presented in *Tai Ji* symbol. The dynamic union of these two forces generates the vital energy, Qi, of all movements, including the life force of all living things. Yin–Yang forces change cyclically, mutually creating, controlling, and penetrating.

Daoism respects nature and emphasizes a harmonic relationship with nature, as do many ancient traditions such as Buddhism, Hinduism, and Native American thought (Ai, 2003). However, corresponding to the first principle, change, historically Daoists were fascinated more by the constant movements in relation to the nonbeing aspect than by the visible (e.g., physical landscape) or invisible (e.g., the spirit) being aspects of nature. The law of nature, therefore, is perceived as in dynamically continuous flow in constant change. The universal principle of all changes is presented by a single word, *Dao*. In its Chinese character, Dao refers to the way or the universal order to be followed in life and in nature (Ai, 2003. In a cosmic sense, it refers to the ultimate, indefinable principle underlying all movements—the process involving every aspect in the universe. The law of nature, not of human logic, is what Daoism intends to comprehend philosophically, to appreciate aesthetically, or to worship spiritually (see Crosby, 2002). Unlike monotheistic religions, however, such law was not created by the Creator but has always been inherent in the universe. The nature of such law is not perceived as a fixed order but in its ever-changing pattern with the movement of both nonbeing and being. Lao Zi said in *Tao Te Jing:*

> When the consistency of the Tao is known,
> the mind is receptive to its states of change. (Ch. 16)
> Man's laws should follow natural laws,
> just as nature gives rise to physical laws,
> whilst following from universal law,
> which follows the Tao (Ch. 25).
> From the principle which is called the Tao,
> the sky, the earth, and creativity are one,
> the sky is clear, the earth is firm,
> and the spirit of the inner world is full. (Ch. 39)

Given its liquid, process-oriented view, Daoism tends not to use a term for the absolute definition of a particular object or structure. Rather, Daoist terms may contain both the depiction of being and the dynamic relationship or energetic interaction among its elements and totality, such as that of humans to sociocultural, geological, and cosmic environments. For example, In *Dao Te Jin,* the term *earth* refers to the nature of the environment that human beings are attached to, rather than to the globe in geological terms. Likewise, the term *sky* or *heaven* tends to involve the nature of the universe and inherent phenomena beyond human comprehension, rather than the place where God lives as in some monotheist perspectives. Likewise, when the *Heart* is referred to as the organ of mind in traditional Chinese medicine (TCM), it is not seen as the neurological organ of thinking, like the brain. Rather, among ancient scholars the Heart concept arises from the perception of the inspiration and passion that accompany intellectual work (e.g., poetry writing, landscape painting, or chess playing), which can be discerned through intuition and through excitement (increased heart rate).

THE INFLUENCE OF DAOIST SPIRITUALITY IN HEALTH CARE AND TRADITIONAL CHINESE MEDICINE

In the history of East Asia, Daoism became the most influential spiritual or philosophical tradition in the development of TCM, affecting its philosophy, theory, terminology, and practice. Literally, TCM, or *Zhong Yi,* means the Medicine of Balanced Energy rather than the Medicine of Middle Kingdom (Ai, 2003; Yuan, 1997). In its over two thousand years of history, TCM had become a popular practice not only among Han Chinese people but among other East Asia populations as well, such as Korean, Mongolian, Tibetan, Vietnamese, and Japanese, and was intertwined with local medicines through cultural exchanges. In a global perspective, TCM may be better referred to as traditional East Asian medicine.

In Daoist philosophy, each person is considered as a cosmos in miniature. According to the first dialectical principle, the manifestation of the Dao within the individual follows the same patterns as does the universe, which can be predicted in changing patterns as registered in the *I Ching.* Stated intellectually, an individual's energy pattern is constantly interacting with that of all beings in one's environment, including that of planets, since one's birth. In theory, TCM is an energetic-function-centered rather than a materialistic-structure-oriented system. In TCM terminology, health and illness are not described in the diagnosis of physical diseases but rather are manifestations of equilibrium or functional imbalance with respect to Qi and Yin–Yang energy patterns. According to the above dialectical principles, TCM differentiates the condition of health not by the absolute absence of disease but rather by the relatively balanced patterns of energy, producing integration, harmony, and vitality.

In practice, TCM focuses on prevention through sensitive recognition and management of energy balance. It emphasizes the treatment of preailment stages and initial manifestations of pathology. A classical medical text, *Nan Jing (Classic of 81 Difficulties with Annotations*, 1970), discussed the many preventive, therapeutic principles of TCM two thousand years ago as the guide for becoming an excellent doctor in preventing substantive illnesses that will eventually lead to mortality. To prevent ailments and promote health, TCM is organized on the dynamic functional system of vital energy, or the movement of Qi. To cultivate one's vital energy, the individual must take the responsibility for one's own healthy lifestyle, harmonic attitude, and energy exercise, called qigong (Ai et al., 2001). Because each person has his or her own pattern of energy movement, the holistic practice of TCM, including its herbal medicine, is more effective when it is delivered in a highly individualized manner rather than following standardized medication formula, as occurs in biomedicine.

The fundamental differences between Daoist TCM and biomedicine stem from their basic observations and their underlying philosophies. For the most part, the operative philosophy of science is embodied in Aristotelian empirical materialism, in which the knowledge of antiquity was systematically organized into the scheme that underlies much of the Western view of the universe. The formulation of a Cartesian mind/matter *(res cogitans/res extensa)* dualism in the 17th century also helped bring about the birth of modern science (Ai, 1996). In this paradigm, matter is lifeless and is completely separated from the scientist as an observer. Biomedicine as the offspring of this outlook focuses primarily on the matter of body, which is further broken down into systems, organs, tissues, cells, chromosomes, genes, and molecules. In this biomedical model, the heart, for example, is treated as a pump—a mechanical organ with regular outputs. The diagnosis and treatment of disease are centered on the material aspect of organs or other levels of structure: physical, physiological, biochemical, or genetic.

In the spirit of Daoism, TCM, in contrast, observes humans in light of an energy web at different levels rather than merely seeing the physical structure. Like early Hippocratic medicine, TCM is psychosomatic and does not follow a soma and psyche dualism (Ai, 2003; Hammer, 1990; Temkin, 1991). According to the holistic dialectic principle, illness is observed in the perspective of mind–body interaction and lifestyle, as well as an individual's context. Both physical health and ailments are inseparable from some psychosocial components. As illustrated earlier, the Heart in TCM means more than an anatomic organ. It contains also the brain–heart relation in modern usage, which is linked to neuroendocrinological functions and the system involving the pituitary-adrenal axis.

The TCM system of diagnosis is built upon a distinctive information system that processes a complicated network of internal and external energetic and pathological factors. The differentiation of syndromes is made according to various principles (eight principal patterns, Qi and blood patterns, viscera patterns, six channel phases, and four phases of febrile illness). All signs of the patient's soma, behavior, emotion, sexuality, psyche, spirit, and contextual factors are accounted for in discerning an energetic effect (Ai, 2003). Based on this mind–body connection, TCM facilitates health grounded in the constant interplay of psyche and soma as well as that of the person and his or her environment, particularly embodied in its theory on Qi and Yin–Yang.

In the Han dynasty about two thousand years ago, the TCM system began to use the five-element system—Wood, Fire, Earth, Metal, and Water—to symbolize functional movement (Maciocia, 1989). Similarly, ancient Greeks used four elements—Water, Fire, Earth, and Air—to represent the basic qualities of natural phenomena. The five-element theory, however, focuses on interrelations among elements rather than on their substantive aspects (Ai, 2003).The interaction among these five elements follows the mutual generating and controlling processes in organic functioning. Organs in pairs, tissues, meridians, some acupuncture points, pulse, tongue status, emotions, sounds, tastes, colors, seasons, stars, herbs, and external pathogenic influences are all interconnected, with various relations coded by these five categories and the Yin–Yang system (Maciocia, 1989; Unschuld, 1985). Seven emotions or psychic elements (joy, anger, anxiety, concentration, grief, fear, and fright) are associated with corresponding functional organs (e.g., Heart, Liver, Lung, Spleen, and Kidney).

From a perspective joining these TCM theories and psychiatric diagnoses, Hammer (1990), an American psychiatrist, devoted an entire book to an explanation of the nature of Qi movement in relation to emotion and illness. TCM views emotions and attitudes as internal responses to stimuli from the environment. When any type of emotion becomes overwhelming, emotions become internal agents of illness. Conversely, the dysfunction of organs will be manifested not only in somatic symptoms but also in certain emotional distresses. For instance, in the Daoist symbolic representation, the Heart is classified as the "Fire" element—an "Emperor" organ that houses the individual's spirit, or *Shen,* and mental energy—and is related to the emotion of joy. From a functional perspective, this connection may be understandable in neuropsychological theory. The heart beats faster due to the increased secretion of adrenal hormone when the person is in an ecstatic emotional status. The energetic activity of another "Fire" organ, pericardium, is to facilitate normal sexual functioning. A defective pericardium may affect this human activity in a variety of ways, ranging from hypo- to hypersexuality, and its related emotion, joy.

In the Daoist relativist view, the energetic balance between mind and body is essential to health and longevity. Unlike the dichotomized solutions in the West, the Daoist view does not propose any type of emotions as either absolutely positive or completely negative. For example, even excessive joy is believed to cause harm to one's energetic balance, as do negative emotions, such as anger. This situation can be understood in today's terms if one considers the case of an older person's sudden death around the time of his or her birthday party, which may lead to excesses of both joy and stress. The key to organic balance and health is the integration of overall aspects, rather than the pursuit of extremity. By the same token, Daoism does not deny sexuality as a human desire, nor does it encourage extreme sexual play in the spirit of hedonism. Rather, sexual energy and behaviors are considered as inseparable parts of health, longevity, and illness. The practice of TCM, including the use of herbs, acupuncture, body manipulation, qigong, and guidance of appropriate sexual life, will readjust dysfunction of both organs and emotions, and will thereby restore the healthy pattern of energy. Following the spirit of Daoism, TCM is the art of life and prevention rather than specified knowledge about or treatment of disease. Although it does not offer the magic bullet of cure, TCM nonetheless provides a valuable holistic perspective on health, healing, and energy promotion for human nature.

THE IMPACT OF DAOIST SPIRITUALITY
ON AGING TODAY

Daoism is one of the Eastern cultural traditions that greatly respect the elderly. Its founder's name, Lao Zi, means "Old Gentleman." It was said that his mother incubated him for 10 years and that he was born as an older person in the fourth century BCE, indicating great respect for an older person who cultivates the knowledge of the Dao and the Te throughout life. The aged person was portrayed as a wise man in *Tao Te Jing*:

> The sage of old (the aged) was profound and wise;
> like a man at a ford,
> he took great care, alert, perceptive and aware . . . . (Ch. 15)

This image of an old wise man is quite different from the negative, demented one commonly perceived in a modern society. The respect for aging in Daoist tradition is particularly due to its appreciation of dialectic thinking and the wisdom accumulated with old age.

Only in more recent decades has modern psychological science begun to accept in theory that dialectical thinking consists of sophisticated approaches toward part–whole relations and seeming contradictions (Peng & Nisbett, 1999, Riegel, 1973). Dialectics is considered to be an important part of adult thought, particularly in creative scientific activities and in cognitive development beyond Jean Piaget's adolescent formal operations stage (Piaget, 1952). Indeed, researchers have found that such thinking becomes more important as people mature and is increasingly used with advancing age (Baltes & Staudinger, 1993; Basseches, 1984; Chandler & Boutilier, 1992; Kramer & Woodruf, 1986). Middle-aged and older persons tend to accept contradictions in reality and to synthesize them into their thinking more than do young people. It would appear, then, that today, when population aging and globalization have become international trends, wisdom and dialectical thinking, along with other late age development, should be more respected and greatly appreciated in Western developed countries, as they are in Daoism.

In practice, Daoism, as the spirit of TCM, also offers a very different but pragmatic philosophy and practice as compared with that of Western medicine for care of the aging and age related chronic conditions. The course of health, illness, and longevity depends on energetic harmony and integration among different parts of physical functions; among body, mind, and spirit; and between the human life and the overall environment. Daoist spirituality may have important implications for care of the aging today, particularly because many chronic illnesses in late life are out of the control of physicians' approaches. To maintain healthy aging, mature persons need to practice self-care and energy exercise rather than solely depending on biomedical care. As suggested by Lao Zi in *Tao Te Jing*:

> Maintaining unity is virtuous,
> for the inner world of thought is one
> with the external world
> of action and of things.
> The sage avoids their separation,
> By breathing as the sleeping babe,
> And thus maintaining harmony. (Ch. 10)
> From constancy, there develops harmony,
> and from harmony, enlightenment.
> It is unwise to rush from here to there.
> To hold one's breath causes the body strain;
> exhaustion follows when too much energy is used,
> for this is not the natural way. (Ch. 55)

One particular healthy-aging practice is the energy exercise qigong, which is heavily influenced by Daoism (Ai, 2003, 2005; Ai et al., 2001). Similar to yoga, this Chinese form of moving or still meditative exercise is practiced in order to achieve the balance and integration of one's wholeness. The nature of still-form meditation, in posture of standing, sitting, or lying, is similar to that of Zen Buddhism. Both emphasize deep breathing, concentration, relaxation, and the detachment of one's mind from disturbing reality, but the two approaches tend to have different techniques and foci. Buddhist practice focuses on the emptiness of the mind, whereas Daoist practice tends to suggest passively following the flow of bodily energy sensation along a certain meridian system, such as Heavenly Circulation, or *Zhou Tian* (Cohn, 1997, pp. 162–165). In terms of objectives, Buddhism stresses the experience of awakening from the illusion of life and enlightenment, whereas Daoism focuses on cultivating energy and promoting longevity through internal and external movements (Cohen, 1997, p. 14).

In part because of its holistic view, the spirituality of Daoism has been pursued and practiced by many mature older people in Chinese history, particularly following their retirement. They practice it daily to regain and develop the spontaneity and vital energy that tends to be damaged in their life-span struggles. Historically, Daoist spiritual practice was often inseparable from the lifelong performance of qigong, which affects all aspects of one's life, attitudes, and spirituality. The primary aim of qigong is not masculine strength but flexibility, integrity, inner strength, energetic harmony, compassion, and longevity (Ai, 2003). One strategy in such practice is the imagery of returning to one's infancy, as indicated in the above excerpt from *Dao Te Jing*—maintaining breath like a sleeping babe. In fact, Lao Zi often mentioned maintaining the softness in body and the simplicity and flexibility in mind evident in an infant. Zhuang Zi, a famous Daoist philosopher, described how to achieve longevity through energy movement and deep breath by practicing the earliest form of qigong, called dao-yin two thousand years ago (cited by Cohen, 1997, p. 16):

> Exhaling through the mouth while exercising the breath,
> Spitting out the old breaths, drawing in the new,
> Moving like the bear, stretching like the bird,
> This is simply the art of longevity!—
> As the aim of those scholars who practice *dao-yin*.

Indeed, qigong seems to be beneficial to one's functional age. The indication of age is associated with the overall decline of mental and physical functioning. An American qigong master, Cohn, described in his book *The Way of Qigong* (1997) many studies done in China on the functional effectiveness of qigong (pp. 73–75). These findings suggest that long-term qigong practice may improve many of the biological markers of aging, such as vital capacity, blood pressure, cholesterol levels, hormone levels, kidney function, mental acuity (including memory), skin elasticity, bone density, reaction time, physical strength, and immune function. A survey of elderly qigong practitioners and nonpracticing seniors showed benefits in hearing, vision, blood pressure, memory, and working capacity among the qigong practitioners. Another group of studies of the antiaging effects of qigong has demonstrated that those practicing it had increased activity of the enzyme superoxide dismutase (SOD) in comparison with the control group. SOD is believed to play a protective role in cell functioning protecting against damage from superoxide, a reactive variety of oxygen that can cause aging and accompanying free-radical damage of tissues and nerves. Still other studies found positive effects in qigong on blood sugar levels, insulin levels, microcirculation, and disease resistance. More such investigation should be replicated in the West with sound research design.

Finally, no matter how long one can live, death is inevitable. To historical and contemporary societies that have had only negative images of death and have not provided holistic care for the dying, Lao Zi offers a Daoist attitude toward death. It implies the image of an immortal soul in the form of spiritual immortality. Lao Zi did not describe any location for the soul after life, whether heaven, as in monotheistic religions, or another form of life, as in Buddhism. Rather, immortality resides in a spiritual unification, integration, or identification of oneself with the universal law, or the Dao. In such imagery, one's spirit becomes alive with all things, even as one's physical body approaches its final natural limitation. In a way, Lao Zi's name has become immortal, identified with the Dao in Daoist spirituality. What he said in *Dao Te Jing* is a fitting conclusion to this chapter:

> He who lives by the way of the Tao,
> travels without fear of ferocious beasts,
> and will not be pierced in an affray,
> for he offers no resistance.
> The universe is the center of his world,
> so in the inner world
> of he who lives within the Tao,
> there is no place
> where death can enter in. (Ch. 50)
> All things are microcosms of the Tao;
> the world a microcosmic universe,
> the nation a microcosm of the world . . .
> from single cell to galaxy . . .
> The virtue of Tao governs its natural way.
> Thus, he who is at one with it,
> is one with every thing that lives,
> having freedom from the fear of death. (Ch. 52)

NOTE

The author gratefully acknowledges Terrence N. Tice, ThD, PhD, and Linda Hendrickson Thurman, BTh, MSEd, for their comments. The author has been supported by the National Institute on Aging Training Grant T32-AG0017, National Institute on Aging Grant R03-AGO-15686-01, National Center for Complementary and Alternative Medicine Grant P50-AT00011, a grant from the John Templeton Foundation, and the John Hartford Faculty Scholars Program.

REFERENCES

Ai, A. L. (1996). Psychosocial adjustment and health care practices following coronary artery bypass surgery (CABG). *Dissertation Abstracts International: Section B: The Sciences and Engineering, 57*(6-B), 4078.

Ai, A. L. (2000). Spiritual well-being, spiritual growth, and spiritual care for the aged: A cross-faith and interdisciplinary effort. *Journal of Religious Gerontology, 11,* 3–28.

Ai, A. L. (2003). Assessing mental health in clinical study on Qigong: Between scientific investigation and holistic perspectives. *Seminars in Integrative Medicine, 1,* 112-121.

Ai, A. L. (in press). Ch. 22, Qigong: Energy-oriented health practice based on an energy-centered world view. In M. S. Micozzi (Ed.), *Fundamentals of complementary & integrative medicine* (3rd ed.). St Louis, MO: Elsevier Health Sciences.

Ai, A. L., Peterson, C., Gillespie, B., Bolling, S. F., Jessup, M. G., Behling, B. A., & Pierse, F. (2001). Designing clinical trials on energy healing: Ancient art encounters medical science. *Alternative Therapies in Health and Medicine, 7,* 83–90.

Ai, A. L., Peterson, C., Tice, T. N., Bolling, S. F., & Koenig, H. (2004). Faith-based and secular pathways to hope and optimism subconstructs in middle-aged and older cardiac patients. *Journal of Health Psychology, 9*(3), 435-450.

Baltes, P. B., & Staudinger, U. M. (1993). The search for a psychology of wisdom. *Current Directions in Psychological Science, 2,* 75–80.

Basseches, M. (1984). *Dialectical thinking and adult development.* Norwood, NJ: Ablex.

Bloom, A. (1968). *The republic of Plato: Translated with notes and an interpretive essay.* New York: Basic Books.

Capra, F. (1991). *The Dao of physics* (3rd ed.). Boston: Shambhala.

Chandler, M., & Boutilier, R. (1992). The development of dynamic system reasoning. *Human Development, 35,* 121–137.

Cohen, K. S. (1997). *The way of Qigong: The art and science of Chinese energy healing.* New York: Ballantine Books.

Crosby, D. A. (2002). *A religion of nature.* Albany: State University of New York Press.

Groth-Marnat, G. (1992). Buddhism and mental health: A comparative analysis. In J. F. Schumaker (Ed.), *Religion and mental health* (pp. 270–280). New York: Oxford University Press.

Hammer, L. (1990). The fundamental energy constructs of Chinese medicine—the traditional five elements system: Emotion and the disease process. In *Dragon rises, red bird flies: Psychology, energy and Chinese medicine.* Barrytown, NY: Station Hill Press.

Kramer, D., & Woodruf, D. S. (1986). Relativistic and dialectical thought in three adult age-groups. *Human Development, 29,* 280–290.

Lao Zi. *Tao Te Jing* (S. Rosenthal, Trans.). Retrieved from http://web.clas.ufl.edu/users/gthursby/taoism

Maciocia, G. (1989). The five elements. In *The foundations of Chinese medicine: A comprehensive text for acupuncturists and herbalists.* New York: Churchill Livingstone.

Nanjjing Institutes of Traditional Chinese Medicine. (Ed.). (1970). *Classic of 81 difficulties with annotations* (in Chinese, *Nan Jing Jiao Yi*). Beijing: People's Press. (First appeared c. 200 CE. Cited as *Nan Jing.*)

Peng, K., & Nisbett, E. N. (1999). Culture, dialectics, and reasoning about contradiction. *American Psychologist, 54,* 741–754.

Piaget, J. (1952). *The origins of intelligence in children.* New York: International Universities Press.

Prebish, C. S. (1998). Introduction. In C. S. Prebish & K. K. Tanaka (Eds.), *The faces of Buddhism in America.* Berkeley: University of California Press.

Riegel, K. F. (1973). Dialectical operations: The final period of cognitive development. *Human Development, 18,* 430–443.

Rubin, J. B. (1996). Psychoanalytic and Buddhist history and theory. In *Psychotherapy and Buddhism: Toward an integration.* New York: Plenum Press.

Temkin, O. (1991). The medicine of the body and the medicine of the soul: Epilogue. In *Hippocrates in a world of pagans and Christians.* Baltimore: The Johns Hopkins University Press.

Unschuld, P. U. (1985). Taoism and pragmatic drug therapy: From antifeudal social theory to individualistic practices of longevity. In *Medicine in China: A history of ideas.* Berkeley: University of California Press.

Verhoeven, M. J. (1998). Americanizing the Buddha: Paul Carus and the transformation of Asian thought. In C. S. Prebish & K. K. Tanaka (Eds.), *The faces of Buddhism in America* (pp. 207–227). Berkeley: University of California Press.

Wilhelm, H. (1967). *Change–selections.* New York: Harper Torchbooks.

Yuan, C. H. (i1997). "Chinese medicine" is not the abbreviation of the medicine of China: *I-Ching* expert Lui Dajun's definition of "Chinese medicine" (in Chinese). *Chinese News, 28,* 23.

CHAPTER NINE

Medical Acupuncture

James K. Rotchford

The field of acupuncture is broad and perhaps in its own way more diverse than conventional Western medicine. In addition to the many types and sizes of needles used, there can be significant variability in the techniques for needling and the models used to decide which points to needle. There are also a variety of ancillary interventions that are frequently associated with acupuncture. Examples include and are not limited to cupping, scraping, electrical stimulation, moxibustion, and massage, as well as the use of Chinese herbs. What's more, acupuncture interventions are rarely standardized, as are interventions in conventional Western medicine. Interventions in acupuncture, although often based on standard diagnostic criteria, are much more likely to be based on individual patient differences and the practitioner's training and style. Historically, acupuncture was taught and learned through prolonged apprenticeships (Eckman, 1996). Until the latter part of the 20th century, there were few textbooks of acupuncture, and the textbooks that did exist were often written in ways that allowed for much interpretation. The Bible would be a Western text comparable to ancient textbooks of acupuncture such as the *Nei Jing* (Huang, 1979. Metaphors, symbols, and contextual issues were highly important in ancient Asian medicine texts. There were no schools of acupuncture per se, and styles and techniques were often passed down from father to son. Consequently, one would expect that through almost all of its history acupuncture differed significantly sometimes within the same community but also across regions of China, Japan, and Korea. It was only under Mao Zedong and his successors that significant strides were made to standardize acupuncture approaches.

Medical acupuncture is acupuncture that has been successfully incorporated into medical or allied health practices in Western countries (Helms, 1998). Some Western clinicians practice very traditional or specific forms of acupuncture, although most practice a hybrid form of acupuncture. Medical acupuncture, like the entire field of acupuncture, is quite diverse (Helms, 1995). In the United States, as well as in most industrialized Western countries, allopathic physicians generally are the providers of medical acupuncture. Indeed, a criterion for membership in the American Academy of Medical Acupuncture is licensure to practice allopathic medicine. The diversity of approaches and the nature of the practice of medicine often cause some practitioners to hold strong opinions about how a patient should or should not be treated with acupuncture. There even remains, understandably, quite a bit of controversy about who is qualified to practice acupuncture. Here political, legal, and financial pressures enter into the picture, further complicating and clouding our understanding of acupuncture's proper role in medicine.

BASIC THEORY

Acupuncture is most often based on the Chinese definition of health that considers health a state in which adequate amounts of energy *(Qi)* flow in a balanced fashion through and around the body. Within the body the Qi flows primarily in meridians, or channels, of which there are 14 primary ones. Illness, then, indicates a breakdown in this balanced flow of energy, brought on either by outside factors (e.g., a virus or an injury) or as the result of long-standing internal imbalances that translate themselves into observable structural or functional abnormalities (e.g., back pain and heart palpitations). For example, a practitioner of Western medicine would approach a case of a stiff, painful back by looking at physical structures-bones out of place, unequal leg lengths, pinched nerves, arthritis, and so on. The medical acupuncturist would also examine the structural problems but would consider that these abnormalities may primarily be the result of an imbalance in the Qi or electrical fields in and around the body.

Western theories abound about how acupuncture might work. Clearly, acupuncture changes levels of endorphins in the brain and spinal cord (Pomeranz, 1996). Some other physiological effects of acupuncture have been measured scientifically. Most recently advances in brain imaging have allowed us to observe how acupuncture effects the blood flow and metabolism in different areas of the brain (Siedentopf et al., 2002; Wu et al., 2002).

MAJOR SCHOOLS OR STYLES OF ACUPUNCTURE

Traditional Chinese Medicine

Traditional Chinese Medicine (TCM) is the most common style or form of acupuncture taught and practiced in the West. It is a style of acupuncture that grew out of reforms in the 1950s in the People's Republic of China. Some complain that TCM is more suited to Asian herbal traditions than to acupuncture. Given the degree of standardization associated with TCM, it has become a popular style to use in Western research related to acupuncture.

TCM practice has many approaches for diagnosis and treatment. Most of these approaches are based, whether overtly or not, on the law of eight principles. With the law of eight principles a patient's overall state is generally defined by four major substates: Yin/Yang, Cold/Hot, Internal/External, and Excess/Deficiency. It is clearly impossible to give TCM, or for that matter any school or style of acupuncture, an adequate synopsis in this brief overview. There are several good references on TCM. For the general public, *The Web That Has No Weaver* (Kaptchuk, 1983) is perhaps the best known. For a more in-depth study into clinical TCM acupuncture, the textbooks by O'Connor and Bensky (1981) Maciocia (1994) can be consulted.

Classical Five Element, or Movement, Acupuncture

This form of acupuncture, which is commonly practiced in the West, was made popular by the late professor J. R. Worsley of England. Some argue that this five element, or movement, acupuncture is a more traditional form in that it involves a "physiology" not formally a part of traditional Chinese herbology and it incorporates more spiritual and Daoist principles. It clearly seems more suited to the exploration of "emotional" issues that may be influencing one's health. Its basic tenets probably date from the period about 200 BCE. If performed in a classical fashion, it requires practitioners to treat patients' constitutions, or basic natures. In the terms of classical five element acupuncture, this is called the causative factor (CF). Patients' natures metaphorically correlate with the seasons, colors, sounds, odors, emotions, and so on. A general reference is by Franglen (2001). The definitive textbooks are by Worsley (1990, 1993).

Auricular Acupuncture

Auricular (ear) acupuncture is considered a part of Chinese acupuncture, but it is usually associated with Paul Nogier (1972) of France, who developed an entire medical approach focusing on acupuncture of the ear.

The Nogier approach is now widely taught and used throughout the West. Nogier's son, Raphael, along with others, continue to develop this school of acupuncture and now call it auricular medicine. One interesting aspect of auricular acupuncture is that it highlights the aspect of Asian medical theory that considers the body as a sort of hologram where the whole can be reflected in any and all of its parts. There are other styles of acupuncture that take advantage of this tenet of Asian medicine. Korean hand therapy and scalp acupuncture are such examples. Pulse and tongue diagnoses are also dependent on the concept that elements of the whole can be found in the parts.

Neuroanatomical Acupuncture

Neuroanatomical acupuncture can be practiced from an entirely Western anatomical and physiological perspective. There are practitioners of this style who maintain that all of acupuncture's effects can be explained by understanding the Western physiology and anatomy of needling specific sites. By causing currents of injury by dry needling muscles, these practitioners relax muscles and can help with a number of musculoskeletal complaints. Stimulation of specific points is also believed to influence the autonomic system in precise ways. There is a large body of evidence demonstrating that electrical stimulation with acupuncture needles at different frequencies can stimulate a variety of neurotransmitters in addition to endorphins and other opiate-like substances. Percutaneous electrical nerve stimulations (PENS) is also gaining popularity among physicians because it does not require them to learn a new model of medicine but simply to apply new techniques to what they already know.

There are a number of articles and textbooks available to help practitioners understand this approach. I particularly recommend the textbooks of Wong (1999, 2002). Gunn (1996) is well known for developing Western physiological explanations of dry needling of points for musculoskeletal complaints. For an introduction to PENS, I recommend the study by Ghoname and colleagues (1999) published in the *Journal of the American Medical Association,* which found it effective in chronic low back pain. A recent study by Weiner et al. (2003) also evaluated this approach in elderly patients and found it to be effective.

As was discussed above, physicians and licensed acupuncturists will often use a hybrid of styles and approaches. The diversity of approaches leads to a questioning of what the term *acupuncture* exactly means. Is PENS something different than electroacupuncture? The need for a more specific definition of acupuncture with appropropriate qualifiers is pressing and is explored in an article by Rotchford and Kobrin (2002). This article would also help those wanting to have a more complete listing of acupuncture approaches.

INDICATIONS FOR ACUPUNCTURE

Historically, indications for medical interventions such as acupuncture were based on expert opinion. The World Health Organization (1980), based on expert opinion, put together a list of conditions suitable for acupuncture (see Table 9.1).

Most clinicians or patients will weigh recommendations on an assessment of risks versus. Benefits (Rotchford, 1998). There is a large body of evidence supporting the relative safety of acupuncture (Ernst & White, 1997; Rotchford, 1999; White, Cummings, Hopwood, & MacPherson, 2001; White, Hayhoe, et al., 2001). Serious side effects are less than 1 in 10,000 sessions.

There are many explanations for the lack of conclusive evidence-based results regarding the benefits of acupuncture. There is often poor methodological quality due to such factors as small trials with insufficient

TABLE 9.1 Conditions Recommended for Acupuncture by the World Health Organization (WHO)

Respiratory diseases
- Acute sinusitis
- Acute rhinitis
- Common cold
- Acute tonsillitis

Bronchopulmonary diseases
- Acute bronchitis
- Bronchial asthma

Eye disorders
- Acute conjuctivitis
- Cataract (without complications)
- Myopia
- Central retinitis

Disorders of the mouth cavity
- Toothache
- Pain after tooth extraction
- Gingivitis
- Pharyngitis

Orthopedic disorders
- Periarthritis humeroscapularis
- Tennis elbow
- Sciatica
- Low back pain
- Rheumatoid arthritis

(continued)

TABLE 9.1 Conditions Recommended for Acupuncture by the World Health Organization (WHO) *(Continued)*

Gastrointestinal disorders
- Spasm of the esophagus and cardia
- Hiccups
- Gastroptosis
- Acute and chronic gastritis
- Gastric hyperacidity
- Chronic duodenal ulcer
- Acute and chronic colitis
- Acute bacterial dysentery
- Constipation
- Diarrhea
- Paralytic ileus

Neurologic disorders
- Headache
- Migraine
- Trigeminal neuralgia
- Facial paralysis
- Paralysis after apoplectic fit
- Peripheral neuropathy
- Paralysis caused by poliomyelitis
- Meniere's syndrome
- Neurogenic bladder dysfunction
- Nocturnal enuresis
- Intercostal neuralgia

power to answer questions, large number of dropouts, improper blinding, and inadequate treatment. There are also theoretical issues related to researching acupuncture as one might a pharmaceutical intervention.

Acupuncture trials frequently poorly resemble standard clinical practice. In contrast, in pharmaceutical clinical trials, the study participants take medication just as they would from a prescribing physician. Because of attempts to determine the specificity and the efficacy of the acupuncture intervention, participants in an acupuncture clinical trial are often subjected to acupuncture that poorly resembles the acupuncture provided during a typical acupuncture session. Asian medicine by its very nature recognizes contextual issues as being very important in determining appropriate interventions and optimizing outcomes. The nature of most pharmaceutical clinical trials is to attempt to minimize contextual issues as factors so that causal attribution to a specific effect of the medicine being taken can be determined. Hence, when a clinical trial of acupuncture attempts to resemble a pharmaceutical trial, the intervention rarely reflects what actually transpires during a typical acupuncture session. Double blinding is always problematic in studies on surgical procedures, and acupuncture is a surgical procedure. There are probably only a handful of standard surgical procedures that have been validated in a true double-blind fashion. Yet this is a common criticism of acupuncture trials.

Although acupuncture research must be designed differently than a standard pharmaceutical trial, it would be helpful if more acupuncture trials went through phase 1 and 2 trials as do new pharmaceutical interventions. Most of the trials in acupuncture have been solely phase 3 trials. As a result, many of the acupuncture trials could be compared to providing a best-guess dose of penicillin to everyone with pneumonia and hoping that the results are positive. Of course, penicillin is only effective against pneumococcal pneumonia at specific doses over a certain period of time. Without attempts to individualize treatment based on individual need, the likelihood of achieving robust findings is severely compromised in a large group of pneumonia patients. Only a small percentage of pneumonia cases is due to penicillin-sensitive pneumococci. What's more, if not enough penicillin is given over enough time, then the therapeutic response is limited. To avoid these types of problems, phase 1 and 2 trials take place. There will be similar problems with acupuncture interventions if there is no attempt to study what is the best acupuncture intervention for a given condition and one continues to depend solely on expert opinion to determine the optimal intervention. Without phase 1 and 2 trials in acupuncture research, we never know if the "best" acupuncture was employed. What's more, using the penicillin analogy again, consider that one school of experts believes that the penicillins are the best class of antibiotics for pneumonia. If we do not do the phase 1 and 2 trials, we will never know if the amount of penicillin used was adequate or whether penicillins were the best antibiotic class to use. This is particularly problematic if the only experts involved all believe that penicillins are the best antibiotics for pneumonia. Furthermore, it would be even more problematic if their training was to never put into question the class of antibiotic, dosage, or route of administration. Unfortunately, many of the clinical trials of acupuncture have been phase 3 studies that depended on experts similarly biased as in the above example of "penicillin" experts. This approach to acupuncture research could understandably result in less than optimal results.

In evidence-based medicine, systematic reviews are often considered the gold standard when it comes to determining efficacy. Systematic reviews of the acupuncture literature are especially problematic because of the "garbage in, garbage out" problem (the formal finding of review of the literature is likely to be of little value if the studies that made up the review have significant design and reporting flaws). Sometimes a decision to include one or another study can make all the difference in the results of systematic reviews and meta-analyses. This is particularly true in acupuncture research because of the heterogeneity of the trials and the often inadequate numbers of patients studied, along with the other methodological problems cited above (Rotchford, 2003).

With these caveats in mind, it is noteworthy that the systematic reviews of acupuncture listed in Table 9.2 found positive efficacy results for acupuncture. Efficacy implies that the specific aspect of the intervention in question was causally related to the positive outcome, whereas effectiveness implies that the intervention was positive compared to the control. It is generally more difficult to demonstrate efficacy than effectiveness.

In most of the conditions in Table 9.2 there have been initial systematic reviews that failed to demonstrate positive effects. The above discussion possibly explains some of the discrepancies commonly found in systematic reviews of the acupuncture literature. Of note, systematic reviews are generally problematic. Ezzo and colleagues (Ezzo, Baussell, Moerman, Berman, & Hadhazy, 2001) examined the reviews to determine readers' consensual rating. That rating never got above 36% despite the conclusions reached in the review.

There are individual studies of sound methodological value that have reported efficacy or effectiveness of acupuncture for a wide variety of other conditions. To list these and discuss these studies is beyond the scope of this chapter. Many of them have been reviewed elsewhere, and reviews of the English literature can be found online at www.acubriefs.com.

In the acubriefs database (www.acubriefs.com), the largest database of references regarding acupuncture in the English language (more than 17,000 references), there were 37 references with *geriatrics* or *gerontology* as a keyword. See Table 9.3 for a list of aging related conditions with at least case reports of acupuncture having a positive effect.

The list in Table 9.3 is not complete, yet it gives the reader a sense of the scope of conditions found in the elderly population that are suitable for acupuncture. Given the safety of acupuncture, it is reasonable to consider it in those patients who have conditions for which standard Western

TABLE 9.2 Positive Efficacy Results Based on Systematic Reviews

1. Low back pain
2. Fibromyalgia
3. Osteoarthritis
4. Acute dental pain
5. Headache showed a positive trend
6. Nausea and vomiting
7. Tobacco addiction

TABLE 9.3 Aging Related Conditions That May Respond Well to Acupuncture

Dementia

Low back pain

Chronic pain

Post herpetic neuralgia

Epigastric pain

Hypertension

Parkinson's disease

Rosacea

Urinary incontinence

Stroke rehabilitation

Peri-operative analgesia

Anxiety and depression

Insomnia

Macular degeneration

Menopausal symptoms

Spinal stenosis

Face lifts

Senile cholecystitis and cholelithiasis

Bell's palsy

Peripheral vascular disease

Peripheral neuropathies

approaches have had little success or for which standard interventions are associated with serious side effects and/or morbidity. Furthermore, if patients are going to respond to acupuncture, 80% start to respond within the first two or three treatments (Rotchford, 1991).

Acupuncture apparently has a significant role in minimizing some of the side effects of chemotherapy, radiation therapy, and other cancer treatments (Johnston, Polston, Niemtzow, & Martin, 2002; Li, 2002; Mak, 2001; Shen & Glaspy, 2001; Wen, 1977; Xie, Zhao, & Li, 2003). Quality of life issues can be especially pertinent in aged populations.

FINDING A REPUTABLE PRACTITIONER

Before going online to find a reputable practitioner, seeking the opinion of your primary care provider (PCP) is perhaps the best first step. If there is resistance or lack of interest on the part of your PCP, then other health care practitioners such as massage therapists or physical therapists may give you their opinion of local reputable practitioners. The online site for the American Academy of Medical Acupuncture (AAMA) (www.medicalacupuncture.org) is the best source to find American physicians qualified to provide medical acupuncture. The phone number is (323) 937-5514. Some AAMA members have demonstrated further competency by becoming certified in medical acupuncture; those who are designated as fellows have made special contributions to the field. In other countries the medical acupuncture society is always a good source for referrals. Links to these societies can be found at www.medical-acupuncture.co.uk/resource.htm#outside.

A listing of licensed acupuncturists can be found at www.acupuncture.com or at the National Certification Commission for Acupuncture and Oriental Medicine's site: www.nccaom.org. The phone number is (703) 548-9004.

CLINICAL EXPECTATIONS FOR MEDICAL ACUPUNCTURE

In China an individual may receive a dozen or so treatments merely as an introduction to an intensive series of treatment sessions. The expense of such an approach is often prohibitive in the West. Patients can choose to have two or three sessions to see if the acupuncture will be effective for them. Some people get relief immediately after a treatment; some notice improvement after a few hours, some after a few days. Usually by the end of the fifth day after a treatment people know if they've been helped. Some conditions require several treatments; some do not respond at all. The number of treatments, then, varies with each person and condition. If one has had a problem for a long time, then a series of 10 to 12 sessions is a reasonable expectation for an initial series of visits. Occasionally symptoms become worse after a treatment and may remain so for a few days before there is any relief. This is a good sign because it indicates that the symptom is treatable and that the acupuncturist has created movement in the vulnerable or affected area. Moreover, people sometimes have fleeting pain in other parts of their body after a treatment and even experience a temporary return of symptoms that they have not had for years.

Before a treatment it is best to be well rested and to eat only a light meal. It is advised to take no alcohol, sedatives, tranquilizers, or painkillers for 4 hours before a treatment unless directed otherwise by a physician. One should continue with other routine medications prescribed by a physician. Treatments generally last at least a half hour, and it is best to schedule at least an hour for each session. After the treatment it is best to take it easy for about 2 hours and to avoid alcohol, painkillers, and so on, during this time. If the treatment is for a painful condition, it is recommended to avoid strenuous activity for 2 days after the treatment, even if one is free of pain.

More and more insurance plans are covering acupuncture. In the United States, Medicare clearly does not cover the costs for any acupuncture. Fees for acupuncture generally range from $50 to $200, depending on the practitioner and services provided.

RESOURCES

For general information, I recommend www.medicalacupuncture.org or www.acupuncture.com. Both of these sites have links to other resources on the Web.

There is also the article "An Overview of Medical Acupuncture" by Joe Helms, MD, at www.medicalacupuncture.org/acu_info/articles/helmsarticle.html.

For research issues I recommend www.acubriefs.com. The site is easy to navigate and has links to other helpful sites pertinent to acupuncture research.

For physicians wondering about integrating acupuncture into their practices, I recommend *Integrating Acupuncture into a Western Medical Practice* by James K. Rotchford, MD, available at www.medicalacupuncture.org/acu_info/articles/incorporating.html.

REFERENCES

Berman, B. M., Ezzo, J., Hadhazy, V., & Swyers, J. P. (1999). Is acupuncture effective in the treatment of fibromyalgia? *Journal of Family Practice, 48*(3), 213–218.

Castera, P., Neguyen, J., Gerlier, J. L., & Sophie, R. (2002). Is acupuncture effective in smoking cessation? A meta-analysis [in French]. *Acupuncture and Moxibustion, 3–4,* 76–85.

Eckman, P. (1996). *In the footsteps of the Yellow Emperor.* San Francisco: Cypress Book Co.

Ernst, E., & Pittler, M. H. (1998). The effectiveness of acupuncture in treating acute dental pain: A systematic review. *British Dental Journal, 184*(9), 443–447.

Ernst, E., & White, A. (1997). Life-threatening adverse reactions after acupuncture? A systematic review. *Pain, 71*(2), 123–126.

Ernst, E., & White, A. R. (1998). Acupuncture for back pain: A meta-analysis of randomized controlled trials. *Archives of Internal Medicine, 158*(20), 2235–2241.

Ezzo, J., Baussell, B., Moerman, D. E., Berman, B., & Hadhazy, V. (2001). Reviewing the reviews: How strong is the evidence? How clear are the conclusions? International *Journal of Technology Assessment in Health Care, 17*(4), 457–466.

Ezzo, J., Hadhazy, V., Birch, S., Lao, L., Kaplan, G., Hochberg, M., et al. (2001). Acupuncture for osteoarthritis of the knee: A systematic review. *Arthritis and Rheumatism, 44*(4), 819–825.

Franglen, N. (2001). *Acupuncture: The five elements.* United Kingdome: Global Books.

Ghoname, E. A., Craig, W. F., White, P. F., Ahmed, H. E., Hamza, M. A., Henderson, B. N. et al. (1999). Percutaneous electrical nerve stimulation for low back pain: A randomized crossover study. *Journal of the American Medical Association, 281*(9), 818–823.

Gunn, C. C. (1996). *The Gunn approach to the treatment of chronic pain: Intramuscular stimulation for myofascial pain of radiculopathic origin* (2nd ed.). New York: Churchill Livingstone.

Helms, J. M. (1998). An overview of medical acupuncture. *Alternative Therapies in Health and Medicine, 4,* 35–45.

Huang, T. N. (1979). *The Yellow Emperor's classic of internal medicine: Simple questions.* Beijing: People's Health Publishing House. (First published c. 100 BCE).

Helms, J. M. (1995). *Acupuncture energetics: A clinical approach for physicians.* Berkeley, CA: Medical Acupuncture Publishers.

Johnstone, P. A., Polston, G. R., Niemtzow, R. C., & Martin, P. J. (2002). Integration of acupuncture into the oncology clinic. *Palliative Medicine, 16*(3), 235–239.

Kaptchuk, T. J. (1983). *The web that has no weaver: Understanding Chinese medicine.* New York: Congdon & Weed.

Li, D. (2002). Acupuncture treatment of vomiting caused by chemotherapy. *Journal of Traditional Chinese Medicine, 20*(4), 272, 273.

Maciocia, G. (1994). *The practice of Chinese medicine: The treatment of diseases with acupuncture and Chinese herbs.* New York: Churchill Livingstone.

MacPherson, H., Thomas, K., Walters, S., & Fitter, M. (2001). A prospective survey of adverse events and treatment reactions following 34,000 consultations with professional acupuncturists. *Acupuncture in Medicine, 19*(2), 93–102.

Mak, E. (2001). Abstract of "Acupuncture: Evidence and implications for cancer supportive care" (Shen, J., et al.). *Acubriefs Newsletter, 2*(7).

Melchart, D., Linde, K., Fischer, P., & Allais, G. (1999). Acupuncture for recurrent headaches: A systematic review of randomized controlled trials. *Cephalalgia, 19*(9), 779–786.

Nogier, P. (1972). *Traite d'auriculotherapie.* Moulins-les-Metz, France: Maisonneuve.

O'Connor, J., & Bensky, D. (Eds., Trans.). (1981). *Acupuncture, a comprehensive text.* Chicago: Eastland Press.

Pomeranz, B. (1996). Acupuncture and the raison d'etre for alternative medicine [interview by Bonnie Horrigan]. *Alternative Therapies in Health and Medicine, 2*(6), 85–91.

Rotchford, J. K. (1991). Medical outcomes research and acupuncture. *American Aacademy of Medical Acupuncture Review, 3*(1), 3–6.

Rotchford, J. K. (1998, October 30). Letting the horses run. *Patient Care,* 123–124.

Rotchford, J. K. (1999). Overview: Adverse events of acupuncture. *Medical Acupuncture, 11*(2), 32–35.

Rotchford, J. K. (2003). Abstract of "Is acupuncture effective in smoking cessation? A meta-analysis" (Castera, P., et al.). *Acubriefs Newsletter, 4*(3).

Rotchford, J. K., & Kobrin, L. E. (2002). The importance of a modern and comprehensive definition for acupuncture in clinical research: Preliminary perspectives. *Medical Acupuncture, 13*(3), 38–40.

Shen, J., & Glaspy, J. (2001). Acupuncture: Evidence and implications for cancer supportive care. *Cancer Practice, 9*(3), 147–150.

Siedentopf, C. M., Golaszewski, S. M., Mottaghy, F. M., Ruff, C. C., Felber, S., & Schlager, A. (2002). Functional magnetic resonance imaging detects activation of the visual association cortex during laser acupuncture of the foot in humans. *Neuroscience Letters, 327*(1), 53–56.

Vickers, A. (1996). Can acupuncture have specific effects on health? A systematic review of acupuncture antiemesis trials [Review]. *Journal of the Royal Society of Medicine, 89*(6), 303–311.

Weiner, D. K., Rudy, T., Glick, S., Boston, J. R., Lieber, S. J., Morrow, L. A. et al. (2003). Efficacy of percutaneous electrical nerve stimulation for the treatment of chronic low back pain in older adults. *Journal of the American Geriatrics Society, 51*(5), 599–608.

Wen, H. L. (1977). Cancer pain treated with acupuncture and electrical stimulation. *Modern Medicine of Asia, 13,* 12–16.

White, A., Cummings, M., Hopwood, V., & MacPherson, H. (2001). Informed consent for acupuncture: An information leaflet developed by consensus. *Acupuncture in Medicine, 19*(2), 123–129.

White, A., Hayhoe, S., Hart, A., Ernst, E., AACP, et al. (2001). Survey of Adverse Events Following Acupuncture (SAFA): A prospective study of 32,000 consultations. *Acupuncture in Medicine, 19*(2), 84–92.

Wong, J. Y. (1999). *A manual of neuro-anatomical acupuncture: Vol. 1. Musculoskeletal disorders.* Toronto: Toronto Pain and Stress Clinic.

Wong, J. Y. (2002). *A manual of neuro-anatomical acupuncture: Vol. 2. Neurological disorders.* Toronto: Toronto Pain and Stress Clinic.

World Health Organization. (1980). Use of acupuncture in modern health care. *WHO Chronicle, 34,* 294–301.

Worsley, J. R. (1990). *Traditional acupuncture: Vol. 2. Traditional diagnosis.* Leamington Spa, Warwickshire, UK: College of Traditional Acupuncture.

Worsley, J. R. (1993). *Traditional Chinese acupuncture: Vol. 1. The meridians and points.* Tisbury, England: Element Books.

Wu, M., Sheen, J., Chuang, K., Yang, P., Chin, S., Tsai, C., et al. (2002). Neuronal specificity of acupuncture response: A fMRI study with electroacupuncture. *Neuroimage, 16*(4), 1028.

Xie, L., Zhao, L., & Li, M. (2003). Zusanli point injection for treating leukopenia induced by radio-chemotherapy. *Journal of Traditional Chinese Medicine, 23*(1), 59–61.

CHAPTER TEN

The Benefits of Qigong

Kevin Chen, Elizabeth R. Mackenzie, and Master FaXiang Hou

WHAT IS QIGONG?

The word *qigong* (pronounced chi kung) is a combination of two Chinese ideograms: *qi,* meaning "breath of life" or "vital energy," and *gong,* meaning "skill or achievement," which implies the application of time and effort. Thus, *qigong* is often defined as "the skill of mastering vital energy (or bioenergy)."

Qigong has over a 3,000 year-old history in China. Qigong as a term has existed for a long time, but it did not become popular until the 1950s, when it gained public acceptance over other traditional and more abstruse terms such as *Daoyin* (conduction), *Tuina* (taking out the stale energy and putting in the fresh energy), *Yangxiou* (health maintenance and cultivation), *Xiounian* (cultivation and practice), and *Yangsheng* (health maintenance and improvement). However, there is still much misunderstanding of qigong due to some conceptual confusion.

Qigong is a general term that covers myriad forms of traditional Chinese energy exercises and therapies. There are over a thousand registered qigong schools or forms in contemporary China, and many more are not registered but are practiced informally. Many meditation forms in the United States could be called qigong in China. For example, Zen is one of the major Buddhist qigong traditions; Japanese Reiki originated from one of the medical qigong traditions in China, and yoga was called "Indian qigong" in China. There is no unvarying definition of qigong. According to the qigong textbook used in the Colleges of Chinese Medicine, qigong is considered to be a self-training method or process in which *qi* (vital energy) and *yi* (mind or intention) are cultivated through adjustment of body posture, breathing, and mental focus to achieve the optimal state of both body and mind (Liu, 1999).

This definition has four basic components: (1) The method is the cultivation of both *qi* and *yi* (mind and intention), not merely a physical exercise. Of course, some forms of qigong may also require physical movement, regulating body posture through movement and gestures, but these are secondary to the cultivation of consciousness or mind. (2) The purpose is to achieve optimal health of both body and mind, as distinguished from so-called hard qigong, which concentrates on qigong as a martial art, and other healing methods that only focus on the health of the body. (3) The process of healing comes through body posture, breathing, and mental focus. Integration of the three into one form or movement corresponds to the integration of body, mind, and spirit. (4) The mode is a form of self-training or a self-care process, not a treatment or quick-fix therapy. Although external qigong therapy (see discussion below) may achieve quick pain relief or improvement, it is not the essence of qigong training. Those who depend on a qigong master or expert to improve their health miss the essence and meaning of qigong. The word *gong* implies the accumulation of skill over time. The benefits of qigong training are mainly determined by the individual's commitment to qigong practice.

BASIC THEORY

Traditional Chinese medicine (TCM) posits the existence of a subtle energy *(Qi)* circulating throughout the entire human body, and existing around all living beings. When the internal qi is strengthened or balanced, it can improve health and ward off or slow the progress of disease. All TCM therapies, including herbs, acupuncture, massage, cupping, and qigong, are based on this perspective or philosophy. The same concept of bioenergy can also be found in many other cultures, such as *Ki* in Japan, *Prana* in India, and *Mana* in Hawaii and the Philippines.

According to TCM, good health is a result of a free-flowing, well-balanced *qi* (energy) system, whereas sickness or the experience of pain is the result of *qi* blockage or unbalanced energy in the body. Acupuncture shares the same *qi*-blood flow and meridian theory with qigong therapy. The meridian system used in acupuncture corresponds to the major channels of *qi* flow. The difference between the two is that acupuncture uses external force (needles or pressure stimulation) to help the *qi* flow and balance, whereas qigong uses mostly internal force (*qi* cultivation and self-practice), and sometimes external *qi,* to help smooth the *qi* flow and clear the *qi* blockage.

In addition to the concept of *qi* or vital energy, the concept of *yi* (mind or intention) plays a key role in qigong practice and qigong healing. TCM believes that most *qi* tends to follow the *yi (qi shui yi xing)*. When a person is under stress or experiencing many random thoughts for a long time, his or her *qi* cannot flow smoothly or normally, and the person will soon experience some *qi* imbalance (emotional disturbance) or *qi* blockage (physical symptom). Therefore, having the consciousness focus on one thing or nothing (mindfulness) is the key training in qigong practice, which is called "empty mind without desire state."

MAJOR QIGONG STYLES OR TRADITIONS

There have been thousands of different qigong forms and schools in Chinese history. Different methods can be used to classify these qigong schools. Traditionally, qigong exercises were passed from generation to generation within families in a private and sometimes secretive manner. Only recently has qigong become a public health practice in China. Although qigong was well known for its healing potential, most qigong forms were not created for the purpose of healing, but for the cultivation of mind and spirituality. Currently, the Chinese government classifies all contemporary qigong into two categories: preventive health qigong and medical (curative) qigong, ignoring its tradition of spirituality.

Historically, qigong can be roughly divided into five major disciplines or traditions: Confucian, Buddhist, Taoist, medical, and martial arts. Each discipline has its own set of goals and methods or forms. The following is a brief overview of the five major traditions in Chinese qigong development (Liang & Wu, 1997).

Confucian qigong was designed to attain a higher moral character and intelligence, and the focus was on education and moral development. This form of meditation was not very popular historically, but it reflects one of the essences of qigong—the focus on consciousness. The typical form in this tradition is a "listen to breathing" or "forgetting self" meditation.

Buddhist qigong, aimed at liberating the mind, emphasizes the cultivation of virtue and enlightening wisdom, and considers the health of the human secondary to spiritual concerns. A pure Buddhist qigong form would view health and healing as a "side effect" of developing a still mind and relaxed state. The Buddhist qigong traditions include Zen, Mi (Tibetan), and Tiantai.

Daoist (or Taoist) qigong, emphasizes the preservation of the physical body, along with spiritual cultivation. Most Daoist qigong consists of training in both the body (*qi,* or *Ming* = life) and the spirit (*yi,* or

Xing = spirituality). Because Daoism puts its emphasis on the current life and explores techniques for preserving long life, many Daoist qigong masters lived to an extremely old age. During a time when the average life expectancy was around 40, most Daoist qigong masters lived 90 or more years, and there are reports of masters living well beyond the normal span of years.

Medical qigong refers to those qigong forms created or practiced for the express purpose of preventing or curing disease. It is influenced greatly by Daoist philosophy but developed independently, shaped mostly by TCM practitioners. Historically, most famous TCM doctors were also good qigong practitioners. Medical qigong taught practitioners how to use the inner *qi* in a dynamic for diagnosis, healing, and preventing disease. Today, medical qigong is still a standard course in many schools of Chinese medicine. The typical medical qigong forms include five-animal qigong (by Hua Tuo), six-sound qigong, brighten-eye qigong, and *taiji* five-element qigong.

Martial arts qigong is intended to train the practitioner in both offense and defense, protecting the body from attacks with weapons and

Tai Chi

Tai chi, or *t'ai chi ch'uan (taiji quan)*, as it is sometimes called, is a form of qigong that is quite well known in the West. In fact, it is more common to find classes in tai chi than qigong, especially for seniors. The movements of tai chi are gentle, slow, and flowing and cultivate serenity in the student; it is thus perfectly suited to an elderly population. Many elderly Chinese practice tai chi daily.

The practice of tai chi consists of a carefully choreographed series of very slow movements designed to harmonize the flow of *qi* (or *chi*) within the body and between the body and the larger environment. From the traditional Chinese perspective, it is as much a meditative technique as a form of exercise.

The word *tai chi (taiji)* refers to the balance point between yin and yang, and one of the most obvious benefits to the practice of tai chi is improved balance. At least one randomized scientific study has found the practice of tai chi to improve balance for older adults (Wolf, 1996). Another more recent study found that the improved functional balance associated with the practice of tai chi reduced the risk of subsequent falls (Li et al., 2004). Many other studies have been conducted, exploring the potential of tai chi for a variety of conditions, including heart disease, stroke rehabilitation, depression, and arthritis.

Tai chi does require practitioners to be able to stand. For extremely frail elders or those confined to wheelchairs, there are forms of qigong that can be practiced seated or even lying down.

strengthening the body for aggressive attacks by powerful fist or foot movement. It also trains the body to deliver fatal blows that are enhanced with *qi,* such as the Burning Palm, or Iron Palm, methods. The cultivation of *qi* is what makes many of the most impressive martial arts demonstrations possible; however, many martial art qigong practitioners have died prematurely due to overexerting their body limits, and this form of qigong is not recommended for health promotion.

Qigong is as complex and rich as Chinese history and culture. As qigong gains in popularity, it is very important for a beginner to know which form of qigong is most appropriate for him or her. The above classification may also help beginners to learn how to determine the authenticity of a qigong form because there are many sham or fake qigong "masters" who do not know what qigong really is, and therefore tend to provide incomplete teachings or misleading instruction. Most qigong practices involve a combination of elements such as relaxation, breath work, guided imagery, slow movement, biofeedback, tranquil state, mindfulness meditation, and mind–body integration.

Medical Qigong

Medical qigong refers to the qigong forms used by traditional medical practitioners with an emphasis on how to use human vital energy for health promotion and disease prevention. Although qigong is considered a self training method through cultivation of *qi* and *yi* to achieve optimal status for both body and mind, the emission of *qi* (or external qigong therapy) has always been part of medical qigong practice in the attempt to help others to regain health. Therefore, one needs to distinguish between internal and external qigong forms in the history and development of medical qigong.

Internal Qigong

Internal training refers to qigong practice or cultivation by oneself to achieve the optimal health status for both mind and body. Self-training of qigong is the major part of qigong therapy.

Internal qigong training, or self-practice qigong, consists of three major forms: movement, standing pole, and static forms.

1. Movement, or active, qigong (mostly an introductory form) uses guided physical movements or gestures (forms) to help practitioners to concentrate on the cultivation and circulation of *qi* (bioenergy) in the body. *Taiji Quan (Tai Chi Kuan)* may be considered a form of movement qigong.

2. Static, or still, qigong is mostly meditation, which may include relaxation, breath work, mindfulness meditation, guided imagery, incantation, seal palm symbols, and a state of mindfulness (the most advanced form). The main purpose of static qigong is the training of intention or consciousness when cultivating *qi* energy. It is said that the intention or consciousness, once well trained, will lead *qi* flow in the body and direct it to where it is needed, thus clearing blocked areas. Blocked or stagnant *qi* is considered the origin of many illnesses and diseases.

3. The standing pole is a form between movement and static qigong, which usually starts with a standing position; as the qi is being cultivated or moved, various spontaneous movements will follow. The magnitude or degree of the movement varies and may even be greater than the movement qigong.

A Description of a Qigong Exercise

Standing pole is one of the most important and well-known qigong exercises. The name refers to the idea that one is like a pole standing upright between earth and heaven (or *yin* and *yang*), somehow connecting the two. Energy is drawn up from the earth, imagined as traveling up the back of the body, and then down the front to return to the earth, forming a complete circuit.

Standing Pole
Breath and movement are combined in this exercise to circulate *qi* throughout the meridian system. All movements should be slow, steady, and deliberate.

To begin, stand comfortably with shoulders relaxed, legs at shoulder width apart, and knees slightly bent. Your head should be slightly bowed, in a relaxed fashion. Keep your arms slightly away from your body. Your body should be totally relaxed: head, neck, arms, stomach, and pelvis.

Next, close your eyes, take a deep breath, and clear your mind. Inhale through your nose, slowly and steadily, and bring energy up the back of your body. As you inhale, imagine *qi,* or energy, entering through the soles of your feet and circulating up your legs and back and then over your head. Exhale through your mouth while imagining the energy moving down the front of your body. Be sure to breathe silently and calmly.

With each inhalation, concentrate on pulling the *qi* up your back. The qi moves through your heels and up the back of your legs. As the *qi* passes your knees, they straighten. When the *qi* reaches the base of the spine, begin to raise your shoulders, imagining that the movement is pulling the *qi* up the spine to the top of your head. Your hips, waist, and spine contract and rise as the *qi* moves through each area.

With each exhalation, concentrate on moving the *qi* down your front side; the movement of your body should follow the energy movement. Follow the movement of *qi* in your imagination from the top of your head as your shoulders move forward; follow it down across your forehead and face, down your chest, and down to your stomach. Here, the *qi* splits off and goes down both legs and your knees bend, then out the balls of your feet, back to the earth.

Repeat this sequence for at least 5 minutes, preferably longer. While doing the standing pole exercise, you may feel warmth in each area the *qi* passes through, or you may experience sensations such as cold or tingling or vibrations. As your practice continues, you may notice heightened sensations in various areas of your body.

Areas of blocked or stagnant qi may feel uncomfortable at first, but this will diminish with continued practice.

The Chinese have practiced various qigong forms for thousands of years to treat various diseases as well as to strengthen health and vitality. Today it is reported that over 100 million people practice qigong in China, and it has become increasingly popular internationally. People practice qigong therapy to treat such diseases as hypertension, arthritis, addiction, cancer, and human immunodeficiency virus (HIV) (Chen & Yueng, 2002; Feng, 1994; Li, Chen, & Mo, 2002; Liu, 1999; Sancier, 1996a,b, 1999). Practitioners credit qigong meditation with improving their daily lives in many ways, including

- A more relaxed, harmonious state of mind and body
- A noticeable reduction in prior ailments and a reduction in feelings of stress
- An increased resistance to illness through a stronger immune system
- A heightened sensitivity to the body's internal organs, with a developed ability to regulate their own health and vitality

Although internal qigong practice has been applied to all age groups, it is probably most appropriate for the elderly to integrate qigong into their daily life. It is never too late to start. Legend has it that Dongbin Lu, a famous Daoist qigong master (b. 798), started his qigong cultivation at the age of 64, and lived a life of more than 100 years.

External Qigong

External qigong therapy (EQT) refers to the process by which qigong practitioners direct or emit their *qi* energy to help others break *qi* blockages and induce the sick *qi* out of body so as to relieve pain, or balance the *qi* flow in the body and get rid of diseases. EQT can be practiced through the use of *qi* (emitting vital energy) or *yi*, the consciousness or intentional therapy, or a combination of the two techniques. Most schools of medical qigong will teach both techniques. Many qigong clinics in Chinese hospitals provide external qigong therapy.

In addition, medical qigong from the Daoism tradition uses bioinformation healing through symbols (Fu), or incantations (Zhou), or their derivatives. There is some reported clinical effectiveness for this therapy, but its mechanism in healing and how the bioinformation is transmitted are far beyond what science can understand at this stage.

Although the physical nature of *qi* remains as yet unproven, there are some intriguing reports that suggest the possibility of physical, biophysical, and/or biochemical alterations induced by qigong therapy or "*qi* emission" (Chen, 2004). For example, *qi* emissions by qigong masters have been reported to be associated with significant structural changes in aqueous solutions; to alter the phase behavior of dipalmitoyl phosphatidyl choline (DPPC) liposomes; to enable the growth of Fab protein crystals (Yan et al., 1999); to inhibit tumor growth in mice (Chen, Li, Liu, & He, 1997); to change the conformation of biomolecules like polyglutamic acid, polylysine, and metallothionein (Chu, He, Zhou, & Chen, 1998); to produce a spectrum shift in heat generation and a lightlike effect on AgBr film (Li et al., 1988); and to reduce phosphorylation of a cell-free preparation (Muehsami, Markow, & Muehsami, 1994). Thus, there is a small but growing body of scientific evidence that suggests the physical existence of *qi*, as well as the healing power of qigong therapy (Agishi 1998; Chen, 2004; Iwao, Kajiyama, Mori, & Ogaki, 1999; Loh, 1999; Sancier, 1996a,b, 1999; Wirth, Cram, & Chang, 1997; Wu et al., 1999).

MEDICAL APPLICATIONS OF QIGONG

Although most qigong forms were not designed for treating a specific disease, qigong practice is very effective in ameliorating the effects of many chronic conditions, such as hypertension, diabetes, allergy, asthma, arthritis, degenerative disk disease, cancer, depression, anxiety, and addiction. Qigong works on increasing the practitioners' self-healing capabilities, including immune functions (the self-defense system), self-recovery capability, and self-regeneration capability. The potential applications of qigong in health and healing are limitless and, to some extent, challenge our current understanding of life and health in general.

Most of the research in this area has been done in China and Japan, but clinical studies are increasingly being carried out in the United States.

The Qigong Institute in California has put together a qigong database, updated every few years, with many scientific studies of qigong around the world. The latest qigong database (version 7.0) contains about 3,400 entries (http://www.qigonginstitute.org/html/database.php).

Qigong Exercise Effectively Reduces Stress

Research has found that 80% of primary care doctor visits in the United States are related to stress. Many common conditions are related to stress, such as headache, hypertension, overweight, lower back pain, asthma, and allergy. Therefore, an effective stress management practice will greatly reduce health problems and increase the quality of life. The relaxation response produced by qigong exercise has been well documented in clinical studies of qigong. For example, He and colleagues (He, Le, Xi, & Zhang, 1999) applied a "stress meter" (equipment measuring skin conductivity) to evaluate the degree of relaxation achieved by qigong meditation versus nonqigong technique (relaxation meditation), and reported that the qigong meditation group achieved significantly deeper levels of relaxation than the control group. Sandlund and Norlander (2000) reviewed more than 20 studies of tai chi quan and stress management, and concluded that tai chi was an effective way to reduce stress; virtually all studies on the benefits of tai chi for seniors have revealed positive results. A randomized controlled study by Lee et al. (2001) reported that qigong therapy could significantly reduce anxiety and cortisol levels, and increase the cellular activities of neutrophil and natural killer cells.

Stroke and Mortality Rates Decreased With Qigong Practice

Sancier (1996b) reviewed a 30-year follow-up study on hypertension patients who were divided into a qigong group and a control group. All subjects were given drug therapy to control their blood pressure. The experimental group also practiced qigong. The mortality rate in the qigong group was nearly 50% lower than the group who did not practice qigong. The incidence of stroke as well as death due to stroke was half for those who practiced qigong. In other words, people who did not practice qigong suffered a stroke or died from stroke at a rate twice that of those who practiced qigong.

Researchers also reported that over the 30-year period, blood pressure of the qigong group stabilized, whereas that of the control group increased. Remarkably, during this period the drug dosage for the qigong group could be decreased and for 30% of the patients, could be eliminated. However, the drug dosage for the control group had to be increased (Sancier, 1996b).

Drug-Free Control of Hypertension

Mayer (1999) reviewed 30 representative studies, mostly in China, that explored the therapeutic effects of qigong therapy for hypertension, including the 30-year longitudinal follow-up study mentioned earlier, and concluded that qigong is an effective way to control hypertension without any adverse side effects.

Sex Hormone Levels Improved With Qigong

One consequence of aging is that the levels of sex hormones change in unfavorable directions. Sancier (1996b) reviewed three studies that indicated the trend of estrogen increasing in males and decreasing in females with age can be reversed by qigong exercise. In an auxiliary study, "changes were accompanied by improvements in symptoms such as soreness, dizziness, insomnia, hair loss, impotence, and incontinence associated with kidney deficiency hypertension (a TCM diagnosis)." (p. 42)

Increased Bone Density and Balance With Qigong

A study related to aging found that bone density was found to increase in male subjects who practiced qigong for 1 year (Sancier, 1996b). Sancier conjectured that qigong therapy also would help restore the bone density of women, especially menopausal women.

Wang, Collet, and Lau (2004) reviewed 12 studies on the effect of tai chi on balance and falls, and reported that long-term tai chi practice had favorable effects on the promotion of balance control, flexibility, and cardiovascular fitness and reduced the risk of falls in the elderly.

Qigong Improves Cardiovascular Conditions

Many studies have documented the improvement of cardiovascular conditions through qigong practice (Sancier, 1996a). For example, Lu, Liu, and Zhuang (1996) compared the treatment outcomes for patients with heart diseases in their clinical studies of qigong therapy with music, and found that the patients treated with qigong and music reported significantly higher rates of complete cure and significant improvement (10% and 32%, respectively) than the conventional medication group (5% and 21%, respectively; $p < .01$).

Wang et al. (2004) reviewed 16 studies of tai chi for patients with cardiorespiratory conditions, and reported that regular practice of tai chi will delay the decline of cardiorespiratory function in older adults and might be prescribed as a suitable exercise for them.

Qigong Therapy in Cancer Treatment

Chen and Yueng (2002) reviewed more than 50 research studies of qigong therapy for cancer preformed in the past 20 years from three different categories: clinical studies on human cancer patients, in vitro studies of cancer cells, and in vivo (animal) studies of cancer with qigong therapy. Most human studies involved clinical observation of cancer patients practicing qigong in comparison with a control group. The typical in vitro study involved randomly dividing the laboratory-prepared cancer cells or other cultures into different groups, with one group being treated with external qigong, plus one or two control groups. Sometimes, one group would be treated by sham qigong as a control. The typical in vivo study involved the injection of tumors or cancerous cells into mice, then randomly dividing the animals into various groups with one group treated by qigong. The control group could be either nontreatment or sham treatment.

No double-blinded clinical trial was found in the literature of human patient study, although many studies had at least one control group. For example, Sun and Zhao (1988) taught self-practice qigong to 93 of the 123 patients with various cancers, and found that the qigong group had significantly more improvement than the control group with conventional drugs only. Zheng et al. (1990) applied a comprehensive qigong therapy to 100 various late-stage cancer patients, and compared their survival rate with those who had other therapies in the same hospital. They reported that 1- and 5-year survival rates were 83% and 17%, respectively, for lung cancer patients (the control was 7% in 5 years), and 83% and 23%, respectively, for stomach cancer (the control was 12% in 5 years). The median survival period for liver cancer patients was 20.7 months in the qigong group, in comparison with 3.5 months in the control ($p < .01$). Fu, Fu, and Qin (1996) observed 186 postsurgery patients of cardiac adenocarcinoma for 8 years, and reported a much better 3- and 5-year survival rates among the patients with qigong therapy (64% and 36%, respectively) than the groups without qigong (36.5% and 20.8%, respectively; $p < .05$).

There seems to be a consistent finding that the group treated with qigong had significant improvement and/or a better survival rate than those treated with a conventional method alone; meanwhile, those who were treated by qigong therapy reported significantly fewer side effects from conventional therapies such as chemotherapy and radiation therapy. The cancer cells used in in vitro studies include human breast cancer cell lines, erythroleukemia (K562), promyelocytic leukemia, nasopharynglioma, nasopharyngeal carcinoma (CNE-2), SGC-7901 gastric adenocarcinoma, spleen cells of mice, and lung tumor cell line (LA-795). Most of the studies have demonstrated the inhibitory effect of qigong on the growth of these cancer cells in comparison with the control groups and sham-treated groups. Most in vivo studies reported that the qigong-treated group often had significantly reduced tumor growth and/or longer survival lives among the cancer-infected animals. In conclusion, there is ample evidence suggesting that qigong therapy brings about an inhibitory effect on cancer growth, both in vitro and in vivo studies. There is room for improvement in these studies, and some studies require replication in order to verify their findings; however, qigong therapy for cancer treatment is an area that is often neglected by mainstream medical research, and it should be seriously examined and considered as an important supplement to conventional cancer treatment (Chen & Yueng, 2002).

There are some anecdotal reports of qigong effectiveness for late-stage cancer patients that indicate that qigong may have powerful curative properties. For example, Yun Liao, a high school teacher from Liuzhou, at age 58 recovered from recurrent breast cancer with post-surgery metastasis to bone using medical qigong therapy alone, after she was told by her doctor there was no effective medical treatment for her condition. Not only her metastatic cancer was gone, but other chronic diseases she had previously suffered (before cancer), such as diabetes, prolapse of lumbar intervertebral disk, and fatty liver, disappeared without any medication (Liao, 1997). M. X. Shen, age 68, the vice principal of Shantou University, used the same qigong therapy to treat his reoccurring liver cancer after three failed surgeries. After 4 months of intensive qigong practice without any drugs or other therapies, his liver cancer disappeared completely; meanwhile, his hepatocirrhosis and hepatitis B disappeared as well without any medication (Shen, 1997).

Cure for Arthritis

Studies involving qigong therapy for arthritis treatment reported that, with qigong practice alone, or combining qigong practice with external qigong therapy and acupuncture, complete remission or marked improvement for rheumatoid arthritis or osteoarthritis could reach 40% to 75% of patients (Feng, Li, & Liu, 1996; Li, 1996).

Chen and Liu (2004) reviewed more than 20 studies of qigong therapy in the treatment of various forms of arthritis, including osteoarthritis, rheumatoid arthritis, scapulohumeral periarthritis, cervical spondylopathy, and arthromyodynia. Most subjects in these studies did not respond to the conventional therapies for their problems. However, qigong therapy (self-practice qigong and/or external qigong therapy) produced significant improvement or complete cure for a large proportion of these patients in many of the reviewed studies.

Recently Chen and Liu (2004) at the University of Medicine and Dentistry of New Jersey (UMDNJ) conducted an open trial of qigong therapy for arthritis to determine if external qigong therapy might be of benefit to patients with chronic arthritis. Ten patients with arthritis participated, and six completed the protocol. All six patients reported reduction in pain, movement difficulty, and anxiety scores. All but one had a decrease in negative mood score and active pain/tender joint count. Two patients reported complete relief, a response that persisted at the 1-month follow-up. Although the results of this pilot study are far from conclusive (due to its design and small size), the positive outcomes suggest that larger, randomized, controlled studies are warranted to confirm benefit from qigong treatment of arthritis (Chen & Liu, 2004).

Complex Regional Pain Syndrome

Wu and colleagues (1999) of UMDNJ studied patients who were taught to practice qigong and patients who were taught an exercise that resembled qigong (the sham group). After 10 weeks, 91% of the qigong patients reported a transient drop in pain compared to only 36% of the control group. A long-term reduction in anxiety in patients suffering from treatment-resistant CRPS-I also was found.

Senility Symptoms Improved With Qigong Practice

In a controlled study by Sancier (1996b) on the mechanism of keeping fit by qigong, 100 subjects were classified either as presenile or with cerebral function impaired by senility. The control group (which did not practice qigong) exercised by walking, walking fast, or running slowly. Criteria for judging outcome were based on measuring clinical signs and symptoms, including cerebral function, sexual function, serum lipid levels, and function of the endocrine glands. The results were that, after 6 months, 8 of the 14 main clinical signs and symptoms in the qigong group had improved more than 80%, whereas none of the symptoms in the control group had improved more than 45%.

Enhanced Activity of Antiaging Enzyme SOD

Superoxide dismutase (SOD) is often called an antiaging enzyme because it is believed to destroy free radicals that may cause aging. However, the activities of this naturally produced enzyme tend to decline as we age. In a study of qigong to treat disorders of retired workers in China (Xu, Xue, Bian, Zhang, & Zhou, 1993), researchers included determinations of plasma SOD, and found that the mean level of SOD was increased significantly by qigong exercise. For example, the SOD level in the qigong group (about 2,700 µ/g Hb) was significantly larger than in the control group (1,700 µ/g Hb; $p < .001$).

Neurological Applications

Sancier (1996b) reviewed two studies where qigong exercise has been shown to increase blood flow to the brain. For subjects with cerebral arteriosclerosis who practice qigong for 1 to 6 months, improvements were noted in symptoms such as memory, dizziness, insomnia, tinnitus, numbness of limbs, and vertigo headache. During these studies, a decrease in plasma cholesterol was also noted. In a study of the effect of qigong on the nervous system, the researcher suggests that qigong meditation may bring about excitatory or inhibitory effects of the central nervous system, thereby unmasking or enhancing the functions that are not part of the normal repertoire of the nervous system.

In the conclusion of the review, Sancier (1996b) wrote, "This review encompasses only a small number of studies from a large collection of research using medical applications of Qigong, mainly in China. The main conclusion from many studies is that Qigong enables the body to heal itself" (p. 44).

Recently, Chen and Turner (2004) published their case study of applying qigong therapy to help a patient recovered from multiple physical symptoms in a short time. In this case, the 60-year-old male patient suffered from a high prostate cancer mark (PSA 12), atrial septal defect, asthma, allergies, multiple injuries from an auto accident, high blood pressure, and edema in the legs. After 2 months of intensive qigong practice, he recovered simultaneously from all these symptoms without any medications. This near miraculous recovery and other documented successes call for formal clinical studies to closely examine the self-healing potential of qigong therapy.

HOW DOES QIGONG WORK?

The mechanism of how qigong works to achieve health benefits is the subject of further scientific exploration. In the review of qigong therapy for cancer, Chen and Yueng (2002) summarized the following scientifically verified mechanism of qigong anticancer features, which may help us to understand qigong healing in general.

1. Qigong therapy improves immune functions. The human body has a powerful immune system to defend itself, but most cancer patients

experience some form of immune deficiency that makes it possible for cancer cells to stay and outlive normal cells. Studies suggest that qigong therapy or qigong practice may help cancer patients increase their immune functions. For example, Feng and colleagues (1988) found that external qi from a qigong healer could enhance the phagocytosis of peritoneal macrophages and increase the activity of acid phosphatase. (Feng et al., 1988). Zhang (1995) reported that qigong practice had significantly increased cancer patients' C_3b rate of red blood cells, the rate of lymphocyte transformation, and phagocytosis of phagocytes. Lei and colleagues (Lei, Bi, Zhang, & Cheng, 1991) examined the in vivo antitumor effect of EQT on the immunologic functions of tumor-bearing mice, and found that the EQT group had significantly higher NK activities, MTC activity, and interleukin-2 (IL-2) levels ($p < .01$). Many studies have shown that the increase of NK cells and many other components of the immune system can significantly reduce the chances of infection or tumor growth (Cai, Banner, Glickman, & Odze, 2001; Feng, Qian, & Chen, 1990). Given the fact that many conventional cancer therapies tend to damage patients' immune functions, which reduces patients' overall capacity for self-recovery, the improvement in the immune system from qigong therapy offers powerful complementary tool in the fight against cancer.

2. Qi energy may directly turn off cancer cells and produce apoptosis. In a study of the inhibitory effect of EQT on transplanted tumor in mice, Chen et al. (1997) found that morphological alterations in the tumor cells from qigong-treated mice include decreased cell volume; nuclear condensation, nuclear fragmentation; decreased ratio of nucleus to cytoplasm; swollen mitochondria, with poorly organized mitochondrial cristae; and some vacuolated and many apoptotic bodies in the extracellular space. These results suggested that EQT might have produced apoptotic effects on the transplanted hepatocarcinoma in mice (Chen et al., 1997). A similar structural analysis was performed by Feng (1994) after EQT studies on cancer cells, who found that the total abnormality rate of chromosomes in the qigong group (5.39%) was significantly higher than that of the control group (1.40%).

3. Qigong therapy increases microcirculation functions. Microcirculation refers to the blood circulation between microartery and microvein (capillary). Qigong practice has been reported to improve the practitioner's microcirculation, changing the viscosity of blood, increasing the elasticity of blood vessels, and controlling the concentration of platelets (Shen & Gao, 1995). Wang et al. (2004) measured the skin temperature before and during qigong practice, and found an increase in facial temperature and increased infrared radiation from the palm. Another study reported a significant increase in microcirculation of nail wrinkles among 19 subjects, from a mean of 8.2 lines/mm prior to qigong practice

to 12.6 lines/mm after qigong ($p < .001$) (Shen & Gao, 1995). The researchers concluded that qigong therapy could adjust the microcirculation function to the optimal state by accelerating blood flow, raising the skin temperature, and increasing the number of microblood vessels, which in turn increases the oxygen and blood supplies to the tissues and cells, strengthens metabolism, and changes the pathological state to a normal biological state.

4. Qigong therapy can raise the pain threshold. Psychologists in China explored the possibility that qigong therapy may raise the pain threshold. Wang (1988) of the China Academy of Science tested the pain threshold at different body locations among 59 cancer patients, found the pain threshold at the right inner joints increased from 122.2 g before to 164.07 g during qigong practice ($p < .01$), and the pain threshold at the left inner joints increased from 100.0 g to 125.76 g during qigong practice. Zhang, Yan, and Zhou (1990) also reported the analgesic effect of external *qi* in a placebo–control study, and they found that external qigong could increase human skin pain threshold, measured by the method of potassium-mediated pain. Yang et al. (1988) reported the analgesic effect of emitted *qi* on rats, which made the psychological effect on pain less likely.

Various traditions of qigong may have different explanations on how qigong works for health and healing. Throughout its whole history, qigong has been employed and developed as a method for prevention, strengthening the mind and body and sometimes curing illness. Qigong's main therapeutic properties may well lie in its regulation of the respiration system, the metabolism system, activity of the cerebral cortex, the central nervous system, and the cardiovascular system, as well as its effect in correcting abnormal reactions of the organs, massaging effect on the organs of the abdominal cavity, and its effect on self-control over the physical functions of one's body. However, there is not enough research or data to document these effects yet. According to TCM and available scientific literature in Chinese, qigong may work to benefit practitioners through the following possible paths.

Motivated qi (vital energy) strikes against sick locations. According to TCM, good health is a result of a free flowing and well-balanced *qi* (energy) system, whereas sickness and the experience of pain are the results of *qi* blockage or unbalanced energy in certain areas of the body. *Qi* imbalance is the precursor of any physical illness. One way to stay healthy and function well is to perform qigong exercises in order to keep the *qi* flowing smoothly in the body so that each cell in the body gets a constant supply of vital energy. Once the supply of *qi* to the cells becomes blocked, blood flow to that area will change, the cells or related organs might start to malfunction, and disease or pain may occur. One possible mechanism of qigong therapy for pain relief and symptom reduction is through motivating *qi* and energy within the body, breaking the *qi* blockage, and balancing the energy system. Therefore, it is common for qigong practitioners to report more serious symptoms or pain on a temporary basis due to *qi* striking against sick locations. These pains or symptoms will go away completely with continued practice.

Cultivation of yi (consciousness and intention) and the emphasis of "empty mind without desire" in qigong practice may help practitioners strengthen their consciousness power and intention energy, release suppressed emotions, and resolve mental disturbances. It is said that qigong training of mind or intention helps practitioners to be released from the socialized self or consciousness (the source of all stress), and returned to the original self or natural consciousness. Many chronic diseases of unknown origin may well be related to mental disturbances, social pressures, or emotional repression. Qigong practice may lead to the release of these emotional disturbances, which may have been the sources of many chronic diseases. It is a common phenomenon for qigong practitioners to cry or laugh during their qigong practice, then feel a sense of complete relief after the practice.

Enhance the body's potential self-healing capability with quality qigong practice. This includes increasing the immune function, the self-repair capability, and the self-regeneration capability. For example, the relaxed and tranquil state achieved during qigong practice can relieve stress, build up vital energy, and rapidly increase the immune function. There is some scientific evidence to connect relaxation and guided imagery with increase immune functioning, whereas stress and depression are implicated in the malfunctioning of the immune system.

HOW TO FIND—AND WHAT TO EXPECT FROM—A QUALIFIED QIGONG MASTER

According to Hou and Wiley (1999), "The only way to judge the skill of a truly qualified master is by the documented results of his treatments." In general, there is a scarcity of qualified qigong healers in the United States who can perform a good external *qi* healing. Therefore, we suggest caution in seeking a qigong master. Because there is no qigong accrediting or licensing system in the United States, one would have to take into consideration the teacher/practitioner's background and training when deciding which qigong form and which instructor to choose. One of the most practical ways is to speak to his or her patients and students to get a sense of their satisfaction. However, there are some other criteria one can use. The Qigong Institute has developed the following guidelines to help scientists who are interested in qigong research to select the appropriate qigong healers or masters in their exploration of qigong. We list these criteria here in an attempt to help the general public identify qualified qigong instructors or healers.

According to the Qigong Institute guidelines, in general, a good qigong healer or master should meet at least three of the following seven criteria:

1. A specially invited member or director of the Chinese Society of Qigong Science (about 1,000 of such members exist in China who have been officially evaluated by the society)
2. A recorded history of scientific research (with published paper(s) or certified report(s))
3. A member of the national or international professional qigong organization(s)
4. A formal disciple of a traceable and renowned qigong master or qigong tradition, such as lineage holder or representative of a special form
5. A solid medical training or background, and preferably belonging to some kind of national organization of medical practitioners
6. Someone who does not currently have any verifiable negative claim against him or her in the field
7. Someone with an established qigong healing practice in this country (some may be visitors with similar qualifications in their home country)

When choosing a qigong class, ask with whom the teacher has studied and what form(s) he or she has mastered, as well as the number of years he or she has studied qigong.

EXPECTATIONS FOR EXTERNAL *QI* HEALING

Some qigong healers may combine medical massage with *qi* healing, and some acupuncturists with qigong training may also perform external *qi* healing in their practice. From the documented success of external qigong therapy, the conditions that can be treated most effectively by external *qi* healing are chronic pain and acute injuries, such as arthritis, lower back pain, degenerative disk disease, fractures, and joint inflammation. EQT can be effective for cardiovascular conditions and chronic fatigue syndrome. It may also be helpful for cancer patients, but the cancer patients should practice qigong meditation themselves to maximize the benefits of qigong therapy.

Before a treatment it is best to be well rested and to eat only a light meal. Anything that may block the *qi* flow in the body, such as a full stomach or strong emotions, is not a good state in which to receive external *qi* healing. The length of EQT varies tremendously by individual healers, which can be as short as 2 minutes or as long as 1 hour. Usually a complete course of treatment needs three to five continuous sessions. For a well-experienced healer on some acute injury, one treatment may make the difference.

No insurance currently covers external qigong therapy. Fortunately, the costs of participating in a qigong class are comparable to any yoga or tai chi class. Fees for external qigong therapy vary by healer, but they generally range from $30 to $500 for each session, depending on the practitioner and the services provided. After a truly good external qigong healing, it may take a long period of qigong meditation for the practitioner to gain his or her energy back, and this limits the number of clients he or she can see in a day.

CONCLUSION

Although the topic of qigong may seem complicated and mysterious, most of the beginning exercises themselves are simple and easily learned. They are also typically not physically strenuous (compared with most types of yoga), and meditative qigong can be practiced by anyone, even those with severe physical limitations. The main challenge is to locate a good teacher or master. Tai chi, a kind of qigong, is fairly widespread in the United States and is a good place to begin to learn about traditional Chinese energy healing if no qigong teachers can be found.

RESOURCES

For general information, we recommend:

The Qigong Institute
561 Berkeley Avenue
Menlo Park, CA 94025
http://www.qigonginstitute.org

National Qigong Association
P.O. Box 252
Lakeland, MN 55043
or http://www.nqa.org

Both of these sites have links to other resources on the Web.

Other organizations with informative Web sites are:

Qigong Research Society
http://www.qigongresearchsociety.org

World Institute for Self Healing
http://www.wishus.org

Qi: The Journal of Traditional Eastern Health and Fitness
http://www.qi-journal.com/qigong.asp

Acupuncture.com: Gateway to Chinese Medicine, Health and Wellness
http://Acupuncture.com/QiKunInd.htm

Books

Cohen, K. S. (1997). *The way of qigong: The art and science of Chinese energy healing.* New York: Ballantine Books.
FaXiang Hou, & Wiley, M. V. (1999). *Qigong for health and well-being.* VT: Journey Editions.
Jahnke, R. (2002). *The healing promise of Qi: Creating extraordinary wellness through qigong and tai chi.* New York: Contemporary Books.

REFERENCES

Agishi, T. (1998). Effects of the external qigong on symptoms of arteriosclerotic obstruction in the lower extremities evaluated by modern medical technology. *Artificial Organs, 22*(8), 707–710.
Cai, Y. C., Banner, B., Glickman, J., & Odze, R. D. (2001). Cytokeratin 7 and 20 and thyroid transcription factor 1 can help distinguish pulmonary from gastrointestinal carcinoid and pancreatic endocrine tumors. *Human Pathology, 32,* 1087–1093.
Chen, K. (2004). An analytic review of studies on measuring effects of external qi in China. *Alternative Therapies in Health and Medicine, 10*(4), 38–50.
Chen, K., He, B. H., Rihacek, G. & Sigal, L. H. (2003). A pilot study of external qigong therapy for arthritis pain. *Journal of Clinical Rheumatology, 9*(5), 332–335.
Chen, K., & Liu, T. J. (2004). Effects of qigong therapy on arthritis: A review and report of a pilot trial. *Medical Paradigm, 1*(1), 36–48.
Chen, K., & Marbach, J. J. (2002). External qigong therapy for chronic orofacial pain. *Journal of Alternative and Complementary Medicine, 8*(5), 532–534.
Chen, K., Shiflett, S. C., Ponzio, N. M., He, B., Elliott, D. K., & Keller, S. E. (2002) A preliminary study of the effect of external Qigong on lymphoma growth in mice. *Journal of Alternative and Complementary Medicine, 8*(5), 615–621.

Chen, K., & Turner, F. D. (2004). A case study of simultaneous recovery from multiple physical symptoms with medical qigong therapy. *Journal of Alternative and Complementary Medicine, 10*(1), 159–162.

Chen, K., & Yeung, R. (2002). Exploratory studies of qigong therapy for cancer in China. *Integrative Cancer Therapies, 1*(4), 345–370.

Chen, X., Li, Y., Liu, G., & He, B. (1997). The inhibitory effects of Chinese Taijing Five-Element Qigong on transplanted hepatocarcinoma in mice. *Asian Medicine, 11,* 36–38.

Chu, D. Y., He, W. G., Zhou, Y. F., & Chen, B. C. (1998). The effect of Chinese Qigong on the conformation of biomolecule. *Chinese Journal of Somatic Science, 8*(4), 155–159.

Cohen, K. (1997). *The way of qigong.* New York: Ballantine Wellspring.

Feng, L. D. (1994). *Modern qigong science.* Beijing: Economic Science Publisher.

Feng, L. D., Li, Q., & Liu, Z. (1996, September). *Therapeutic effects of emitted qi on rheumatoid arthritis.* Paper presented at the Third World Conference on Medical Qigong, Beijing.

Feng, L., Qian, J., & Chen, S. (1990). *Research on reinforcing NK-cells to kill stomach carcinoma cells with waiqi (emitted qi).* Paper presented at the Third National Academic Conference on Qigong Science, Guangzhou, China.

Feng, L. D., Qian, J. Q., Chen, S. Q., et al. (1988, October). *A study of the effect of the emitted Qi of Qigong on human carcinoma cells.* Paper presented at the First World Conference for Academic Exchange of Medical Qigong, Beijing.

Fu, J. Z., Fu, S. L., & Qin, J. T. (1996, September). *Effect of qigong plus anti-cancer body-build herbs on the prognosis of postoperative patients with cardiac adenocarcinoma.* Paper presented at the Third World Conference on Medical Qigong, Beijing.

He, H. Z., Li, D. L., Xi, W. B., & Zhang. C. L. (1999). A "stress meter" assessment of the degree of relaxation in qigong vs. non-qigong meditation. *Frontier Perspectives, 8*(1), 37–42.

Hisamitsu, T., Seto, A., Nakazato, S., Yamamoto, T., & Aung, S. K. H. (1996). Emission of extremely strong magnetic fields from the head and whole body during oriental breathing exercises. *International Journal of Acupuncture and Electro-Therapy Research, 21,* 219–227.

Hou, F. X., & Wiley, M. (1999). *Qigong for health and well-being.* Boston and Tokyo: Journey Editions.

Iwao, M., Kajiyama, S., Mori, H., & Ogaki, K. (1999). Effects of qigong walking on diabetic patients: A pilot study. *Journal of Alternative and Complementary Medicine, 5*(4), 353–358.

Kiang, J. G., Marotta, D., Wirkus, M., & Jonas, W. B. (2002).External bioenergy increases intracellular free calcium concentration and reduces cellular response to heat stress. *Journal of Investigative Medicine, 50*(1), 38–45.

Lee, M. S., Huh, H. J., Hong, S. S., et al. (2001). Psychoneuroimmunological effects of Qi-therapy: Preliminary study on the changes of level of anxiety, mood, cortisol and melatonin and cellular function of neutrophil and natural killer cells. *Stress Health, 17,* 17–24.

Lee, M. S., Lee, M. S., Kim, H. J., & Moon, S. R. (2003). Qigong reduced blood pressure and catecholamine levels of patients with essential hypertension. *International Journal of Neuroscience, 113,* 1707–1717.

Lei, X. F., Bi, A. H., Zhang, Z. X., & Cheng, Z. Y. (1991). The anti-tumor effects of Qigong-emitted external Qi and its influence on the immunologic function of tumor bearing mice. *Journal of Tongji Medical University, 11*(4), 253–256.

Li, M., Chen, K., & Mo, Z. X. (2002). Heroin detoxification with Qigong therapy. *Alternative Therapies in Health and Medicine, 8*(1), 50–59.

Li, S. H. (1996, September). *Treating rheumatoid arthritis with qigong: Clinical observation of 120 cases.* Paper presented at the Third World Conference on Medical Qigong, Beijing

Li, S. P., Meng, X. Y., & Tsui, Y. H. (1988). The effect of qigong on the electron magnetic resonance spectrum of AgBr. P.81. In *Proceedings of the 1st World Conference for the Academic Exchange of Medical QiGong* (Chinese). Beijing.

Li F, Harmer P, Fisher KJ, McAuley E Li F, Harmer P, Fisher KJ, McAuley E. (2004). Tai Chi: Improving functional balance and predicting subsequent falls in older persons. *Medicine and Science in Sports and Exercise, 36,* 2046–2052.

Liang, S. Y., & Wu, W. C. (1997). *Qigong empowerment: A guide to medical, Taoist, Buddhist, and Wushu energy cultivation.* East Providence, RI: The Way of the Dragon Publishing.

Liao Y. (1997). Taiji Five-Element Qigong saved my life from the terminal metastatic cancer. *China Qigong Science, 8,* 20–21.

Lin, Z., & Chen, K. (2002). Exploratory studies of external qi in China. *Journal of International Society of Life Information, 20*(2), 457–461.

Litscher, G., Wenzel, G., Niederwieser, G., & Schwarz, G. (2001). Effects of QiGong on brain function. *Neurological Research, 23*(5), 501–505.

Liu, T. (1999). *Qigong study in Chinese medicine.* Beijing: People's Health Publisher.

Loh, S. H. (1999). Qigong therapy in the treatment of metastatic colon cancer. *Alternative Therapies in Health and Medicine, 5*(4), 111–112.

Lu, L. T., Liu, Y. K., & Zhuang, Y. B. (1996, September). *The clinical study of coronary heart disease treated by Qigong with music.* Paper presented at the Third World Conference on Medical Qigong, Beijing.

Lu, Z. Y. (1997). *Scientific qigong exploration: The wonders and mysteries of qi.* Malvern, PA: Amber Leaf Press.

Mayer, M. H. (1999). Qigong and hypertension: A critique of research. *Journal of Alternative and Complementary Medicine, 5*(4), 371–382.

McGee, C. T., with Chow, E. P. Y. (1994). *Miracle healing from China: Qigong.* Coeur d'Alene, ID: Medipress.

Muehsami, D. J., Markow, M. S., & Muehsami, P. A. (1994). Effects of Qigong on cell-free myosin phosphorylation: Preliminary experiments. *Subtle Energies, 5,* 103–104.

Sancier, K. M. (1996a). Anti-aging benefits of Qigong. *Journal of International Society of Life Information Science, 14*(1), 12–21.

Sancier, K. M. (1996b). Medical applications of qigong. *Alternative Therapies in Health and Medicine, 2*(1), 40–45.

Sancier, K. M. (1999). Therapeutic benefits of qigong exercises in combination with drugs. *Journal of Alternative and Complementary Medicine, 5,* 383–389.

Sancier, K. M., & Chow, E. P. Y. (1989). Healing with Qigong and quantitative effects of Qigong measured by a muscle test. *Journal of the American College of Traditional Chinese Medicine, 7*(3), 13–19.

Sandlund, E. S., & Norlander, T. (2000). The effects of Tai Chi Chuan relaxation and exercise on stress responses and well-being: An overview of research. *International Journal of Stress Management, 7*(2), 139–149.

Singh, B., Berman, B., Hadhazy, V., & Creamer, P. (1998). A pilot study of cognitive behavioral therapy in fibromyalgia. *Alternative Therapies in Health and Medicine, 24*(2), 67–70.

Shen, G. X., & Gao, J. X. (1995). Exploration of the mechanisms of Qigong anticancer therapy [in Chinese]. *Zhongguo Qigong kexue (China Qigong Science), 2*(8), 30–31.

Shen, M. X. (1997). Qigong is an effective way to defeat cancer [in Chinese]. *China Qigong Science, 5,* 8–10.

Sun, Q. Z., & Zhao, L. (1988, October). *Clinical observation of qigong as a therapeutic aid for advanced cancer patients.* Paper presented at the First World Conference for Academic Exchange of Medical Qigong, Beijing.

Tsang, H. W. H., Mok, C. K., Yeung, Y. T.A., & Chan, S. Y. C. (2003). The effect of qigong on general and psychological health of elderly with chronic physical illnesses: A randomized clinical trial. *International Journal of Geriatric Psychiatry, 18,* 441–449.

Wang, C. C., Collet, J. P., & Lau, J. (2004). The effect of Tai Chi on health outcomes in patients with chronic conditions. *Archive of Internal Medicine, 164,* 493–501.

Wang, J. M. (1988, October). *On the Anti-tumor mechanism of Qigong.* First World Conference Acad. Exch. Med. Qigong. Beijing, China.

Wirth, D. P., Cram, J. R., & Chang, R. J. (1997). Multisite electromyographic analysis of therapeutic touch and Qigong therapy. *Journal of Alternative and Complementary Medicine, 3*(2), 109–118.

Wolf, S. L., Barnhart, H. X., Kutner, N. G., McNeely, E., Coogler, C., Xu, T., & Atlanta FICSIT Group. (1996). Reducing frailty and falls in older persons: An investigation of Tai Chi and computerized balance training. *Journal of the American Geriatric Society, 44,* 489–497.

Wu, W. H., Bandilla, E., Ciccone, D. S., Yang, J., Cheng S. S., Carner, N., Wu, Y., & Shen, R. (1999). Effects of Qigong on late-stage complex regional pain syndrome. *Alternative Therapies in Health and Medicine, 5*(1), 45–54.

Xu, H. F., Xue, H. N, Bian, M. G., Zhang, C. M., & Zhou, S. Y. (1993). *Clinical study of the anti-aging effect of qigong.* Paper presented at the Second World Conference for Academic Exchange of Medical Qigong, Beijing.

Yan, X., Fong, Y. T., Wolf, G., Wolf, D., & Cao, W., (2001). Protective effect of XY99-5038 on hydrogen peroxide induced cell death in cultured retinal neurons. *Life Science, 69,* 289–299.

Yan, X., Lin, H., Li, H., Traynor-Kaplan, A., Xia, Z. Q., Lu, F., et al. (1999). Structure and property changes in certain material influenced by the external Qi of Qigong. *Material Research Innovation, 2,* 349–359.

Yan, X., Lu, F., Jiang, H., Wu, X., Cai, W., Xia, Z., et al. (2002). Certain physical manifestation and effects of external Qi of Yan Xin Life Science Technology. *Journal of Scientific Exploration, 16*(3), 381–411.

Yu, W. P., & Bi, Y. S. (1990). Medical Qigong. In *The English-Chinese Encyclopedia of Practical TCM* (Vol. 8). Beijing: Higher Education Press.

Zhang, L., Yan, X. Z., & Zhou, Y. (1990). *Study of enhancement in inducing anti-tumor lymphokines by Qigong Waiqi on immunosuppressed mice.* Paper presented at the Third National Academy Conference on Qigong Sciences, Beijing.

Zhang, R. M. (1995). Clinical observation and experimental study of Qigong therapy for cancer. *Chinese Qigong Science, 2*(8), 24–29.

Zheng, R. R., et al. (1990). Observation of 100 cases with comprehensive Qigong therapy for treating later-stage cancer [in Chinese]. *World Qigong, 1990,* 3, 19.

CHAPTER ELEVEN

Yoga:
An Introduction

Robert Butera

> It might surprise you to learn that traditionally, the ideal age to begin the practice of Yoga was said to be fifty-three, the age marking one's passage into a new stage of life, one of contemplation and self-discovery.
> —Alice Christensen, *Easy Does It Yoga*

Yoga is an original and ancient holistic art of living that includes physical, mental, moral, and spiritual spheres of human existence. A Sanskrit word, *yoga* means "to join" or "union," and the practice of yoga brings this union to all levels of one's self. Popular usage of the term focuses primarily on exercises beneficial for physical health, and many people have experienced yoga in stretching classes. As the past 2 decades have witnessed, yoga has increasingly become an accepted practice. Medical doctors, psychotherapists, chiropractors, and nurses are recommending yoga to help reduce stress. More people spend their vacations at retreats and seek to discover their happiness by spiritually motivated living. The further one explores the depths of yoga practice and tradition, the more one integrates its holistic and transforming qualities.

BACKGROUND

Yoga originated in India thousands of years ago. The authoritative text on classical yoga is *The Yoga Sutras* by Patanjali, written around 2,000 years ago (ancient Indian texts have no reliable dates). Mountain ashrams were founded by yogis who wished to learn more about themselves and reality by reaching *Samadhi*, or perfect concentration. The yogis studied nature and lived simply as an aid to reaching higher states of consciousness. Patanjali edited the forms of yoga being practiced at these ashrams in 300 to 500 CE, and is believed to have formulated 195 short sentences or "rules" that explain yoga in terms of the Samkhya philosophy of the time (Dasgupta, Vol. 1, p. 339).

Although yoga is one of the six philosophical systems of India, it is not a religion but rather a philosophy of living. A religion defines God in terms of a specific faith, whereas a philosophy guides one's lifestyle. Classical yoga is any pursuit that leads to complete mastery of one's self by uniting the lower self with the higher self, or the individual self with the universal self. Some call this self-actualization or enlightenment. Yoga encourages a personal experience of the divine, but it does not adopt any one religion or exclude those who do not believe in God.

The Reverend J. M. Dechanet, who wrote *Christian Yoga,* explains that the purpose of yoga is to purify the human mind so that the individual may gain a clearer experience of reality. Classical yoga does not define this "experience of reality," nor does it define God or the experience of God. For an open-minded person who wishes to learn from all religions, even most guru-centered institutions do not pose any threat to one's religion. As in any field, there may be groups using yoga in their name that follow extreme principles. One does not have to have a guru or change one's name or job in order to do yoga. Under most circumstances, classical yoga recommends that one remain in the same job and learn from the situation.

Patanjali noted eight "limbs" of yoga for the beginning student, which are used as a foundation for classical yoga programs. The first two steps create moral awareness: *Yama,* or restraint, consists of five virtues—nonviolence, truth, nonstealing, self-restraint, and nongreed; while the *Niyamas,* or observances to be cultivated, are purity, contentment, discipline, study of scriptures, and devotion to God. With a background in virtuous conduct and virtuous aim, a person will approach yogic techniques with the attitude of personality transformation. The physical aspect of yoga now has a context to be expressed in a way that leads to faith and higher consciousness.

These virtuous qualities then serve as the intentions for doing yoga postures or *Asanas,* the third step. Yoga postures can be grouped into six categories: standing, balancing, sitting, backward bending, forward bending, and twisting and inverted, all of which should be demonstrated first in a class. Yoga postures promote increased blood circulation, internal organ massage, improved digestion, limber muscles and joints, oxygen increase, improved lymphatic circulation, and overall better mood.

As a result of stretching with awareness, one becomes better acquainted with the body and can learn to notice problems before aches escalate into injuries.

Asanas prepare the body for the fourth step, *Pranayama,* or breath control, which includes simple breathing techniques aimed to slow and deepen the breath, consequently bringing the mind to a state of deep concentration. There are many types of breathing exercises, all of which intend to bring greater awareness and integration of the mind, body, and spirit. Pranayama helps to balance the emotions and has also been documented to boost immune function by increasing oxygen metabolism, stimulating lymph propulsion and generation, and improving the nervous system's interface with the immune system.

Fifth is the *Pratyahara,* or sensory withdrawal, a technique of quieting the mind and learning to consciously ignore sensory information. Often sounds, feelings, and images may cause the mind to be disturbed. Therefore, by learning to consciously disregard sensory information, meditation is facilitated. These first five steps are considered Hatha Yoga, and prepare the body for the final three steps of concentration, meditation, and perfect concentration. All eight steps together are Raja Yoga, also termed Ashtanga Yoga.

Ayurveda

A sister science to yoga is Ayurveda, an ancient healing system that also stems from the Vedas in ancient India, among the oldest bodies of knowledge in human culture. Ayurvedic medicine respects the "lore of life" *(Ayur Vidya)* or the power of Nature to cure disease and promote health. In this sense doctors cannot cure illness themselves but rather assist Nature's healing efforts. Ayurvedic medicine incorporates the six philosophies of India, one of which is yoga. According to Lad (2002), Ayurveda states that "the purpose of life is to know or realize the Creator, both within and without, and to express this Divinity in one's daily life." Ayurveda incorporates modern techniques with ancient wisdom to provide a uniquely personalized treatment for the individual, including elimination of the cause of illness, treatment, and rejuvenation of the body (Lad, 2002).

Yoga in the United States

The first documented group in the United States to study Indian philosophy and religion was the Transcendental Club in Concord, Massachusetts, founded by Ralph Waldo Emerson and Henry David Thoreau. The ideas of yoga entered America notably in 1843, when Emerson received a copy of the Bhagavad Gita (Leviton, 1993, p. 67), a religious text combining India's earliest literature with Samkhya philosophy and yoga. The Bhagavad Gita describes yoga as a form of practice leading to the highest truth. In Europe, Indian scriptures were translated as early as 1809, and circulated widely among the intellectual communities of France and Germany (Schwab, 1984). Asian philosophical ideas have influenced the West in the philosophy of Emerson and Thoreau's writings and in psychology through Carl Jung's works (Coward, 1985).

Popularly noted as the introduction of yoga to America was Swami Vivekananda's address to the World Parliament of Religions in Chicago in 1893. The force and clarity of Vivekananda's lecture surprised many, as India was considered a backward and poor society. The first Vedanta Society was founded in New York City by Vivekananda, who lectured throughout the United States (Leviton, 1993, p. 68). His popular text, *Raja Yoga,* which included a translation of the *Yoga Sutras,* was published by 1901 (Vivekananda, 1901). Vivekananda introduced yoga as a means for spiritual evolution, and this tradition is continued by numerous Vedanta Centers around the United States.

The number of yoga activities in the United States blossomed in the early 1900s. An attempt to document each group that introduced yoga would be an interesting survey that could investigate the various interpretations of yoga, including the successes and failures of yoga in America. The various interpretations of yoga philosophy and types of practice is a subject in and of itself. The word *yoga* is a general term that may include the psychophysical-spiritual practice of any type of group, from religious and philosophical to the physical culturist. Yoga could mean any technique that unites the lower self with a higher reality. As a person's experience of the divine is completely subjective, there is no way to discount any form of yoga outside of those that are blatantly dishonest or violent in some fashion.

Schools of Yoga

There are hundreds, if not thousands, of schools of yoga, and there are pearls of wisdom in all of them. The different schools often contradict themselves regarding physical techniques, but each one has a system that works to some end. One group may teach a stretch with the arm turned in and the other out, or breathing techniques may differ. Remember that the means must equal the ends in yoga. The fitness adage "No pain, no gain" is unrelated to yoga. You do not bring stress into your body to release the stress: Yoga for personal growth is an experience that brings steadiness to the mind. Values stated by yoga's traditional philosophy are a good common denominator for all schools to follow. Such practices are guided by the virtues mentioned above. Classical yoga transforms the deepest aspects of the mind. The psychophysical yoga health practices in classical yoga bring relaxation to the body and concentration to the mind. The yoga practices of posture, breathing, and relaxation serve to quiet the mind for contemplation of deeper issues, such as the roots of suffering, internal peace, and spiritual insight. Yoga becomes a lifestyle. One does not immediately change one's outward life; however, attitudes may shift. Numerous people who learn relaxation begin to notice that they react to stressful situations with a deep breath instead of panic. Others start to read uplifting books and eat a more wholesome diet. In time, one's behavior becomes aimed toward balance and peace of mind, and this in turn enriches life.

HEALTH BENEFITS OF YOGA

Although much remains unknown with regard to the scientific understanding of the effects of yoga practice on health, a growing body of evidence shows yoga to have significant and measurable health benefits.

Musculoskeletal Disorders

The use of yoga postures to treat musculoskeletal disorders (e.g., osteoarthritis) is an area of growing interest to medical researchers. Garfinkel and colleagues (Garfinkel, Schumacher, Husain, Levy, & Reshetar, 1994) found that yoga practiced once a week for 8 weeks was beneficial in the treatment of osteoarthritis of the hands, and a similar program was found to relieve the symptoms of carpal tunnel syndrome (Garfinkel et al., 1998). Sharon Kolaskinski, MD, a rheumatologist at the University of Pennsylvania, is heading up a study to evaluate the practice of yoga as a treatment for osteoarthritis of the knee (personal communication, 2003). Although many smaller studies have been conducted that point to yoga as a promising intervention for musculoskeletal disorders, larger well-controlled clinical trials are needed to confirm these findings (Luskin et al., 2000; Raub, 2002).

Coronary Artery Disease

Manchanda et al. (2000) conducted a 1-year, prospective, randomized, controlled trial of 42 men with coronary artery disease (CAD). Participants in the experimental group ($n = 21$) received a program of risk factor control, dietary changes, moderate aerobic exercise, and yoga. The control group ($n = 21$) received risk factor control and the American

Heart Association step I diet (standard care). Those in the experimental group were less likely to require revascularization, had less angina, and showed greater reductions in body weight, cholesterol (total and low-density lipoproteins [LDL]) than those in the control group. Other similar studies suggest that a lifestyle program that includes yoga practice can reduce risk factors for persons with coronary artery disease (Mahajan, Reddy, & Sachdeva, 1999; Ornish et al., 1998; Schmidt, Wijga, Von Zur Muhlen, Brabant, & Wagner, 1997).

Hypertension

A randomized study of 33 persons ages 36 to 65 with documented hypertension found that yoga (practiced twice a day for 11 weeks) was as effective as standard medical treatment for controlling hypertension (Murugesan,Govindarajulu, & Bera, 2000). Twenty men with essential hypertension were treated with yoga asanas or a tilt table for 3 weeks to restore normal baroreflex sensitivity. Both groups exhibited a significant reduction in blood pressure (Selvamurthy et al., 1998). Slow, deep breathing (similar to the breathing of some pranayama exercises) was shown to have significant effects on reducing hypertension in a group of 81 persons (ages 57–59) with chronic heart failure (Bernardi et al., 2002). Although there is a lack of large-scale clinical trials in this area, several other studies conducted over the 30 thirty years suggest that yoga can be an effective tool in controlling hypertension (Haber, 1983; Patel & North, 1975; Sundar et al., 1984). Evidence is accumulating that yoga is among the growing list of nondrug interventions for hypertension prevention and control (Labarthe & Ayala, 2002).

Asthma

Studies conducted to evaluate the effectiveness of yoga techniques at ameliorating the symptoms of asthma have shown some positive results. In a group of 53 asthmatics (compared to a matched control group), the daily practice of slightly over 1 hour of yoga asanas was found to improve peak expiratory flow rate (PEFR), reduce medication use, and decrease the frequency of attacks (Nagarathna & Nagendra, 1985). A follow-up study (n = 570) found that yoga and meditation significantly improved PEFR, with the greatest benefit experienced by those who practiced yoga most (Nagendra & Nagarathna, 1986). A randomized, double-blind, placebo-controlled, crossover trial (n = 18) found that pranayama breathing techniques are an effective treatment for mild asthma (Singh, Wisniewski, Britton, & Tattersfield, 1990). However, more and better studies are needed to confirm these effects (Raub, 2002).

NIH-FUNDED STUDIES ON YOGA

Among the yoga studies funded by the National Institutes of Health are:

- Yoga and exercise for low back pain (Group Health Cooperative; Sherman, primary investigator [PI])
- Yoga and relaxations exercises for insomnia (Brigham and Women's Hospital; Khalsa, PI)
- Yoga for multiple sclerosis (Oregon Health and Science University; Oken, PI)
- Yoga for chronic obstructive pulmonary disease (University of California–San Francisco; Carrieri-Kohlman and Stulbarg, PI) (source: http://nccam.nih.gov/research/)

YOGA PRACTICE, PHILOSOPHY, AND LIFESTYLE

Yoga concerns physical, mental, moral, and spiritual health, studying each facet of life in order to raise consciousness. Due to numerous applications of yoga to health conditions, one may think that yoga is concerned only with physical health. But as one studies yoga, an emphasis on mastering the mind becomes a means for yoga practice. Yoga practice takes one beyond personal thoughts and egocentric conceptions, wherein one nears spirituality, the nonsectarian term for the study of reality. Considering the needs of another person for no gain of one's own is a spiritual act. Meditation to quiet one's thoughts to go beyond the ego is a spiritual act.

Our attitudes and values are considered in each aspect of yoga. What we eat expresses values, thinking patterns, and attitudes. We may have deep values and attitudes, but living our values is very difficult. Yoga helps practitioners experience the values they do live so that they may understand how to improve themselves. Yoga brings into alignment values and lifestyle.

With help from yoga's philosophy, one is motivated to follow the yoga lifestyle, which includes healthy diet, exercise, yoga postures, breathing, meditation, study, and positive attitude. As one balances one's life by minimizing stress, the body weight and metabolism may normalize. Once the mind is mastered, the health may be improved. However, it is possible that a health condition does not improve, but a person masters the mind. Yoga helps with health but is not limited to the physical level.

A yoga lifestyle means that yoga does not stop at yoga exercises. Most community yoga classes cover yoga's stretching movements, relaxation, and possibly breathing exercises. The yoga lifestyle applies the principles of yoga to one's daily life by adopting healthy attitudes. For example, yoga emphasizes a nonviolent attitude beginning with behavior and ending with subtle thoughts. When you remember to act nonviolently while driving in a car or during a heated discussion, then you are practicing the yoga lifestyle. Any way of living that aims at increasing consciousness while performing daily activities is the yoga lifestyle. This includes diet, rest, spiritual practice, relationships, yoga exercises, study, work, and hobby. Because yoga helps cultivate a concentrated mind, it helps one develop a strong will for making lifestyle changes such as smoking cessation or the avoidance of unhealthy foods.

Yoga is not a pill or a miracle cure. The scientific medical model often views cure in terms of pills. Some medical protocols recommend "alternative medicine" like yoga for stress management. This type of piecemeal usage of yoga reduces yoga to some stretching, relaxation, and breathing. The profound emphasis of cultivating a personality that is immune to disease is lost. An overall lifestyle cannot be prescribed. Lifestyle education has a philosophical basis and is a long-term pursuit.

The "miracle cure" belief is found in popular literature where people are healed of incurable diseases like multiple sclerosis, cancer, asthma, and heart disease by using a yoga lifestyle approach. The enthusiasm of those who healed themselves is often attributed to yoga, and yoga is touted as a miracle cure. This type of enthusiasm causes false hopes for some people, and in others it causes an attachment to the techniques of yoga. The body is an amazing and mysterious entity, and the miraculous claims are never explainable in intellectual arguments. Thus, it is best to do whatever you can and remain unattached to the results of your effort.

As a means of understanding how the mind works, yoga has a complete psychology. In its psychology, yoga views ignorance as the root of disharmony in the human condition (Aranya, p. 117). The ignorance consists of misapprehending the true reality for the changing reality; wrong beliefs cause suffering. When one invests heart and soul in material pursuits like fame, wealth, or even health for security, there is inevitable disappointment. The fame, wealth, and health all eventually pass due to changes like old age. A life based on material qualities is beset with unrest. Yet most of us live as if the changing material reality is all that exists. Yoga teaches one to have faith in an unchanging aspect of reality, notably God, a higher power or a larger reality that transcends the ego.

As the yoga practitioner understands the essence of reality, the sufferer is removed from the equation. If you think that you are only a body and something happens to the way you look, a great deal of unhappiness follows. However, if you value your spirit first and foremost, the changing aspects of your life such as looks and money have less effect on your happiness. Yoga teaches one to remove ignorance by detachment and practice (Aranya, p. 35). As the mind is stabilized and an enlightened worldview dawns, a person is both undisturbed by pain and pleasure and full of willpower that cultivates a healthy way of life. According to the Upanishads, India's earliest literature, one in the highest state of consciousness cannot suffer. (This type of mind has positive benefits on health and is the source of balance in mind–body healing.)

The Upanishads inspire one to practice meditation where understanding happens as an experience beyond words, yet one that the soul comprehends. The teaching of the Upanishads is to concentrate the mind in order to know the profound depths of the soul. This objective view to life leads to clarity of mind. However, notice that this includes a higher Self that is united to the body, senses, and mind. The common ascetic understanding of the spiritual as good and the body as bad is not taught in yoga. The body and mind are to be integrated and thereby mastered.

BEGINNING YOGA

Yoga is an excellent practice for all ages: "The ancient yogi's have affirmed that not only the young and the old but even the very old, the sick and the infirm can undertake the practice of yoga with success and, thus, achieve the highest fruit thereof" (Yogendra, 1993, p. 49). The practices vary according to need; thus, one may utilize any beneficial yoga practice. As a health practice, yoga helps energize the body and mind and is an excellent exercise for older adults. Often, as one gains life experience, the meditative aspects of yoga are more appreciated.

You do not need to stop working and move to the Himalayas to practice yoga. In time, you may choose to change your lifestyle if you are overworked or out of balance in some area of your life. However, this change can be as small as watching less television or finding some quiet time each day where you reflect on your life. You may continue working with the openness to make healthy changes at a slow pace. Changes in diet are best performed slowly, unless a doctor orders otherwise.

You can start daily yoga practice slowly. No two people will do an identical practice; thus, be creative and let yoga mold to your life at first. Later, you may make choices to change behaviors. Use discipline for regularity, and try to do yoga because of a desire from within. Forcing yourself to get up early in the morning or perform some other sacrifice may cause harm unless you are compelled from within and it is fun. Do no yoga pose or yoga practice that causes pain. Yoga should leave you feeling invigorated and positive.

Find a teacher that you like as a person. Investigate the teacher to make sure you receive proper guidance. However, be careful of your idealistic projections onto the instructor, which can make some teachers appear greater than they are. The well-educated, simple-living teacher with a warm heart is your safest choice.

In a beginning yoga class the union being developed is the union of mind and body. To facilitate this union of the mind and body, it is important in practicing yoga that the postures are held only to a comfortable stretching position. If you stretch beyond your limit of comfort, it is very difficult to keep your mind on the experience of the pose. The mind will tend to wander and become distracted as a way of avoiding the discomfort and thus eliminating the practice of mind–body union. Also, holding a posture to a point of pain may cause injury.

Comfort and awareness are integral on so many levels to yoga practice. In class a posture may be demonstrated as an ideal, and students are encouraged to move toward that ideal posture within the bounds of their own physical ability. Many poses are practiced with the eyes closed to help students keep an internal focus and to assist in minimizing competition with others. Yoga is not about how far your body can stretch; it is about what you do with your mind while maintaining a yoga asana. Someone may hold a perfected yoga pose, but their body is uncomfortable, and their thoughts are either about when the discomfort will end or about something totally unrelated to their experience. This student is not practicing yoga (union). Another student may be holding a very moderate variation of the pose, but their mind is completely immersed in the awareness of the experience, and union (yoga) is achieved.

Diaphragmatic breathing promotes a natural, even breath movement that strengthens the nervous system and relaxes the body. This is the way we were born breathing. If you ever watch a baby breathe, you will notice how the lower rib cage area expands outward with each inhalation and relaxes back with each exhalation. Practicing diaphragmatic breathing regularly will keep it familiar to you. As it becomes more familiar, you will be able to remember to shift your breathing to the diaphragmatic breath when you notice a rapid, shallow breath due to tension in your life.

In order to use yoga in your life, it is essential to practice what you learn in class. Developing a home practice can take some thought and contemplation initially so that you can work the practice into your life in a gradual and smooth way. It is helpful to understand that beginning a regular yoga practice is growing a positive habit in your life.

Choose a space large enough to lie down, one that is well ventilated and offers a comfortable temperature and is free from distraction during your practice time. Choose a time of day when you have an empty stomach. A realistic goal for a beginner is 15 to 20 minutes per day. Ideally, you should practice around the same time of day every day, but do not become overly concerned or annoyed if you miss days or have to practice at a different time. Remember, real change happens slowly.

A yoga practice should begin with a centering exercise, including relaxation techniques, breath awareness, or prayer. Include at least one asana (posture) from each category: standing, balancing, sitting, backward bending, forward bending, twisting, and inverted. For a beginning student, it is best to practice only those postures that have been demonstrated in class. Students should follow each posture with a brief pause to reflect and release any unnecessary tension. The pause and letting go can be just as important in a yoga practice as performing the posture. Perform standing poses first, followed by sitting, lying, and inverted poses. The entire process follows a pattern toward stillness of mind; thus, begin standing and move to relaxation.

Following an asana practice is relaxation, pranayama, and meditation. To spend even a couple of minutes deeply relaxing, even if you simply take a few deep, relaxing breaths in the corpse pose, is important and helpful. Regular practice of pranayama, or breath control (e.g., diaphragmatic breathing), provides a greater awareness of energy flow, improves stamina, and promotes a sense of well-being. It is also important for beginning students to try to cultivate the regular habit of sitting in meditation, even if just for 5 minutes. Simply sitting quietly on a pillow or in a chair and observing the breath can be considered meditation.

Many people ask how long it will take before they see the results of yoga, but this question is flawed according to an important aspect of yoga philosophy. Yoga is to be performed without attachment to the results. If you are focused only on results, then you may be thinking more about the end of your practice and not enough about your practice. The more effort you put into your yoga practice, the more benefits you will experience. Also, the results are relative to who you are as an individual. Issues like emotions and health are beyond our control to a certain degree. "Do your best and let go of the results" is a helpful quote taught by the Yoga Institute.

As one begins to practice yoga regularly, an awareness arises. Usually within a few weeks one notices correct posture as well as varying levels of tension in the body. This growing awareness that begins with the body gradually expands to cover all aspects of one's self-emotions, thoughts, desires, aspirations, and spirituality. Ultimately, the heightened awareness allows one to balance or strengthen areas of one's personality and lifestyle that need adjustment. Yoga becomes an ultimate form of health promotion for the mind and body. Later in yoga practice, meditation becomes an essential means of understanding the mind and expanding yoga's union to include mind, body, and spirit.

One does not have to become a vegetarian to practice yoga. Nonviolence is a central theme of yoga, and many people who practice yoga find that a vegetarian diet serves them better for a variety of reasons. Eating lower on the food chain is good for the earth, and science shows that a plant-based diet lowers health risks. Others believe that killing animals is violent or that meat is not good for the health. A third issue from yoga is that foods influence one's mind. Certainly, if you overeat any food, the mind suffers. You may notice a lighter feeling in the mind when eating vegetarian. However, it is not recommended to make sudden dietary changes, and if you choose to become vegetarian, make sure you receive balanced nutrition.

Yoga is not contortionism or acrobatics. In yoga magazines or on television, you may have seen a so-called yogi tying his body in extraordinary configurations. This type of circuslike performance belongs under a big tent and has no relation to classical yoga. Those acrobats who use yoga for achieving great physical strength also misunderstand the essence of yoga. The simple idea to remember is that if you control the body, there is no guarantee that you will control the mind. Who is to know if the flexible contortionist is happy or not? However, when the mind is understood, there surely is control over the body (Aranya, pp. 234–235). From peace of mind, it is easy to follow a healthy discipline for the body. Although some so-called yogis revere yoga postures as "the" cure-all and "the" pathway to higher consciousness, any authentic student of yoga realizes that the physical level must be integrated with the emotional, moral, and spiritual aspects of life. (A yoga of intellect only, can equally lose balance by neglect of the physical.)

Western culture sees philosophy for the mind, religion for the spirit, and exercise for the body. Thus, yoga taught in the United States is often akin to aerobics. Yoga is perceived to be a sport adopted from India. Little or no association to mind or spirit happens due to a Western mindset. Ideally, yoga postures should be taught with benefits for all levels of a person (i.e., forward bends to stretch the hamstrings, massage the intestines, develop an attitude of surrender; relaxation focuses on a letting-go feeling and develops faith in a larger reality). This sacred way of living becomes accepted as common sense, and people begin to see how to maintain a higher awareness when doing simple actions. Practitioners learn that all aspects of life, from washing to work to meditation, are pathways to healthy living.

Maintaining yoga as a spiritual lifestyle in a materialistic society is increasingly difficult. Yet the reward for preserving the integrity of yoga satisfies the deepest levels of one's being. If you are fortunate enough to have a nice yoga community in your area, contribute to that group, as the students make the yoga center thrive.

RESOURCES

Books

Aranya, Swami Hariharananda. *Yoga Philosophy of Patanjali*. Calcutta: U. of Calcutta Press, 1963–1981.
    A classical translation of The Yoga Sutras fit for the intermediate or advanced student. Some understanding of advanced yogic concepts may be necessary for studying this text.

Christensen, A. *Easy does it yoga*. American Yoga Association. 1999.
Christensen, A. *The easy does it yoga trainer's guide*. American Yoga Association. 1995.
    These books offer easy yoga poses as well as "chair yoga" techniques.

Coward, Howard. *Jung and Eastern Thought*. State University of New York Press. 1985.
    An interested treatise on famed psychotherapist, Carl Jung and his view on Eastern thought. Some of his thinking exposes various problems when integrating Eastern and Western thought.

Dasgupta, Surendranath. *A History of Indian Philosophy Vol. 1-5*. Delhi: Motilal Banarsidass, 1922–1975.
    A comprehensive history of Indian philosophy may be appropriate for the scholar and student versed in a more intellectual study.

Dechanet, J. M. *Christian Yoga*. Harper & Row Publishers. 1960.
    A monk in the order of St. Benedict, this Catholic priest shares his own Yoga practice shedding light on the Hindu-Christian dialogue.

Leviton, R. Celebrating 100 Years of Yoga in America. *Yoga Journal,* May/June 1993. Issue 110, pp. 116–150. Berkeley, CA: California Yoga Teachers Association, pp. 67–71.

Ornish, D. *Dr. Dean Ornish's program for reversing heart disease*. 1990
    Offers an entire lifestyle approach based on yogic teachings for those with heart ailments. The information in this text is well researched and clinically proven.

Schwab, R. *The Oriental Renaissance*. New York: Columbia University Press, 1984.
    Very detailed explanation of the spiritual aspects of Eastern thought.

Stewart, M. *Yoga over 50*.
    Illustrated guide to home practice. Some of the poses are more advanced and are better suited for the experienced practitioner. There is a brief overview of yoga and some tips for relaxation, breathing, and meditation.

Vivekananda, S. *Karma Yoga*. New York: Baker & Taylor Co., 1901.
Raja Yoga. New York: Longmans, Green, and Co., 1901.

Winter Ward, S. *Yoga for the young at heart*.
Gentle stretching exercises for vitality, strength, and flexibility, for beginners, baby boomers, and seniors. Includes sections on restorative, menopause, and seated yoga. Also available: *Joy of Rejuvenation* audio-tape and videos (found at www.yogaheart.com).

Web Sites

American Yoga Association (www.americanyogaassociation.org)
Offers classic work on seniors yoga as well as a yoga system based on the philosophical context of yoga. The site also offers a teacher's guide to instructing seniors. The association is based in Ohio and Florida.

(www.yrec.org) Yoga Research and Education Center
Offers resources and links to all branches of yoga, including scholarly pursuits as well as yoga therapy. The association is based in Northern California; however, offers a nationwide contact list.

Yoga Heart (www.yogaheart.com)
Based in Colorado, Yoga Heart offers products and workshops.

REFERENCES

Bernardi, L., Porta, C., Spicuzza, L., Bellwon, J., Spadacinia, G., Frey, A. W., et al. (2002). Slow breathing increases arterial baroreflex sensitivity in patients with chronic heart failure. *Circulation, 105,* 143–145.

Garfinkel, M. S., Schumacher, H. R., Husain, A., Levy, M., & Reshetar, R. A. (1994). Evaluation of a yoga based regimen for treatment of osteoarthritis of the hands. *Journal of Rheumatology, 21,* 2341–2343.

Garfinkel, M. S., Singhal, A., Katz, W. A., Allan, D. A., Reshetar, R., & Schumacher, H. R. (1998). Yoga-based intervention for carpal tunnel syndrome: A randomized trial. *Journal of the American Medical Association, 280,* 1601–1603.

Haber, D. (1983). Yoga as a preventive health care program for white and black elders: An exploratory study. *International Journal of Aging and Human Development, 17*(30), 169–176.

Labarthe, D., & Ayala, C. (2002). Nondrug interventions in hypertension prevention and control. *Cardiology Clinics, 20*(2), 249–263.

Lad, V. D. (2002). *Textbook of Ayurveda: Fundamental principles*. Albuquerque, NM: The Ayurvedic Press.

Luskin, F. M., Newell, K. A., Griffith, M., Holmes, M., Telles, S., DiNucci, E., et al. (2000). A review of mind/body therapies in the treatment of musculoskeletal disorders with implications for the elderly. *Alternative Therapies in Health and Medicine, 6,* 46–56.

Mahajan, A. S., Reddy, K. S., & Sachdeva, U. (1999). Lipid profile of coronary risk subjects following yogic lifestyle intervention. *Indian Heart Journal, 51,* 37–40.

Manchanda, S. C., Narang, R., Reddy, K. S., Sachdeva, U., Prabhakaran, D., Dharmanand, S., Rajani, M., & Bijlani, R. (2000). Retardation of coronary athcrosclerosis with yoga lifestyle intervention. *Journal of the Association of Physicians of India, 48,* 687–694.

Murugesan, R., Govindarajulu, N., & Bera, T. K. (2000). Effect of selected yoga practices on the management of hypertension. *Indian Journal of Physiology and Pharmacology, 44,* 207–210.

Nagarathna, R., & Nagendra, H. R. (1985). Yoga for bronchial asthma: A controlled study. *British Medical Journal, 291,* 1077–1079.

Nagendra, H. R., & Nagarathna, R. (1986). An integrated approach of yoga therapy for bronchial asthma: A 3–54 month prospective study. *Journal of Asthma, 23,* 123–137.

Ornish, D., Scherwitz, L. W., Billings, J. H., Brown, S. E., Gould, K. L., Merritt, T. A., Sparler, S., et al. (1998). Intensive lifestyle changes for reversal of coronary heart disease. *Journal of the American Medical Association, 280,* 2001–2007.

Patel, C., & North, W. R. (1975). Randomised controlled trial of yoga and biofeedback in management of hypertension. *Lancet, 2*(79250), 93–95.

Schmidt, T., Wijga, A., Von Zur Muhlen, A., Brabant, G., & Wagner, T. O. (1997). Changes in cardiovascular risk factors and hormones during a comprehensive residential three month kriya yoga training and vegetarian nutrition. *Acta Physiologica Scandinavica, 640*(Suppl), 158–162.

Selvamurthy, W., Sridharan, K., Ray, U. S., Tiwary, R. S., Hegde, K. S., Radhakrishan, U., & Sinha, K. C. (1998). A new physiological approach to control essential hypertension. *Indian Journal of Physiology and Pharmacology, 42,* 205–213.

Singh, V., Wisniewski, A., Britton, J., & Tattersfield, A. (1990). Clinical practice: Effect of yoga breathing exercises (pranayama) on airway reactivity in subjects with asthma. *Lancet, 335,* 1381–1383.

Sundar, S., Agrawal, S. K., Singh, V. P., Bhattacharya, S. K., Udupa, K. N., & Vaish, S. K. (1984). Role of yoga in management of essential hypertension. *Acta Cardiologica, 39*(3), 203–208.

Yogendra, J. (1993). *Cyclopedia yoga 1.* Santacruz, India: The Yoga Institute.

CHAPTER TWELVE

Ayurveda: Mother of Traditional Medicine

Mari Clements

Scholars have traced the origins of Ayurveda as far back as 5000 BC, when the teachings of Ayurveda began as an oral tradition in India. The earliest form of instruction was taught using spiritual songs, or hymns. The earliest written form of Ayurveda as a medical text evolved from the Vedas, which are religious writings consisting of philosophical principles and healing verses. The Vedas are regarded as the oldest written record of knowledge. The basic eight branches of Ayurveda are documented in the *Atharva-Veda*, one of the four Vedas. Three authentic texts written in Sanskrit remain available today, and they are at least 1,200 years old. During the period 300 BCE to CE 600 Ayurveda and Indian culture flourished. Buddhist missionaries helped to spread Ayurveda throughout the Middle East and Asia and to the European continent. It is believed by many that the imprint of Ayurveda can be recognized at the core of many traditional medicines.

During British colonial rule in India, until around 1920, there was a sharp decline in the teaching of Ayurveda. The British did not allow Ayurveda to be taught in medical schools and prohibited all Ayurvedic teaching institutions. Recently there has been a revival in the teaching of Ayurveda in India. It has been a struggle to create a uniform school system for Ayurveda, however, that would maintain standards of education that match the allopathic system. The World Health Organization has recently expressed interest in and support of Ayurveda as a primary medicine in India. The Indian government has helped to form research organizations, and studies are ongoing to help promote the acceptance and understanding of Ayurveda worldwide.

THE HEALING PRINCIPLES OF AYURVEDA

The word *Ayurveda* is from *Ayur* ("life") and *Veda* ("knowledge" or "science"). Ayurveda, then, is the knowledge or science of life. Within Ayurveda there is a unique blend of philosophies that span spirituality, astrology, lifestyle regimens, medicine, and psychology. The purpose of Ayurveda is to promote longevity, rejuvenation, and self-realization within any person who participates in the recommended practices. Ayurvedic healing modalities include surgery, yoga, herbal medicine, diet, psychology, massage, and cleansing therapies, as well as color, gem, and aromatherapy. Food as medicine is considered one of the foremost approaches to health and longevity in Ayurveda. The diet and lifestyle recommendations of Ayurveda can be incorporated into any formulation of a patient's medical plan. As an Ayurvedic practitioner, I have found that there are an enormous number of therapies to choose from that are safe and sensible. An important aspect of Ayurveda is that it sees each patient as an individual, with individual needs; those needs require individually determined recommendations.

Ayurveda offers principles in the art of daily living that can help us to maintain the quality and longevity of our lives. Within these principles there is a "formula" that can be applied to our daily life habits to help reestablish balance in our lives. The foundation of Ayurveda aims to restore our basic individual nature, that which we were born with. The premise is that we are healthiest and happiest when we live in harmony with our own true nature. The qualities of our nature are reflective of the universe around us. We can use these qualities to both determine our imbalances and illnesses as well as to heal ourselves. To learn to apply the Ayurvedic principles, we need to first understand these qualities and the way that they manifest in our anatomy and physiology. These qualities provide us with the basic language of Ayurveda.

A fundamental belief in Ayurveda is that there is an innate intelligence that exists within each and every cell. The biochemistry of our body is shaped by that same intelligence. We can observe the work of this intelligence in our immune system, nervous system, and endocrine system. Genetics has taught us that our deoxyribonucleic acid (DNA) passes on its programmed information to ribonucleic acid (RNA), which in turn passes this information to cells throughout the body. Ayurveda believes that this innate intelligence is affected by all of our thoughts and memories. Awareness, what we are aware of, what we perceive to be true, becomes the driving force behind this intelligence. As we age, this flow of intelligence becomes altered by our emotional and physical experiences. By old age all our cells will be reflecting the unique experiences we have processed and metabolized from all our senses. These unique experiences will be manifested in our tissues and organs. This reflects the adage "We are as old as we think we are."

THE COSMIC PRINCIPLES OF AYURVEDA

Ayurveda looks to nature to find the representation of qualities that define us and the world around us. Within these qualities we discover a polarity that can be used to establish balance in our lives and produce the richness of health and happiness.

There are five great elements within nature that represent the core qualities found in the human body. These five elements are earth, water, fire, air, and ether. Each of these elements contains the qualities of solid, liquid, radiant, gaseous, and etheric forms of matter. These qualities also represent the shifting state of density within matter and within fields of expression from solid to etheric. These elements represent a particular quality that can be applied, in a descriptive sense, to just about anything.

> *Earth* manifests the idea of solidity, stability, and giving resistance to action.
> *Water* manifests the idea of liquidity, a flowing motion, and bringing forth life.
> *Fire* manifests the idea of light, perception, movement, and transformation
> *Air* manifests the idea of subtle movement, of direction, velocity, and change.
> *Ether* manifests the idea of connection, communication, and self-expression.

These five elements correspond with both the function and the form of the human body. Earth is represented in the bones and promotes structure and stability in the body. Water is represented in the plasma, blood, urine, sweat, saliva, and mucus. Fire manifests in the metabolic process and in the production of bodily heat. Air relates to any kind of movement in the body. Ether manifests as our emotions, thoughts, and communication within the body.

Within these five elements there are 20 attributes, and within those attributes there are 10 qualities and their opposite counterparts. Ayurveda, like traditional Chinese medicine that uses yin and yang, utilizes the science of opposite qualities to promote balance. The science of opposites presupposes that like increases like and that opposites cure or balance each other, particularly when there is a condition of excess. Disease and dis-ease of the mind or body can manifest as an excessive amount of a certain quality or qualities that have accumulated in the body or mind. Disease can also manifest from a lack of or a deficiency in a certain quality. Where there is an accumulation or a deficiency, aggravation results, and this leads to disease. When these opposite qualities are also assigned to food, herbs, exercise, and lifestyle activities, they can be used to eliminate or reduce the accumulation that is promoting the imbalance and causing the illness.

The 20 attributes are cold/hot, heavy/light, dense/flowing, soft/hard, smooth, rough, wet/dry, gross/subtle, static/mobile, dull/sharp, and cloudy/clear.

THE THREE METABOLIC BODY TYPES

Ayurveda circumscribes the qualities from the five elements and the 20 attributes into a system or model referred to as the science of the three biological humors, called *doshas*. The doshas represent physiological principles of structure and function in the body. Each dosha governs a different aspect of the body. Learning the differences and essences of each dosha helps to simplify the application of Ayurveda.

Vata

Vata is ruled by the elements of air and ether. It is represented by the attributes of dry, light, cold, rough, clear, subtle, and mobile. Vata governs enthusiasm, inspiration, expiration, elimination, and all movement. It is increased by the tastes of bitter and pungent and slightly by astringent.

Pitta

Pitta is ruled by the elements of fire and water. It is represented by the attributes of somewhat oily, sharp, hot, light, mobile, and liquid. Pitta governs vision, digestion, heat, hunger, thirst, softness in the body, luster, cheerfulness, and intellect. It is increased by the tastes of salty and pungent and slightly by sour.

Kapha

Kapha is ruled by earth and water. It is represented in the attributes of wet, cold, heavy, dull, sticky, cloudy, dense, soft, and firm. Kapha governs unctuousness, binding, firmness, heaviness, potency, strength, and restraint. It is increased by the tastes of sweet and salty and slightly by sour.

Using the qualities of the three doshas, born of the five elements of nature and the 20 attributes, we can reestablish balance by increasing or reducing these qualities of which we have either too little or too much. We can locate these qualities in the foods that we eat, the activities that we participate in, and the emotions that we express. These qualities also predominate during certain life stages, with Kapha governing childhood, Pitta governing middle age, and Vata governing old age. Generally, Ayurveda recommends reducing whatever qualities we are excessive in. If we are too Kapha in nature, we would participate in Kapha-reducing activities and eat Kapha-reducing foods. We are an amalgam of all three doshas, but generally we are predominate in one or two doshas that we need to balance by applying the science of opposite qualities. What we crave and like most we should avoid or at least limit in our diet and in our life.

> When Vata dosha is in balance, we are mentally alert, energetic, enthusiastic, imaginative, artistic, and optimistic.
> When Pitta dosha is in balance, we have strong digestion, keen intellect, and a bright complexion. We are energetic, goal-oriented, and decisive.
> When Kapha dosha is in balance, we are calm, rational, prudent, compassionate, and dependable. We have a strong immune system and good endurance.

Table 12.1 lists the mental, behavioral, and physical symptoms that indicate imbalances for the three doshas. Table 12.2 gives suggestions on restoring balance, as well as appropriate diets.

AYURVEDA AND PSYCHOLOGY

Ayurveda provides us with a specific language we can use to understand the mind. There are three primal qualities in nature that compose the main essence of Cosmic Intelligence. This Cosmic Intelligence exists both outside us and inside our minds. The three primal qualities, or *gunas* (Sanskrit for "what binds"), are Sattva, Rajas, and Tamas. They represent the qualities and energies of our mental state, both the conscious and the deep unconscious.

> Sattva: inner peace, compassion, receptivity, clarity, discrimination, endurance, selflessness
> Rajas: anger, desire, irritability, discontent, judgmental, aggressive, ambitious, arrogant
> Tamas: deep attachment, addictive, passive, fearful, depression, ignorance, delusional, lazy, dependent, low self-esteem

TABLE 12.1 Dosha Imbalances

	Mental Symptoms	Behavioral Symptoms	Physical Symptoms
Vata	Worry, anxiety	Inability to relax	Poor appetite
	Overactive mind	Restlessness	Fatigue
	Impatience	Impulsiveness	Constipation
	Poor concentration	Insomnia	Dry or rough skin
	Short attention span		Low stamina, loss of energy
	Depression, psychosis		Intestinal gas
			High blood pressure
			Lower back pain
			Menstrual cramps
			Irritable bowel
			Chapped skin, lips
			Intolerance to cold and wind
			Aching or arthritic joints
			Unintentional weight loss
			Acute pain (especially nerve pain)
			Muscle spasms, seizures
Pitta	Anger, hostility	Outbursts of temper	Skin inflammations, acne
	Self-criticism	Argumentative	Excessive hunger or thirst
	Irritability	Tyrannical	Bad breath
	Impatience	Critical of others	Hot flashes
	Resentment	Intolerance of delays	Heartburn, acid stomach
	Jealousy	Addictions	Ulcers

Sour body odors
Rectal burning, hemorrhoids
Patchy, florid complexion
Intolerance to heat
Red-rimmed eyes
Sunburn, sunstroke

Drowsiness
Intolerance to cold and damp
Sinus congestion
Fluid retention in tissues
Chest congestion
Skin pallor
Loose or aching joints
High cholesterol
Heaviness in limbs
Frequent cold
Weight gain, obesity
Allergies, asthma
Excess phlegm, cough
Sore throat
Cysts and other growths
Diabetes

Kapha

Dullness
Lassitude
Stupor
Depression
Overattachment

Procrastination
Resistance to change
Greed
Stubbornness
Possessiveness
Lethargy

TABLE 12.2 Approaches to Restoring Balance

	To Restore Balance	Dosha-Reducing Diet
Vata	Adequate rest	Eat sweet, sour, and salty foods
	Adhere to daily routines	Choose warming, moist, lubricating, and heavy foods
	Cultivate calmness	Eat primarily cooked foods
	Moderate to light noncompetitive exercise	Warm drinks
	Meditation	Eat adequate amounts of fat and protein
	Warm weather	Limit dry foods and bitter tastes
		Eat three scheduled meals
		Limit bitter, astringent, and pungent foods
Pitta	Establish clear purpose for lifestyle routines	Eat sweet, bitter, and astringent foods
	Cultivate serenity	Choose cooling, heavy, and dry foods
	Cultivate an even temperament	Limit fatty foods
	Cultivate kindness	Eat plenty of complex carbohydrates
	Avoid competition	Limit spices
	Moderate, noncompetitive exercise that does not overheat	Cool (not cold) food and drinks
	Exercise for enjoyment	Two to three regularly scheduled meals, on time
	Cool weather	Substantial-size meals
		Limit sour and pungent foods
Kapha	Maintain an attitude of adaptability	Eat pungent, bitter, and astringent foods
	Stay open to change	Choose light, dry, stimulating foods
	Vigorous exercise	One noontime meal or two meals a day
	No more than 8 hours of sleep	Eat a big lunch and small dinner
	Stay active	Avoid sugar, fats, dairy, and salt
		Avoid cold foods and drinks
		Limit sweet, sour, and salty foods

How can we affect our own mind and establish the qualities of Sattva as a predominant mental state? Ayurveda recommends looking at a variety of aspects in our life, our food choices, lifestyle choices, and relationships. How do the foods we eat make us feel? Do we feel energized or exhausted, heavy or light, satisfied or still craving? What are our senses taking in? What impressions are being made as we watch a violent film versus a Disney cartoon? What impressions are being made if we live in an inner-city ghetto versus a wealthy suburb or life in a loving family versus life with an abusive family? These physical and mental impressions become a food that either nourishes us or depletes us in some way. Our lifestyle choices, our environment, and our food choices can help to create a change of mind. Relationships have a huge influence on the gunas, with like increasing like. One Tamas person can increase a Tamas-like mind in another. It would be the same for Rajas and Sattva. So choose your friends carefully.

Sattvic foods: vegetarian, organic fresh foods, whole foods, small, light meals.

Rajasic foods: excessively spicy, salty, or sour foods and stimulants like coffee and alcohol

Tamasic foods: stale, old, rancid, very cold, artificial and canned, greasy or heavy foods; all animal flesh and organs, sugar, and white flour

AYURVEDA AND PERFECT HEALTH

According to the principles of Ayurveda, the causative factors for disease are repressed emotion, stress, trauma, lifestyle, diet, bacteria, genetic factors, and weather. We can see how applicable Ayurveda is to the modern medicine setting when we apply this philosophy to recent research showing that approximately 80% of all physician office visits are stress related. The goal of Ayurveda is to remove the causative factor of the disease rather than just placate the symptoms. Ayurveda also believes that these causative factors can be prioritized according to the degree of affect it will have on your health: (1) Your innate dosha constitution outweighs environmental influences if you maintain a balanced constitution through proper food and lifestyle choices. (2) Mind and emotions will outweigh physiological factors. Depression and worry will cause illness in the body, and a calm and cheerful mind will promote health and wellness.

Age can be measured in three ways. First, there is our chronological age, which measures how old we are in years. Then there is our physiological age, which determines the condition of our health using the same type of biomarkers that are outlined in the book *Biomarkers: The 10 Determinants of Aging You Can Control* (Evans & Rosenberg). These biomarkers include lean body mass, strength, basal metabolic rate, percentage of body fat, aerobic capacity, blood pressure, insulin sensitivity, cholesterol ratios, bone density, and body temperature regulation. The condition of these biomarkers determines our physiological age. So a 66-year-old man could have the physiological age of a 50-year-old or an 80-year-old, depending on the condition of his biomarkers. The psychological or emotional age is the age that you feel. The only fixed or unchangeable age here is the chronological age. To quote Deepak Chopra from his book *Ageless Body, Timeless Mind* (1993), "Aging is nothing but a set of misguided transformations, processes that should remain stable, balanced, and self-renewing but deviate from their proper course." Ayurveda seeks to rebalance, restabilize, and rejuvenate the aging body. Using diet, herbs, lifestyle recommendations, and an intervention called Pancha Karma, Ayurveda has many therapies to help slow the aging process.

Strong digestive ability is considered to be the cornerstone of health. Symptomatic imbalances often show up initially in a person's digestive profile. Proper digestion, assimilation, and elimination of the food we eat will provide the foundation for all the other functions of the body. The key to digestion in Ayurveda is through the maintenance of *agni* ("biological fire") that governs metabolism. When agni is low or too high, our whole system is affected. When agni is low, there is a buildup of *ama* ("toxins") from poorly digested food in the body; when agni is too high, too much heat, dryness, and acid will accumulate. The food that we eat becomes our most important medicine because it has such a direct affect on our agni and because we put more food than any other substance into our body. Paying attention to our digestion and elimination becomes an excellent indicator of our well-being. Problems in these areas are usually the first stage of a disease process. Digestive problems such as heartburn, nausea, and bloating and elimination problems such as gas, constipation, and loose stools become useful indicators. There are specific eating guidelines within Ayurveda that can be applied along with the dosha-recommended food lists and lifestyle recommendations. Table 12.3 lists guidelines for the promotion of healthy digestion.

AYURVEDIC THERAPIES

Herbal Therapy

The pharmacology of Ayurveda contains thousands of medicines, and many of them are herbal combinations. These remedies are used to support the physiological condition of the patient and reestablish harmony

TABLE 12.3 Guidelines for the Promotion of Healthy Digestion

Eat in a quiet environment: no television, loud music, or other distractions.

Do not eat when emotionally disturbed or upset.

Eat slowly and chew your food well.

Eat sitting down and with good posture.

Eat when hungry: allow 4 to 6 hours between meals.

Avoid icy cold beverages and milk with meals.

Drink warm beverages, sipped slowly and in small amounts, with meals.

Eat lightly cooked, fresh and warm foods most of the time.

Eat until two-thirds to three-quarters full.

Walk or sit quietly for 30 minutes after meals.

and balance. Herbs are classified according to the qualities they contain as well as the qualities they produce in the body. For example, an herb may be classified as having heating or cooling properties, sweet or bitter taste, dry or damp qualities. These same qualities will be increased in the person ingesting the plant. In this way herbs can be used to increase or decrease these qualities in the body. Ayurveda is very practical in its application of botanical medicine.

Various carriers are also used depending on the condition of the patient. Herbal teas, tinctures, herbal ghee, medicinal wines, powders, and tablets are used. Herbal preparations are to be taken at different times also according to constitution, condition of agni or digestive ability, and severity of disease.

Pancha Karma

The human body requires regular cleansing to ensure long and proper functioning. Accumulated toxins from poor diet and environmental pollution need to be removed to prevent blockages and malfunctioning. Pancha Karma is a detoxification therapy that uses a variety of purification techniques and procedures to eliminate or neutralize the accumulation of ama (toxins) in the body. These techniques serve to (1) remove excess dosha and ama and (2) provide tonification to strengthen and renew the body. Pancha Karma also serves to enhance vital energy and prevent the occurrence of disease. The palliation therapy that can be applied includes adjustment of food and liquid, exercise, exposure to sun, and exposure to fresh air. Supportive herbal therapy may be used to either increase digestive power or promote detoxification. Purification techniques include the following:

Vamana: an herb-induced emesis
Virechana: an herb-induced purgation
Anovasana Basti: a medicated enema with oil
Niruha Basti: decoction used for a cleansing enema
Nasaya: a nasal medication usually consisting of a medicated oil

There are also preparatory procedures that need to be applied before these purification techniques can be administered. These procedures include special diet, oilation therapy, and swedena, or sweating therapy. The special diet usually consists of eating a mono-food diet of kitchari. Kitchari is a single-dish meal composed of yellow split mung beans and basmati rice that is cooked until soft. Spices and vegetables compatible to your dosha can also be added to this dish. This dish is considered very easy to digest as well as nourishing. A person is encouraged to eat as much as he or she needs. This mono-food diet allows the body to have a rest while maintaining its strength.

Oilation therapy includes ingesting enough fat in the form of ghee (Indian clarified butter) or oil to thoroughly lubricate the digestive track for proper elimination of toxins. Oilation therapy is also applied externally through massage, or abhyanga, using copious amounts of medicated oils. This massage is applied by two practitioners using rhythmical strokes and is designed to deeply moisturize the skin, break up toxins, and stimulate circulation. Shirodhara is a process that consists of pouring warm sesame oil over the third eye in a steady stream lasting about 20 to 30 minutes. This oilation process expands consciousness, synchronizes brain waves, nourishes the brain cells, and coordinates the mind and body.

Swedna, or sweating therapy, is an herbal steam therapy that removes mental, emotional, and physical toxins that are lodged deep in the tissues. The usual therapy format is to apply the abhyanga massage first to increase circulation, break up toxins, and improve the skin's elimination ability, then apply the swedena therapy to draw out the toxins and end with the Shirodhara treatment to induce a final balancing between the mind and body.

Meditation

Meditation is an integral part of Ayurveda. Meditation promotes a Sattvic mind, calm, rational, and accepting. It promotes a balanced disposition. Stress, as we know, affects us physiologically in a very negative way. Meditation is a very direct technique that helps us to mediate this stress response. One marker for greater exposure to stress is lowered dehydroepiandrosterone (DHEA) hormone levels. DHEA is the precursor to the stress hormones adrenaline and cortisol, and it is also the hormone that is associated with the aging process. Levels of DHEA begin to decline naturally after the age of 25. There have been studies that have shown that meditation helps to bolster DHEA levels. Studies have also shown that people who meditate regularly go to their physicians' offices less often, have lower blood pressure, and have less incidence of cardiac disease. Meditation has been referred to as a "hypometabolic wakefulness" by researcher R. Keith Wallace, who has studied the effects of meditation.

There are various types of meditation taught by Ayurvedic practitioners. Dr. Vasant Lad teaches So-hum meditation, using the breath as the focal point. The Maharishi Mahesh Yogi teaches transcendental meditation (TM), which uses a specific Sanskrit word or mantra as the focal point. At Deepak Chopra's center in California, instructors teach primordial sound meditation, which also uses a specific Sanskrit word or mantra as the focal point. These focal points provide sound vibrations that gradually lead the mind out of its stuck patterns of thinking and into the silence that lies beneath thought. Pure awareness and integration with the Cosmic Intelligence can be found in this silence. Your consciousness will empty itself, and as it does, there is an expansion of awareness that extends out beyond yourself.

Pranayama

Pranayama is similar to qigong in Chinese medicine. They are both breathing techniques to energize the body, increase metabolic activity, and promote healing. The breathing techniques that would be recommended to you would depend on your constitutional dosha and its current condition.

Yoga

Yoga is another branch of Ayurveda that has its own highly developed philosophy. It has been practiced in India for hundreds of years and plays an integral part in Ayurveda as a healing practice. Different yoga postures, or *asanas*, would be recommended according to a person's constitution and imbalances. Table 12.4 lists yoga, herbal, diet, and lifestyle changes to promote balance of the three doshas.

AYURVEDIC ASSESSMENT

Ayurvedic practitioners assess for basic or original constitution, current constitution and its imbalances, and disease states. There are a variety of techniques available, including reading pulses and visual cues, such as the

TABLE 12.4 Recommended Changes for Promoting Balance

	Vata	Pitta	Kapha
Yoga	Postures that promote relaxation, rejuvenation, grounding, and centering; gentle, slow movements that are relaxing and restorative	Postures that are moderately vigorous and cultivate relaxation and serenity; calm, slow, noncompetitive yoga that promotes a cooling in the body	Vigorous yoga that promotes an increased heart rate and sweating; a yoga that stimulates and invigorates the whole body
Herbal	Tonic, supportive herbs such as ashwaghanda	Cooling and cleansing herbs such as neem, aloe vera, and milk thistle	Stimulating and cleansing herbs such as hot spices, guggul, and turmeric
Diet	Dairy, nuts, fats, moist grains, root vegetables, and mild spices	Sweet fruits, raw vegetables, rice, wheat, leafy greens; no hot spices; limit salt and fat	Hot, bitter-tasting foods such as hot peppers and bitter greens; dreamed vegetables, light grains; and legumes; limit all fluids and fats
Lifestyle	A calm routine that allows for plenty of rest and limited stress	An independent lifestyle with a slightly challenging but noncompetitive job	A stimulating and challenging life with lots of change; hard work and less sleep

face, tongue, lips, and nails. Urine analysis is also used for checking color, smell, and viscosity. A self-evaluation questionnaire is also administered. The most important is noticing the patient's overall appearance and how the person presents himself or herself. Also important is listening carefully to the patient's "story" and picking up any visual or auditory clues he or she has to offer.

Radial pulse is felt on the left wrist for women and on the right wrist for men. There are three positions and as many as seven depths for each of the three positions. The organs can also be assessed through palpation of the pulses, which is very similar to the Chinese medicine practice of pulse reading. This method palpates both wrists, with three positions on each wrist and a superficial and deep touch at each position. This gives us six readings on each wrist, 12 in all.

Dr. Lad's Daily Routine

This daily routine is adapted from *Ayurveda: The Science of Self-Healing* (1984), by Dr. Vasant Lad.

- Awaken before sunrise.
- Evacuate bowels and bladder upon awakening.
- Bathe every day.
- Perform 12 pranayamas in the morning and evening to create a fresh mind and body.
- Do not eat breakfast after 8:00 A.M.
- Wash your hands both before and after eating.
- Brush your teeth after all meals.
- Take a short, leisurely walk after each meal (about 15 minutes).
- Eat in silence, with awareness of the food.
- Eat slowly and chew well.
- Massage your gums, applying sesame oil with your finger every day.
- Fast 1 day a week to reduce toxins in the body.
- Sleep before 10:00 P.M.

AYURVEDA CASE STUDIES

Kapha Case Study

A 55-year-old, large boned, obese client presents with newly diagnosed type 2 diabetes and a Syndrome X profile, with hypertension, insulin resistance, and high low-density lipoprotein (LDL) cholesterol.

She describes herself as a happily married housewife for 30 years. Her physician sent her to the Ayurvedic practitioner for diabetes education.

Her present lifestyle includes no exercise, taking care of grandchildren during the week, skipping meals, and snacking on sugary foods instead. The Kapha nature is represented by her obesity, large frame, high cholesterol, insulin resistance, diabetes, a preference for sweet foods, and her resistance to exercise. Her mental nature is that of Kapha, with her continued role as a caretaker and her desire to stay at home rather than go out into the world. Skipping meals is also part of the Kapha nature. To reduce Kapha, she will need to change, and Kaphas do not like change. She needs to follow both the Kapha diet and the Kapha-reducing lifestyle that includes avoidance of sweet foods and vigorous exercise. Kaphas need mental and physical stimulation in their life, and they prefer to be couch potatoes.

Pitta Case Study

A 45-year-old male presents with a long history of GERD; he was recently diagnosed with angina. He is 5 feet, 10 inches and 180 pounds. He works as a supervisor for a large construction company. He eats on the run, smokes cigarettes, and loves drinking beers with his coworkers after work. He loves to play competitive squash in the winter and tennis in the summer. His wife recently left him, and he is fighting for joint custody of their children. He referred himself to the Ayurvedic practitioner because his GERD had gotten worse and he is having trouble getting to sleep at night. The Pitta nature is represented in his capacity to work and play hard. He loves the heat of competition, alcohol, and smoking. His GERD is representative of this heat and his poor eating habits. Pittas thrive on stress, but it eventually takes its toll as represented by both the GERD and angina. Pittas are independent and will self-refer themselves more than others. This patient also has a mental Vata imbalance due to the anxiety from the divorce. He would need to follow the Pitta diet to reduce the heat in his body, while also following a Vata nurturing lifestyle of routine, rest, and calming activities to reduce the Vata imbalance in the mind.

Vata Case Study

A 55-year-old woman presents with mild osteoporosis, irritable bowel syndrome (IBS), and newly diagnosed chronic fatigue. She is medium boned, 5 feet, 6 inches and 120 pounds. She lives alone and works at an advertisement agency as a graphic designer. She found the name of the Ayurvedic practitioner in the phone book and has come because she desperately wants help to keep working despite her present illness. The Vata nature is represented by her low body weight, osteoporosis, IBS, and fatigue. Her creativity and living alone are also suggestive of the Vata nature.

However, her mental nature is that of Pitta, with her drive to keep on working despite the low energy and her love of the competitive environment of advertising. She needs to follow a Vata diet to reduce the IBS symptoms and to replenish the body. To calm the Pitta mind, she will need to participate in a Pitta-calming lifestyle that includes avoiding competition and participating in an exercise program such as strength training that does not require too much energy. The strength training provides the Pitta mind with something to focus on. She needs to be encouraged to take time away from work to participate in fun activities.

LOCATING A PRACTITIONER

There is no standardized credential for Ayurvedic practitioners in the United States. Ayurveda is a fairly new import into this country, and there are not many qualified practitioners available at this time. An Ayurvedic doctor will have a bachelor or doctor of Ayurvedic medicine and surgery (BAMS or DAMS) degree and will have been trained in India. There is also a diploma degree offered by some institutions in India as well as the now defunct New England Ayurvedic Institute. This is the Diploma of Ayurveda (DAy), which is more like a status of certification.

For more information, see the list of sources in Resources.

RESOURCES

American Institute of Vedic Studies, P.O. Box 8357, Santa Fe, NM; telephone: (505) 983-9385; fax: (505) 982-5807; Web site: www.vedanet.com

The Ayurvedic Institute, 1311 Menual Blvd NE, Albuquerque, NM 87112; telephone: (505) 291-9698; fax: (505) 294-7572; Web site: www.ayurveda.com

Ayurvedic and Naturopathic Medical Clinic, 2115 112th Ave. NE, Bellevue, WA 98004; telephone: (425) 453-8022; Web site: www.ayurvedicscience.com

California College of Ayurveda, 1117A E. Main St., Grass Valley, CA 95945; telephone: (800) 541-6699; Web site: www.ayurvedacollege.com

The Himalayan Institute, 952 Bethany Turnpike, Honesdale, PA 18431; telephone: (800) 822-4547; Web site: www.himalayaninstitute.org

The Maharishi College of Vedic Medicine, 2721 Arizona St. NE, Albuquerque, NM 87110; telephone: (888) 895-2614; Web site: www.maharishi-medical.com

National Ayurvedic Medical Association (NAMA), Web site: www.ayurveda-nama.org

National Institute of Ayurvedic Medicine, 584 Milltown Rd., Brewster, NY 10509; telephone: (888) 246-6426; Web site: www.niam.com

Additional Resources

www.ayurveda.com
www.ayurvedacollege.com
www.ayurveda-nama.org
www.ayurveda-foryou.com
www.banyontrading.com
www.chopra.com
www.mapi.com
www.niam.com
www.theraj.com

Books

The Ayurvedic encyclopedia. (1998). Bayville, NY: Ayurveda Holistic Center Press.
Chopra, D. (1989). *Quantum healing.* New York: Bantam Books.
Chopra, D. (1993). *Ageless body, timeless mind.* New York: Three Rivers Press.
Frawley, D. (1989). *Ayurvedic healing.* Salt Lake City: Passage Press.
Frawley, D. (1996). *Ayurveda and the mind.* Twin Lakes, WI: Lotus Press.
Lad, V. (1984). *Ayurveda: the science of self healing.* Twin Lakes, WI: Lotus Press.
Lad, V. (2002). *Textbook of Ayurveda: fundamental principles.* Albuquerque, NM: Ayurvedic Press.
Tiwari, M. (2000). *The path of practice: a woman's book of healing.* New York: Ballantine Books.

REFERENCES

Chopra, D. (1993). *Ageless body, timeless mind.* New York: Three Rivers Press.
Lad, V. (1984). *Ayurveda: the science of self healing.* Twin Lakes, WI: Lotus Press.

CHAPTER THIRTEEN

Meditation and Healthy Aging*

Elaine J. Yuen and Michael J. Baime

Meditation is one of the oldest and most widely practiced mind–body therapies. Meditation practices drawn from the Buddhist and Hindu traditions have become frequently used in a variety of settings by caregivers and care recipients alike. A large body of knowledge suggests meditation supports an understanding of the subjective experiences, quality of life, and psychosocial variables that play a central role in health and healing. Most of the current research in meditation has not focused on elderly age groups in particular, but the utility of meditation practice has been well established for the general population. However, the utility of mindfulness, engendered by meditation practices, may be salient for elderly populations as they face issues of control and survival, memory loss, and outgrowing previous life patterns (Langer, 1989, pp. 81–114).

Elders face substantial life stresses: They must often cope with decreasing physical and mental abilities, increased dependence within their living situations, and changing family dynamics. Depression, anxiety, personality traits, social support, and spirituality have all been associated with disease incidence and outcomes (Achterberg et al., 1995). Research has shown that elders may prefer mind–body strategies that are self-administered and include both physical and cognitive elements, as they wish to remain involved in their self-care as long as possible (Lansbury, 2000; Robichaud & Lamarre, 2002).

*Parts of this chapter have been adapted from Baime, M. J. (1999). Meditation and mindfulness. In W. B. Jonas & J. S. Levin (Eds.), *Essentials of complementary and alternative medicine.* Philadelphia: Lippincott Williams & Wilkins.

Meditation practices have the potential to benefit both elderly care recipients and their formal/informal caregivers. The underlying view of meditation, drawn from Buddhist and Hindu teachings, gives caregivers and care recipients alike perspectives that address impermanence, death, and dying. This view has been incorporated into treatment and caregiving approaches, particularly in hospice and palliative care settings where elders face daily experiences of loss and change within their lives (Cason & Lindbergh, 2001; Collett, 1999; Ostateski, 1994). Practitioners of meditation have discovered that meditation can be done concurrently with their existing religious traditions, and that it is not necessary to become a Buddhist. Rather, contemplative seekers from many traditions have benefited from the practices and understandings of meditation (Arnis, 1989; Bair, 1998; Fox, 1998, 2000; Kaplan, 1997; Keenan, Keenan, & Kasimow, 2003).

Evidence that the mind has a meaningful role in health maintenance and disease recovery has fueled interest in meditation as a treatment in medical settings. Meditation has been used as primary therapy to treat specific diseases, as injunctive therapy in comprehensive treatment plans, and as a means of improving the quality of life of individuals with chronic or debilitating illnesses. Meditation can teach patients how to cope more successfully with the stresses of illness and treatment (Achterberg et al., 1995), as well as give them an increased sense of control and spiritual experiences (Astin, 1997). The causal relationship between improvement of psychosocial variables and disease prevention is unknown. However, ongoing research has examined relationships between mind–body practices and clinical treatment in areas as diverse as cancer treatment (Brown & Ryan, 2003; Carlson, Ursuliak, Goodey, Angen, & Speca, 2001; Kabat-Zinn, 1998), depression and anxiety in patients as well as family caregivers (Ducharme, 2002; Kabat-Zinn, 1992; Kabat-Zinn et al., 1992), and heart disease (Luskin, Reitz, Newell, Quinn, & Haskell, 2002). The National Institutes of Health concluded the following:

> More than 30 years of research, as well as the experiences of a large and growing number of individuals and health care providers, suggests that meditation and similar forms of relaxation can lead to better health, higher quality of life, and lowered health-care costs . . . . Most important, meditation techniques offer the potential of learning how to live in an increasingly complex and stressful society while helping to preserve health in the process. Given their low-cost and demonstrated health benefits, these simple mental technologies may be some of the best candidates among the alternative therapies for widespread inclusion in medical practice and for investment of medical resources. (Achterberg et al., 1994, p 16)

In this chapter, we will first describe meditation, its physiological and psychological effects, and practices of frequently available meditation disciplines, such as mindfulness and transcendental meditation (TM). Documented benefits and potential applications of these meditation practices will then be outlined. A resource list of readings and Web sites is included for those interested in learning more about meditation.

WHAT IS MEDITATION?

There is a plethora of practices that are considered to be "meditation" disciplines, including physical disciplines such as yoga, or Christian contemplative practices (Merton, 1996). Many techniques originated as spiritual practices within traditional religious contexts, such as the contemplations of St. Thomas Aquinas or the Buddhist practice of sitting meditation. The meditation techniques discussed in this chapter will focus on those used in silent sitting meditation, where a focal point such as breathing or a mantra is used. These meditation techniques use awareness of ordinary physical processes, such as breathing and attention to one's mind states, as a focal point that allows for the integration of one's physical being, emotional impulses, and conscious thoughts.

Meditation experiences have been described in some texts as a "sacred state of consciousness." However, there is nothing inherently religious about these practices. Meditation practices can be taken from their traditional cultural or religious setting and used as tools to improve health and quality of life. The same techniques that are used to promote personal or spiritual growth may be directed toward the relief of stress or physical discomfort. Meditation teacher Sakyong Mipham Rinpoche notes that the state of mindfulness could be viewed as an ordinary, and often neglected, aspect of our natural mind:

> The practice of mindfulness/awareness meditation is . . . inherent in all human beings. In meditation we are continuously discovering who and what we are. That could be quite frightening or quite boring, but after a while, all that slips away. We get into some kind of natural rhythm and begin to discover our basic mind and heart. Often we think about meditation as some kind of unusual, holy spiritual activity. As we practice, that is one of the basic beliefs we try to overcome. The point is that meditation is completely normal; it is the mindful quality present in everything we do. (Sakyong Mipham Rinpoche, 2003)

Old age is a naturally contemplative time of life. The slowing down and attention to detail that characterize old age can be seen as analogous to the mindfulness practices of meditation. For elders, rather than focusing on a singular meditation technique, it may be helpful to work with them to understand that these contemplations and mindfulness practices are already inherent in their lives. This perspective allows them to view their daily routines and domestic rituals in a new light.

Sitting meditation techniques all share a structured mental process that deepens awareness by bringing it to rest on a stable focus. A traditional analogy of meditation often refers to taming the mind in a way that is similar to the practice of a sport or a musical instrument. This process may include resting the attention

1. On a physical sensation, such as breathing (this is used as a focus in some forms of traditional Buddhist or mindfulness meditation)
2. On a thought or word that is silently repeated (this is used as some yoga practices and in transcendental meditation).
3. On an external object, such as a candle's flame or a statue
4. On simply being with what is, as in the Tibetan Buddhist tradition of Dzogchen

By intentionally directing and regulating the attention of one's mind, the meditator modifies the mind's function and its relationship to the body. One learns to rest awareness in the present moment without struggle or wandering. This cessation of struggle is often experienced as mental and physical relaxation. Herbert Benson documented this as the "relaxation response," a naturally occurring contemplative state where relaxation and focus of the mind can affect physical and mental health and alleviate stress (Benson, 1985, p. 5).

Individuals who practice meditation regularly have significant reductions in anxiety and depression; these reductions have been documented with many commonly used psychometric tools. There is also evidence that the regular practice of meditation improves a person's functional status and quality of life. Meditation has been shown to significantly reduce the number of somatic symptoms reported by a broad range of patients with medical diagnoses. Meditation also benefits individuals without acute medical illness or stress. People who meditate regularly report they feel more confident and more in control of their lives. They say that their relationships with others are improved, and they experience more enjoyment and appreciation of life (Baime & Baime, 1996; Kabat-Zinn, 1996).

COMMONLY TAUGHT TYPES OF MEDITATION

There are a host of meditation practices available to health care practitioners and the general public today, drawing upon a number of different

Eastern and Western traditions. An Internet search yielded over 4 million sites using the keyword "meditation." In some medical texts, meditation practices have been distinguished as being expansive (e.g., mindfulness, which uses the entire field of attention as a focal point), or concentrative (e.g., TM, which uses a word or mantra as a focal point). However, meditation as it has been taught in Buddhist and other contemplative traditions includes both expansive and concentrative techniques as a means to train the mind, often alternating them as the practitioner modulates their awareness. Training the mind has been compared in traditional analogy to tuning a musical instrument: as being not too loose and not too tight. If the string (or the mind) is too loose or relaxed, it will not sound or reverberate. If it is too tight, it will break.

Therefore, when considering the many meditation techniques available through classes, tapes, the Internet, and books, it is equally important to consider how an individual may benefit from the various types of meditation, as well as the environment or context in which it is taught. Elders may connect with some types of meditation but not others; for instance, highly devout Christians may find the repetition of a singular prayer that focuses their mind to be most calming; whereas others may desire to rest their attention on whatever arises. Others may desire to combine sitting meditation practices with contemplative exercises, such as chi-qong or tai-chi. Below we discuss two frequently taught "schools" of meditation stemming from the mindfulness and TM traditions.

Mindfulness Meditation

Mindfulness meditation has its origins in traditional Buddhist practice and was originally taught as having four foundations, or components, referring to the physical body, emotions, mental contents, and transcendent awareness (Thera, 1962). In the modern context, mindfulness can be seen as a tool by which we understand the mind and create a sense of being in the most profound sense. Mindfulness brings an awareness of the mind's cognitive and emotional processes by observing them in meditation with nonjudgmental awareness (Trungpa, 1976, pp. 17–22). Meditation master Chogyam Trungpa Rinpoche comments:

> In order to experience this state of being, it is necessary to practice what is known as mindfulness. You simply pay attention to your breath, as you breathe in and out, and to every detail in your mind, whether it is a thought pattern of aggression, passion, or ignorance, or just insignificant mental chatter. Mindfulness also means paying attention to the details of every action, for example, to the way you extend your hand to reach for a glass. You see yourself lifting it, touching it to your lips, and then drinking the water. So every detail is looked at precisely—

which doesn't make you self-conscious, particularly, but it may give you quite a shock; it may be quite real. When mindfulness begins to grow and expand, you become more aware of the environment around you, of something more than just body and mind alone. And then, at some point, mindfulness and awareness are joined together, which becomes one open eye, one big precision. (Trungpa, 1987, p. 200)

Mindfulness meditation was introduced in medical settings by Jon Kabat-Zinn, who founded The Stress Reduction Clinic at the University of Massachusetts Medical Center in 1979. Since that time, Kabat-Zinn has been instrumental in promoting the use of meditation as a treatment in Western medicine. Mindfulness meditation has been used in medical centers and hospital-based stress management programs throughout the United States and Europe (Majumdar, Grossman, Dietz-Waschkowski, Kersig, & Walach, 2002); currently, mindfulness-based stress reduction programs are sponsored by hospitals, medical schools, and clinics. Mindfulness programs have also been taught in the workplace to lawyers, judges, and managers (Riskin, 2002; see also www.shambhalainstitute.org) and in prisons (Whitney, 2002). Kabat-Zinn was one of the first researchers of the effects of meditation on mental and physical health (Kabat-Zinn, 1982; Kabat-Zinn et al., 1992), and his research has helped to set the stage for its broad acceptance as a mind–body treatment modality. A recent review of the scientific literature showed that there were over 60 studies that examined the effects of the mindfulness-based stress reduction program and improving mental and physical health (Grossman, Niemann, Schmidt, & Walach, 2004).

Mindfulness teaches its practitioners to cultivate a nonjudgmental state of openness and relaxation that can be maintained throughout activity. In formal mindfulness meditation, practitioners are taught to place their attention on a simple event, such as breathing, and to stabilize and evenly rest the awareness in the present moment. Mindfulness is the practice of resting steadily with "clear and single-minded awareness of what actually happens to us and in us at the successful moments of perception" (Thera, 1962). During this time, wandering thoughts and shifts in attention are noticed as they occur without suppressing, resisting, or commenting on them. Mindfulness meditation cultivates "an intentionally non-reactive, nonjudgmental moment-to-moment awareness of a changing field of objects" (Kabat-Zinn, Ohm Massion, Herbert, & Rosenbaum, 1998, p. 768).

Informal meditation practice, described as the application of mindfulness outside formal meditation sessions, is also emphasized. Meditators are taught to rest their awareness on any event that occurs. This is said to cultivate both a balanced equanimity and a fuller and richer experience of life. Kabat-Zinn (1993, pp. 262–263) says:

The key to mindfulness is not so much what you choose to focus on but the quality of the awareness that you bring to each moment. It is this investigative, discerning observation of whatever comes up in the present moment that is the hallmark of mindfulness and differentiates it from other forms of meditation. The goal of mindfulness is for you to be more aware, more in touch with life and with whatever is happening in your own body and mind at the time it is happening—that is, the present moment. By fully excepting what each moment offers, you open yourself to experience life much more completely and make it more likely that you will be able to respond effectively to any situation that presents itself.

Mindfulness meditation provides cognitive learning as well as relaxation. Meditators are taught to recognize the repetitive patterns of their stressful thoughts and emotions and to inquire into them. Discovering that the thoughts and feelings accompanying stress reactions are often maladaptive or inaccurate leads one to more adaptive and skillful responses to stress.

Transcendental Meditation

Transcendental meditation is one of the most widely practiced forms of meditation in the West; somewhere between 2 million and 5 million individuals have been taught the technique (Achterberg et al., 1995; Alexander, 1994; see also www.tm.org). Numerous research studies have been performed to investigate its efficacy in physiological, psychological, and social domains, and much of what is known about the physiology of meditation comes from the study of TM. TM has its origins in the Vedic tradition of India and was introduced to the West by the Maharishi Mahesh Yogi.

In TM, the meditator sits with his or her eyes closed for 20 minutes, twice a day, and effortlessly attends to a syllable or word (i.e., a mantra). Whenever thoughts or distractions arise, the attention is directed back to the mantra. One report states that TM "is said to allow the individual to experience increasingly refined levels of mental activity until a state of 'pure consciousness' is experienced in which the mind is fully alert, yet completely silent and settled. This distinctive experience of 'restful alertness' has been distinguished from the aroused state of ordinary waking and the restful but inert state of sleep" (Alexander et al., 1993). The late Charles Alexander, a prominent TM researcher, wrote that "during TM, ordinary waking mental activity is said to settle down, until even the subtlest thought is transcended and a completely unified wholeness of awareness beyond the division of subject and object is experienced. In this silent, self referential state of pure wakefulness, consciousness is fully awake to itself alone with no objects of thought or perception" (Alexander, 1994, p. 545).

Early work by Herbert Benson utilized the focusing techniques of TM to develop the "relaxation response," which has been documented to be effective in reducing heart rate, lowering blood pressure, reducing metabolic speed, and alleviating stress (Benson, 1982; Caudill, Friedman, & Benson, 1987; Domar, Noe, & Benson, 1987). More recently, programs developed by the Mind–Body Medical Institute at Harvard have sought to integrate techniques found in TM with mindfulness and other modalities to evoke the relaxation response, and to improve health in general (Deckro et al., 2002; see also www.mbmi.org).

Research documenting the use of TM studying many different medical conditions and patient populations has been compiled by the TM-sponsored Institute for Scientific Research at Maharishi University of Management (see http://www.tm.org/research/508_studies.html). There have been over 500 studies to date, finding positive healing relationships between TM and improved physiological and mental functioning in patients, schoolchildren, prisoners, and employees in the workplace.

The TM program also includes another technique: the TM-Siddhi. This more active form of meditative yoga also has its roots in Vedic tradition. More recently, the Maharishi Mahesh Yogi has also recommended Ayurvedic medicine, the traditional health care system of India, and has promoted the use of Ayurvedic food supplements and products as a complement to TM (Sharma & Alexander, 1996), as well as developed a series of short health education courses that include topics on preventive health, diet, and nutrition (see http://www.tm.org/main_pages/programs.html).

PSYCHOLOGY OF MEDITATION

Meditation has been used for millennia as a way to calm and stabilize the mind. Initially, formal meditation periods provide respite from the speed and turmoil of everyday life. Later, the meditator learns to remain in a state of relaxation even in the midst of activity or stressful surroundings. Meditators consistently report that they can handle difficult situations more easily as they become more adept at meditation. Ultimately, the path of meditation becomes a larger journey toward greater psychological stability and health. The initial need to deal with a stressful medical condition may be subsumed into the larger goal of learning to cope more skillfully with all the stresses of life. Although life has undeniably always been stressful, present-day culture has its own unique stressors and demands. Many people think that these demands are more than they can reasonably manage. Elders in particular often feel marginalized by the rapid pace of our society, and often struggle to "keep up" producing chronic stressors (Schacter-Shalomi, 1995).

Numerous studies have shown that meditation practices support coping with distress and disability in daily life, as well as address depression, anxiety, and affective disorders. Mindfulness meditation has been found to decrease stress by reducing overall psychological symptomatolgy, increasing a sense of control in one's life; and increasing one's spiritual experiences (Astin, 1997). For elders, meditation practices may help to give perspective to their life as physical and mental abilities operate at a slower pace. Deeper goals of meditation include liberating the spirit from the egocentric self, developing a sense of harmony within the universe, and nourishing the ability to increase compassion. These values may be increasingly important to elders as they work to understand physical declines, impending death, and the loss of friends (Helpard, 1998).

While elders cherish good physical health as much as other age groups, they also broadly define quality of life. In old age quality of life has been described as having dimensions of well-being, meaning, and value (Sarvimaki & Stenbock-Hult, 2000). Through the nonjudgmental acknowledgment of thoughts, feelings, hopes, and fears, meditation practice provides a context where anxieties about physical and mental functioning may be faced, felt, and understood. A challenge that elders face is social isolation, and working with meditation practices in a social context of a group or with a facilitator may optimally provide a way to work with these issues (Bishop & Scurlock, 1992).

Elders and their caregivers often face concerns of memory loss and inability to concentrate, and integrative medicine may have the ability to prevent and even reverse memory loss (Branin, 2001; Khalsa, 1998). Elders in nursing homes who are engaged in mindful learning have been shown to be more active, alert, and happy than those who are not allowed to make as many decisions or who may not be as engaged in their lives. Through mindfulness exercises, a group of nursing home residents were able to improve their memory and attention (Langer, 1989, pp. 88–89).

Perlmutter and others (Perlmutter, 1988; Perlmutter & Hall, 1992; Smitt, 1997, 1999, 2000) have posited that there are three dimensions of cognition to consider in adults:

1. Fluid intelligence (this type of cognition is related to the speed of processing within the brain and typically diminishes with aging)
2. Crystallized intelligence (this type of cognition forms our "knowledge base" and may increase as people age

3. Metacognition (this type of cognition is related to strategic thinking and understanding how the mind works, and is a developed ability at any age)

Mindfulness practices, which aim to bring enhanced awareness to ordinary day-to-day events, may support the strategic thinking capacities of metacognition. For instance, if elders are aware that they keep misplacing their glasses, enhanced metacognition may help them to develop a mental strategy to address this problem, such as putting the glasses in the same place all of the time.

In addition to improving cognitive abilities, the cultivation of a nonjudgmental perspective found in meditation practices may help elders to have a nonstereotypical view of themselves. Research has shown that those who are haunted by a stereotypical or preconceived notion of being less able have lower levels of performance (Hess, Auman, Colcombe, & Rahhal, 2003; Steele, 1997). Meditation practices are able to help elders free themselves from the many stereotypes our culture holds about the aged, such as being frail, infirm, and chronically ill (personal communication, T. Lhamo, July 31, 2003; personal communication, V. Howard, July 12, 2003).

Traditional Buddhist beliefs have as their foundation an understanding and acceptance of life transitions of birth, old age, sickness, and death. Contemporary practitioners have taken these views and applied them to the fears of impermanence and aging that we experience in a modern society whose priorities are to maintain youth. Larry Rosenberg (2001, p. 13), a sociologist and Insight Meditation teacher, writes:

> We harbor a huge amount of unfelt fear about sickness, aging, and death, and that fear robs us of vitality, partly because we expend so much energy avoiding and repressing it. Bringing up this fear and facing it is a great enhancement to our lives. Really facing death enables us to appreciate and make the best use of our life in a whole new way.

For elders and their caregivers, fear and hesitation to directly face the personal inevitability of their own impermanence are often paramount. Even for those who may not be acutely ill, there is often an unarticulated awareness of their diminishing abilities, be it as ordinary as not being able to drive, or to depend on others for help in ordinary activities of living. Elders often require support to be able to grieve these smaller functional losses, as well as to work through larger issues of sickness and death.

PHYSIOLOGY OF MEDITATION

Western medical science began an organized study of physiological changes associated with meditation in the early 1960s, and by 1970 there was a growing body of evidence that meditation alters physiology as well as the psyche (Wallace, 1970). In some cases, specific findings varied among early studies and among different meditation techniques (Woolfolk, 1975), although it was apparent that the physiological state produced during meditation differs from that which occurs during rest or sleep (Dillbeck & Orme-Johnson, 1987). Subsequent research has clarified many of these differences and has begun to show a consistent set of physiological changes that accompany meditation. It is hypothesized that meditation creates a unique physiological state that maintains a high level of central nervous system functioning and alertness while simultaneously allowing for rest and relaxation (Jevning, Wallace, & Beidebach, 1992). A conference at the Massachusetts Institute of Technology brought together psychologists, neuroscientists, Buddhist teachers, and practicing meditators to discuss and understand further the nexus of how the physiology of meditation could affect states of consciousness (see http://www.investigatingthemind.org/).

Meditation affects many different physiological systems, and these biological changes provide part of the theoretical rationale for the use of meditation as a medical treatment. Most studies have found that physiologic markers decreased during meditation and that these changes were more marked than those that occurred during other types of rest. In Benson's work on the "relaxation response," he documented changes in oxygen consumption, respiratory rate, heart rate, alpha waves, blood pressure, and muscle tension using different meditation techniques, including TM, Zen, and yoga, progressive muscle relaxation, and hypnosis (Benson, 1976, pp. 98–99).

Many recent studies have focused on the interrelationships between the cognitive changes that meditation practices bring, brain chemistry, and the neuroendocrine system. There is compelling evidence that the neural structures involved with attention and control are affected by meditation (Lazar et al., 2000). The effects of meditation on the pituitary adrenal axis are particularly well studied. Numerous studies show an acute decrease in cortisol secretion during meditation (Jevning, Wilson, & Davidson, 1978; Michaels, Parra, McCann, & Vander, 1979; Sudsuang, Chentanez, & Veluvan, 1991), and a preliminary study found that meditators had reduced cortisol, thyroid-stimulating hormone, and growth hormone secretion in response to an experimental stress (MacLean et al., 1994). Other research has shown alterations in concentrations of beta-endorphin and corticotropin-releasing hormone (Harte, Eifert, & Smith, 1995), melatonin (Massion, Teas, Hebert, Wertheimer, & Kabat-Zinn, 1995), dehydroepiandrosterone sulfate (DHEA-S; Glaser et al., 1992), and SYMBOL-aminobutyric acid (GABA; Elias & Wilson, 1995).

Extensive research has explored electroencephalogram (EEG) changes during meditation. Most of this work shows increases in high-voltage theta wave burst activity and frontal alpha wave coherence in tracings obtained during meditation. EEG coherence, a measure of simultaneous phase EEG activity at different cortical locations, is also increased during meditation and may be associated with some of the subjective experiences of meditation (Aftanas & Golocheikine, 2002; Farrow & Hebert, 1982; Lehmann et al., 2001); however, the significance of these changes is unknown. Functional brain scanning, a newer technique that directly measures brain activity or central nervous system blood flow, has been used to quantify changes in regional brain function during meditation. Meaningful changes in the activation of focal brain regions have been documented during meditation (Herzog, 1990–1991; Newberg et al., 2001). Increased blood flow has been observed in areas of the brain that involve focusing attention, as well as decreased activity in the orientation area, believed to be related to a sense of openness and loss of self-reference point (Newberg et al.2001; see also www.andynewberg.com/qna.asp). Research into the physiology of perception and meditators has also found changes in sensitivity to stimuli and in sensory evoked potentials (Becker & Shapiro, 1981; Brown, Forte, & Dysart, 1984; McEvoy, Frumkin, & Harkins, 1980).

Meditation practices have been related to metabolic changes. One study documented a 50% decline in respiratory rate and a 40% decrease in oxygen consumption during meditation in experienced meditators (Farrow & Hebert, 1982). This study also describes brief periods of complete respiratory cessation that correlate with the meditators' report of peak meditative intensity. Another report documented that three Buddhist monks were able to vary oxygen consumption markedly using different advanced Tibetan Buddhist meditation techniques: Oxygen consumption decreased as much as 64% and, during a different meditative practice that attempts to increase "inner heat," increased as much as 61% (Benson et al., 1982).

It has been difficult to demonstrate a consistent effect from meditation on autonomic nervous system function. There is little evidence for a reproducible effect on heart rate that differs significantly from other types of rest; however, galvanic skin resistance seems to increase reliably during meditation, suggesting decreased sympathetic activity (Jevning et al., 1992). A preliminary study found that meditators experienced no changes in circulating catecholamines but did experience significant decreases in beta-adrenergic receptors (Mills et al., 1990). Another study found decreases in autonomic activation among inexperienced meditators but increased activation in more proficient meditators (Corby, Roth, Zarcone, & Kopell, 1978). This disparity possibly explains some of the inconsistent results in other studies.

APPLICATIONS OF MEDITATION

Clinical Evidence

Studies have established myriad benefits of meditation practice on health. Although there are few singular studies of meditation in an elderly population, research has shown that elders are interested in mind–body therapies, especially as complementary therapies to existent medical practices (Astin, Pelletier, Marie, & Haskell, 2000; Luskin et al., 2000). TM, mindfulness meditation, and general relaxation techniques were studied in a group of nursing home residents, showing favorable outcomes for both the TM and mindfulness groups in both behavioral and physiological dimensions (Alexander, Langer, Newman, Chandler, & Davies, 1989). Anecdotal evidence of teaching meditation to elders has indicated that they benefit from these techniques, although ongoing support from trained instructors is often required. Elders may most beneficially combine stress reduction techniques with other modalities of care, incorporating modifications that account for changes due to aging (Weinberger, 1991).

Practitioners of all types of meditation consistently report some common effects. All forms of meditation generate a state of relaxation. This relaxation appears to be different from that induced by other more active or physical methods of relaxation, such as exercise or progressive muscle relaxation. Another frequently reported benefit is a sense of psychological balance or equanimity. Meditation cultivates an emotional stability that allows the meditator to experience intense emotions fully while simultaneously maintaining perspective on them. As described in the tradition of mindfulness meditation, "the practitioner of their attention (i.e., mindfulness) becomes able to contain any reaction: making space for it, but not completely identifying with it because of the consummate and presence of nonjudgmental awareness" (Epstein, 1995, p. 111). TM also describes the development of this type of emotional balance and suggests that it is a consequence of that relaxation that meditation provides.

Proponents of meditation—particularly mindfulness meditation and TM—claim that it enhances psychological insight or understanding. Through the sustained application of nonjudgmental awareness, the meditator sees repetitive patterns of behavior and cognition more clearly. In mindfulness meditation, individuals are taught to experience and explore thoughts and feelings as events that are allowed to occur without invoking habitual patterns of response; this allows the meditator to gain insight into the nature of his or her involuntary habitual reactions. Kabat-Zinn et al. (1998, p. 769) write that "the element of constant inquiry characteristic of mindfulness practice, promoted not through thinking but through bare attending and a continual non-discursive questioning about what one is actually experiencing, lays the foundation for such insight to arise." Although insight is not emphasized as strongly in TM as in other types of meditation, enhancement of autonomy and freedom from unhealthy patterns of behavior are frequently described. One prominent investigator of TM writes that "meditators become better able to see another person's perspective, yet they cannot easily be swayed by social pressure to do something which they judge to be wrong" (Orme-Johnson, 1995).

In summary, elders and caregivers would potentially benefit from the emotional and cognitive support that meditation practices bring. There is evidence that for elders there is a relationship between stress levels, coping strategies, and "life review" techniques (Puentes, 2001). Although anecdotal evidence shows that meditation practices are able to give elders insight into their losses and grieving by allowing these conflicting emotions to surface (Van Tilburg, 1991), more formal research investigating the outcomes and mechanisms of how meditation works with elders and their caregivers is needed.

Major Applications

Despite the inherent challenges of designing conclusive clinical studies of meditation, there is a considerable amount of evidence that details benefits of meditation practice. Recent studies funded by the National Center for Complementary and Alternative Medicine (NCCAM) include investigations of the relationship between meditation and eating disorders (Kristeller & Hallett, 1999), hypertension, chronic back pain, and heart disease (see CRISP: Computer Retrieval on Scientific Projects, crisp.cit.nih.gov/crisp). In general, meditation practice decreases the number of symptoms reported by patients with a wide variety of physical problems, as well as increases experiences of well-being.

Psychotherapy

Meditation has long been used as a psychological therapy, and some of the earliest proponents of meditation in the West were psychologists. During a lecture at Harvard University in the early 1900s, the renowned psychologist William James is said to have recognized a visiting Buddhist monk in the audience and exclaimed, "Take my chair! You are better equipped to lecture on psychology than I. This is the psychology every-one will be studying 25 years from now" (Fields, 1981). Although his pre-diction was premature, in the last 20 years many clinicians have reviewed the use of meditation as an adjunct to psychotherapy and explored its psychotherapeutic benefits (Bogart, 1991; Carpenter, 1977; Craven, 1989; DelMonte, 1987, 1989; Goleman, 1976; Kutz, 1985; Kutz, Borysenko, & Benson, 1985; Shapiro, 1982; Shapiro & Giber, 1978).

In *Thoughts without a Thinker* (1995), Epstein explores the uses of mindfulness meditation and psychotherapy. He examines meditation from the perspective of Western psychology and claims that

> the meditative practices of bare attention, concentration, mindfulness, and analytic inquiry speak to issues that are at the forefront of contem-porary psychodynamic concern; they are not about seeking some other-worldly abode . . . . I hope to make clear how potent a force they can be in conjunction with more traditional Western psychotherapies. (p. 111)

Other researchers have noted that Eastern psychology provides a fresh perspective on the nature of the mind and its workings. An aca-demic conference entitled "Investigating the Mind: Exchanges between Buddhism and Biobehavioral Science" explored the interface between the traditional Buddhist values and modern Western psychology (see http://www.investigatingthemind.org).

At a symposium sponsored by Harvard Medical School, Daniel Goleman (1991) remarked:

> Buddhist psychology offers modern psychology the opportunity for genuine dialogue with a system of thought that has evolved outside of conceptual systems that have spawned contemporary psychology. Here is a fully realized psychology that offers the chance for a complemen-tary view of many of the fundamental issues of modern psychology: the nature of mind; the limits of human potential for growth; the possibil-ities for mental health; the means for psychological change and trans-formation. (p. 4)

Clinical research into the psychotherapeutic benefits of meditation clearly suggests that regular meditation results in decreased anxiety (Gaylord, Orme-Johnson, & Travis, 1989; Goldberg, 1982; Kabat-Zinn, 1992; Miller, Fletcher, & Kabat-Zinn, 1995; Puryear, Cayce, & Thurston, 1976; Reibel, Greeson, Brainard, & Rosenzweig, 2001; Rosenzweig, 2001; Shapiro, Schwartz, & Bonner, 1998; Smith, Compton, & West, 1995) and depression (Baime & Baime, 1996; Smith et al., 1995; Teasdale, Segal, & Williams, 1995; Teasdale et al., 2000).

Mindfulness has also been hypothesized to improve attention in old age (Langer, 1989). Studies have shown that attention decreases with aging, as the tendency for attention to wander begins. A mindfulness technique was shown to assist elders' cognitive abilities by helping them to notice the details and texture of their experience (Levy, 2001). The insight resulting from mindfulness meditation is similar to what is described during cognitive therapy, in which patients are taught to objectively see their faults and feelings to learn where cognitive and emotional distortions arise (Beck, Rush, Shaw, & Emery, 1979). Some therapists have suggested that the antidepressant effects of cognitive therapy can be maintained with meditation (Teasdale et al., 1995). Meditation also has similarities to the process of psychodynamic psychotherapy (Epstein, 1995).

Spiritual and Emotional Support for Elders and Caregivers

Elders often struggle to find articulate meaning and value in their life as their physical and mental abilities change (Hines, Babrow, Badzek, & Moss, 2001; Jacobzone, 2000; Kraaij, Pruymboom, & Garnefski, 2002; Schimmel-Spreeuw, Linssen, & Heeren, 2000). Mindfulness has been shown to support psychological well-being through its facilitation of being in the present moment (Brown & Ryan, 2003). Vicki Howard, a therapist trained in meditation who has worked with elders in life review, commented, "The challenge of old age is to allow the dissolution of form, to open to that. Elders cannot do it alone, our culture is so unsupportive, people go to pieces in despair"(personal communication, July 12, 2003). Meditation practice provides an environment that allows elders to experience fully their physical and mental impermanence, and perhaps to develop a larger view of their lives beyond the fear of loss of control or dying.

Caregivers, often focused on addressing elders' problems, may neglect self-care issues, and caregiver strategies for coping may include support, adaptive activities, spiritual means, and avoidance (Brinson & Brunk, 2000; Clarke, 2001; Evers, Tomic, & Brouwers, 2001; Sawatzky & Fowler-Kerry, 2003; Schmall, 1995; Toseland, Labrecque, Goebel, & Whitney, 1992; Zimber, 1998). Although there are few formal studies that have documented meditation practices as a coping strategy for caregivers, there is a plethora of anecdotal evidence that describes how meditation has helped caregivers understand their loved one's mental state(s) and work with their own losses as they care for their ailing family member. The benefits of mindfulness meditation, often described as beneficial for both professional and family caregivers, may address burnout and compassion fatigue (Ko-I Bastis, 2000; Stone, 2001; see also http://www.caregiver.com/articles/mindfulness.htm), working with death and dying (Longaker, 1997; Ostateski, 1994), and establishing mindful home care environments (Cason & Lindbergh, 2001; Collett, 1999).

Pain and Fibromyalgia

Meditation is a generally accepted therapy for chronic pain (National Institutes of Health [NIH], 1995; Kabat-Zinn, 1982; Kabat-Zinn, Lipworth, & Burney, 1985). Studies found significant reductions in measures of present-moment pain, negative body image, inhibition of activity by pain, symptoms, mood disturbance, and psychological symptomatology, including anxiety and depression. Drug utilization related to pain decreased, and activity levels and feelings of self-esteem increased (Kabat-Zinn et al., 1985). A technology assessment statement of the National Institutes of Health reviewed the evidence for the use of different relaxation treatments for chronic pain, including meditation, autogenic training, and progressive muscle relaxation. The statement concluded that "the evidence is strong for the effectiveness of this class of techniques in reducing chronic pain in a variety of medical conditions" (NIH, 1995).

A study of patients with the symptoms of fibromyalgia, a difficult-to-treat syndrome of chronic pain and fatigue, reported significant improvement in symptoms in over one-half of participants (Kaplan, Goldenberg, & Galvin-Nadeau, 1993). Another study reported that fibromyalgia patients had increased positive mood and decreased anxiety, feelings of connectiveness to others, ability to relax and enjoy life, and more positive coping responses after a mindfulness training program (Tiefenthaler & Grossman, 2002).

Hypertension and Cardiovascular Disease

Meditation has been shown to be helpful as an adjunctive therapy for cardiovascular disease, as there is a close relationship between stress, anxiety, and the symptoms of cardiovascular disease (Esch, Stefano, Fricchione, & Benson, 2002; Tacon, McComb, Caldera, & Randolph, 2003). Meditation has long been recommended as an effective treatment for hypertension, but controversy exists over the magnitude of the benefit it provides. Some studies have documented only small decreases in blood pressure as compared with medication (Eisenberg et al., 1993; Mathias, 1991; Silberberg, 1990). Much of the published research has inadequate study design and sample size. One review identified more than 100 published studies and concluded that only 26 were well designed enough to be useful (Eisenberg et al., 1993). Despite these methodological problems, most of the studies show reductions in blood pressure with meditation (Alexander et al., 1996; Schneider et al., 1995). Antihypertensive drugs are clearly more effective than meditation, but because of a high prevalence of hypertension, even a relatively small treatment benefit could be expected to have a meaningful impact on both public health and the overall cost of medical care. Meditation is likely to be a highly cost-effective and efficacious treatment of mild hypertension when the risk and cost of pharmacological treatment outweigh the benefits. It might also be a useful adjunct to drug treatment.

Meditation, in conjunction with standard medical care, has been used to treat coronary artery disease. A review of mind–body therapies in the treatment of cardiovascular disease noted that mindfulness triggered a "relaxation response" where bodily calm, rather than a fight-or-flight response, was evoked (Luskin et al., 1998). Another study documented a significant decrease in exercise-induced cardiac ischemia measured with standard treadmill exercise testing (Zamarra et al., 1996). Dean Ornish and his group at the University of California have demonstrated significant regression of coronary artery stenoses as measured by both coronary angiography and positron emission tomography with a lifestyle regimen that included at least 1 hour of stress management, including meditation, daily (Gould et al., 1992; Koertge et al., 2003; Ornish, 1998; Ornish et al., 1990). Preliminary findings suggest that cardiovascular mortality in the elderly is also decreased by meditation (Alexanderet al., 1996). Accumulating data about the psychosocial factors associated with coronary heart disease have fueled interest in this area (Kabat-Zinn, 1992).

Cancer

Mindfulness meditation programs have been used with cancer patients to address the psychological disturbances and stress that they may experience during cancer treatment. Numerous case reports have documented regression of various cancers with intensive meditation, but there are no well-designed prospective clinical trials. Cancer outpatients with a wide variety of cancer diagnoses, stages of illness, and ages were found to have reduced mood disturbance in anxiety, depression, anger, and confusion scales, as well as fewer symptoms of stress (Carlson et al., 2001; Shapiro, Bootzin, Rigueredo, Lopez, & Schwartz, 2003; Speca, Carlson, Goodey, & Angen, 2000). Stress reduction programs combined with dietary changes have been piloted as a possible preventive measure in the recurrence of prostate cancer (Saxe et al., 2001). There is ongoing research on meditation used in conjunction with art therapy to help cancer outpatients enhance both the supportive and expressive aspects of the group therapy experience (personal communication, Caroline Peterson, July 1, 2003), and meditation practices have been combined with other complementary therapies to treat cancer (Alferi, Antoni, Ironson, Kilbourn, & Carver, 2001).

Other Applications

Meditation has been studied as a treatment for many other physical and emotional problems, but in most areas the studies are too small or too few to allow meaningful conclusions. A small prospective study used stress management techniques that included meditation for a group of men found positive for human immunodeficiency virus (HIV), and improvements were found in T-cell counts as well as in several psychological measures of well-being (Taylor, 1995). Meditation has been reported to improve function or reduce symptoms in patients with several neurological diseases, including epilepsy in patients resistant to standard treatment (Deepak, Manchanda, & Maheshwari, 1994; Panjwani et al., 1995), as well as patients with parkinsonism (Szekely, Turner, & Jacob, 1982), patients with multiple sclerosis who experienced fatigue (Freal, Kraft, & Coryell, 1984), and those with psoriasis (Benhard, Kristeller, & Kabat-Zinn, 1988).

Limitations

Research on meditation as a medical therapy has been complicated by some of the same problems confronting research of other alternative and complementary therapies: It may not be optimal for the investigation of meditation and similar mind–body therapies using the prospective, randomized, placebo-controlled double-blind study. Furthermore, it is difficult to create a suitable placebo for a meditation-based intervention, especially when a research design requires using a blinded control group that cannot be told if it is receiving the active treatment, as well as to design a convincing placebo that is presented as meditation.

It can be argued that meditation works by the same mechanism as does the placebo effect. This point does not diminish the effect of meditation, but rather suggests that treatments that enhance the mind's capacity to heal the body (with low cost and little risk) may provide meaningful clinical benefits. A placebo may be an effective treatment because it provides a focus through which the mind can affect the body; meditation may provide or heighten the same benefit.

Even if a suitable placebo can be devised, it may be difficult to randomize participants to a nontreatment group. Individuals who will commit the time and effort to practice meditation regularly are usually convinced of its benefits and may not consent to be part of an untreated control group. The cultivation of a regular meditation practice demands more active participation from the patient than do most medical treatments. Some studies compare meditators to a demographically similar nonmeditating control population; even when this is done prospectively, significant differences in lifestyle or personality between two such groups are likely. These differences weaken the findings of any such comparison.

A few reports describing deleterious psychological effects of meditation have been published. There is no prospective study of the adverse effects of meditation, although in the face of the millions of individuals who practice meditation regularly, such problems seem uncommon. Individuals with severe preexisting psychopathology, such as schizophrenia, are probably at the highest risk of experiencing adverse effects; one report suggests that meditation precipitated acute psychotic breaks in patients with chronic schizophrenia (Walsh & Roche, 1979). Episodes of depersonalization are also reported, although they may not create any problems for the individual; it is difficult to interpret them outside the context of the individual's experience (Castillo, 1990; Kennedy, 1976).

Shapiro (1992) canvassed 27 participants of an intensive meditation retreat and found that, although subjects reported many more beneficial than negative effects, 63% of them experienced at least one adverse effect at some time. Adverse effects were described as including "increased awareness of negative qualities and emotions within myself"; increased disorientation, "such as becoming aware of how low my self-image is, how often I get down on myself"; addiction to meditation; and boredom or pain. The same study found that 92% of the subjects reported positive effects, including "greater happiness and joy; more positive thinking; more self-confidence; better ability to get things done; better problem solving . . . more relaxed; less stressed" (Shapiro, 1992). Finally, one researcher reported an increased incidence of what were described as "complex partial epileptic-like signs" in regular meditators, although symptoms included "profound meaning from reading poetry/prose" and "religious phenomenology" (Persinger, 1993). For us it is possible that individuals predisposed to such experiences are more likely to pursue meditation in the first place. In general, most proponents of meditation in a medical setting would not recommend meditation to individuals with severe personality disorders, psychotic disorders, or severe depression (especially with suicidal ideation or intent) unless concomitant psychotherapeutic or medical treatment is obtained.

RESOURCES ON MEDITATION

Where to Learn More

The practices and benefits of meditation are now documented in the lay as well as academic literature (Begley, 2001; Stein, 2003). Classes, workshops, books, and tapes on the meditation practices are readily available in stores and on the Internet. Meditation practices are sometimes taught alone, that is, as a stress reduction technique; however, in many wellness programs and integrative medicine centers, they are combined with other modalities, such as yoga, qiqong, dietary or herbal supplements, and spiritual healing (Alferi et al., 2001; Benson, 1996, 1997; Lantz, Buchalter, & McBee, 1997; Ornish et al., 1983; Standish et al., 2001). Although meditation may have its roots in Buddhist and Hindu traditions, it is also often used as a modality to enhance a personal spirituality, which in the West has Christian or Jewish roots. Sociologist E. Burke Rochford (2003, p. 219) comments on a series of group interviews:

> Traditional ways of thinking suggest that, when faiths collide, commitments to an existing religion are jeopardized . . . . Yet a sizeable portion of those I interviewed told a different story. Rather than being corrosive to their faith, the encounter with Buddhism deepened and enriched their understanding of Christianity, as well as their identity as Christians. In other cases, Buddhist practice served to reinvigorate commitment to a dormant or even rejected Christianity.

Many programs offer intensive 1- or 2- week training programs in meditation practices, supplemented by discussion of specific clinical and psychosocial issues. For caregiver support groups, these issues may include working with compassion fatigue, dealing with changing family roles, and stress reduction. For elders, issues may address memory loss, life review and acceptance of simplicity, and clarifying life priorities. Other programs, such as Frank Ostateski's, Zen Hospice Project are longer and geared for in-depth training in the integration of meditation practices with caregiving issues and a person's existent spiritual traditions. All programs may offer time-delimited courses, or also offer formats for ongoing support, such as weekly or monthly meetings.

Other meditation programs may be more generic and not targeted specifically to elders or to a medical audience. These programs may be beneficial to those who simply would like to learn more about meditation, bringing their experience along for processing with a more generalized group of participants. We have included a short list of contemplative centers that sponsor short- and longer-term meditation programs.

In the Resources section we have included a list of books, tapes, magazines, and Internet-based resources on some of the meditation techniques and programs that we have mentioned in this chapter. Although not by any means a comprehensive list, these resources are listed to give readers an outline of what is available if they wish to learn more about meditation for their elderly clients, for family caregivers, or for themselves as care providers.

Training and Credentialing

One of the challenges caused by the more widespread use of meditation in health care is the lack of formal credentialing or licensure for meditation instructors. There are many traditions of meditation, and individuals with widely varying degrees of training and experience teach meditation in many different contexts. Although this means that there are numerous opportunities to learn how to meditate, there is no consensus about what constitutes the necessary training for a meditation teacher. There is no certification for Western instructors who wish to teach meditation as a medical or mind–body therapy. Traditional religions or organizations, such as Buddhism and TM, that include meditation as a core component of their activity have specific requirements for formal training and explicit credentialing for new teachers. Usually extensive experience and a high level of expertise are required for authorization as a teacher within such traditions, but such teachers may not have extensive experience with medical patients.

At the University of Pennsylvania Program for Stress Management, we suggest that an individual have at least 10 years of personal practice and formal instruction in mindfulness meditation before receiving additional training to teach meditation. For individuals with appropriate training, we have offered a 4- to 6-month internship that addresses some of the specific issues that arise when meditation is practiced as a medical therapy. Our teachers are also expected to spend at least 2 weeks out of each year in intensive meditation retreats. There are exceptions to these guidelines, but we encourage individuals with less experience to work wholeheartedly to deepen their own practice and study.

The Stress Reduction Clinic at the University of Massachusetts also provides several types of professional training programs. Five- to 7-day residential programs are offered at sites throughout the United States. These programs are highly experiential and require no previous training or experience. Further study is also available at a professional internship program held at its Massachusetts clinic. These programs provide basic training in the practice and principles of mindfulness meditation and explore how it might be applied to an individual's own personal or professional situation. Jon Kabat-Zinn's book *Full Catastrophe Living* (1990) details the University of Massachusetts program and is an excellent introduction to the use of mindfulness meditation in medicine.

CONCLUSION

Meditation practices have been established as a treatment that is helpful in addressing anxiety and depression, alleviating physiological symptoms, and reducing the effects of stress. Many meditation practitioners have documented an improved quality of life. All meditation practices have in common a goal of calming and stabilizing the mind, thereby increasing an awareness of internal, psychological events as well as external, phenomenological experiences. Meditation practices are available to health care practitioners and the general public, and draw upon Eastern and Western traditions. In this chapter we have discussed two frequently taught types of sitting meditation, those in the mindfulness and transcendental meditation traditions.

Elders and their caregivers may find meditation practices support coping with decreasing physical and mental abilities, and increased physical dependence on others. Elders may find that meditation practices allow them to simplify their lives in the midst of cognitive declines, whereas caregivers may appreciate the facets of stress reduction that meditation practices can bring to their busy lives. Meditation practices have also been shown to reduce symptoms of chronic pain, hypertension, cardiovascular disease, and the stresses of cancer patients.

The presentation of meditation has evolved to meet the needs of each culture it has entered. Meditation is entering the West as a secular and scientifically validated psychological and medical therapy. In keeping with the inclinations and goals of Western culture, meditation will be used because of its practical and concrete benefits. Elders and their caregivers may be able to benefit from the stress reduction and physical benefits of meditation, as well as its ability to support life changes and losses. Meditation will likely be shown to be an efficacious treatment for many social and medical problems, and potentially be an effective way to decrease health care costs and utilization. Ultimately, however, meditation will be practiced here for the same reason that it has flourished in so many cultures for thousands of years: because it helps people to feel better and to enjoy life more fully.

NOTE

The authors would like to thank Timothy Brigham, PhD, Victoria Howard, PhD, Karma Trime Lhamo, and Ken D. Smith, PhD, for their helpful comments and suggestions.

RESOURCES

Books

Meditation Practice in General

Chodron, P. (2000). *When things fall apart: Heart advice for difficult times*. Boston: Shambhala.

Kabat-Zinn, J. (1990). *Full catastrophe living: Using the wisdom of your body and mind to face stress, pain, and illness.* Delta.

Merton, T. (1996). *Contemplative prayer.* New York: Image Books, Doubleday.

Mipham, S. (2002). *Making your mind into an ally.* New York: Riverhead.

Nhah Hahn, T. (1987). *The miracle of mindfulness: An introduction to the practice of meditation.* Boston: Beacon Press.

Salzberg, S. (2002). *Lovingkindness: The revolutionary art of happiness.* Boston: Shambhala.

Caregiving, Death, and Dying

Cason, A. & Lindbergh, R. (2001). *Circles of care: How to set up quality home care for our elders.* Boston: Shambhala.

Collett, M. (1999). *At home with dying: A Zen hospice approach.* Berkeley, CA, and London: Shambhala.

Dalai Lama, & Hopkins, J. (2002). *Advice on dying: And living a better life.* Atria Books.*

Ko-I Bastis, M. (2000). *Peaceful dwelling: Meditations for healing and living.* Tokyo: Charles E. Tuttle.

Levine, S. (1989). *Healing into life and death.* New York: Anchor Books.

Levine, S., & Levine, O. (1989). *Who dies?: An investigation of conscious living and conscious dying.* New York: Anchor Books.

Lief, J. L. (2001). *Making friends with death: A Buddhist guide to encountering mortality.* Boston: Shambhala.

Longaker, C. (1998). *Facing death and finding hope: A guide to the emotional and spiritual care of the dying.* New York: Doubleday.

Nhat Hanh, T. (2003). *No death, no fear.* New York: Riverhead Books.

Rosenberg, L. (2001). *Living in the light of death: On the art of being truly alive.* Boston: Shambhala.

Shalomi-Schacter, Z., & Miller, R. S. (1997). *From age-ing to sage-ing: A profound new vision of growing older.* New York: Warner Books.

Sogyal Rinpoche. (1992). *The Tibetan book of living and dying.* San Francisco: Harper.

Stone, S. (2001). *At the eleventh hour: Caring for my dying mother.* Present Perfect Books.

Meditation, Buddhism, Christianity, and Judiasm

Kasimow, H., Keenan, J. P., & Keenan, L. K. (Eds.). (2003). *Beside still waters: Jews, Christians and the way of the Buddha.* Boston: Wisdom.

Nhat Hahn, T. (1995). *Living Buddha, living Christ.* New York: Riverhead.

Magazines and Tapes

Inquiring Mind, P.O. Box 9999, Berkeley, CA 94709; http://www.inquiringmind.com

Shambhala Sun Magazine, 1345 Spruce St., Boulder, CO 80302; 1585 Barrington St., Suite 117, Halifax, NS B3J 1Z8 Canada; http://www.shambhalasun.com

Snow Lion Newsletter, P.O. Box 6483, Ithaca, NY 14851; http://www.snowlionpub.com

Sounds True; http://www.soundstrue.com
   Sounds True sells tapes and videos, offering more than 500 titles about spiritual traditions, meditation, psychology, creativity, health and healing, self-discovery, and relationships. Sounds True disseminates spiritual wisdom that embraces the world's major spiritual traditions and the arts and humanities, as embodied by the leading authors, teachers, and experts of our times.

Tricycle: The Buddhist Review, 92 Vandam St., New York, NY 10013; http://www.tricycle.com

Web Sites

For Caregivers

Living/Dying Project, Educational Services; http://www.livingdying.org/education.html
   The Living/Dying Project was founded in 1977 by Stephen Levine and is the outgrowth of the Hanuman Foundation Dying Center in Santa Fe, New Mexico. The project offers spiritual support for persons facing life-threatening illness and for those who care for them, as well as educational services.

Rigpa Spiritual Care Program; http://www.rigpa.org/WIR/SPC/
   The compassion and wisdom of the Buddhist teachings are applied to help those facing illness or death, their families and caregivers. For people of any faith, the Spiritual Care Program has been designed to augment the professional's training with a comprehensive and practical approach to end-of-life care. It provides education and training to doctors, nurses, social workers, therapists, volunteers, and clergy of all denominations.

Upaya Foundation, Service and Programs; http://www.upaya.org/programs/death_dying.html

Founded by Joan Halifax. Programs are based on Eastern and Western psychology, philosophy, and contemplative practices. Contemplative practices are found in many spiritual traditions; those of the Project on Being with Dying are inspired by the long and rich tradition of Buddhism.

Zen Hospice Project; http://www.zenhospice.org
Inspired by a 2,500-year-old Buddhist tradition, Zen Hospice Project (ZHP) is a fusion of spiritual insight and practical social action. Begun in 1987, ZHP is now nationally recognized as an innovative model in the movement to improve end-of life care. ZHP provides a spectrum of collaborative services including residential hospice care, volunteer programs, and educational efforts that foster wisdom and compassion in service.

Places to Learn Meditation

Center for Mindfulness in Medicine, Health Care, and Society; http://www.umassmed.edu/cfm/
Founded by Jon Kabat-Zinn at the University of Massachusetts, this center is dedicated to furthering the practice and integration of mindfulness in the lives of individuals, institutions, and society. These initiatives include the Stress Reduction Program—the oldest and largest academic medical center–based stress reduction program in the country—as well as a range of professional training programs and corporate workshops, courses, and retreats.

Insight Meditation Society; http://dharma.org
The Insight Meditation Society (IMS) was founded in 1975 as a non-profit organization to provide an environment conducive to the practice of vipassana (insight) and metta (lovingkindness) meditation, and to preserve the essential Buddhist teachings of liberation. IMS now operates two retreat facilities—the Retreat Center and the Forest Refuge—which are set on 160 secluded wooded acres in the quiet country of central Massachusetts. The Web page also lists IMS centers in the United States and worldwide.

Maharishi University of Management; http://www.mum.edu/
This private college in southeast Iowa was founded by the Maharishi Mahesh Yogi in 1971. Students practice the transcendental meditation and TM-Sidhi program, techniques shown to increase creativity and awaken latent reserves in the brain. The curriculum includes bachelor's, master's, and doctoral programs in the arts, sciences, humanities, and business. In addition to the traditional majors, they offer such special

programs as Sustainable Living, Digital Media, Maharishi Vedic Medicine, and Maharishi Vedic Science.

Mind and Life Institute; http://www.mindandlife.org

The Mind and Life Institute is a collaboration between the Dalai Lama and Western scientists who seek to understand the interrelationships between higher consciousness, psychology, and physiology. The institute sponsors conferences and maintains a Web page describing books, publications, and research initiatives.

Mind/Body Medical Institute; http://www.mbmi.org

Under the direction of Herbert Benson at Harvard University, the Mind/Body Medical Institute's work is based on the inseparable connection between the mind and body—the complicated interactions that take place between thoughts, body, and the outside world. Mind/body medicine integrates modern scientific medicine, psychology, nursing, nutrition, exercise physiology, and belief to enhance the natural healing capacities of body and mind. The Mind/Body Medical Institute sponsors workshops and training sessions for the general public as well as for health care professionals.

Naropa University; http://www.naropa.edu/contemplativecare/

Naropa University in Boulder, Colorado, sponsors a degree program in Engaged Buddhism, as well as a certificate program for health care professionals in end-of-life care. These programs emphasize the nexus between meditation and contemplative action. Naropa encourages the integration of world wisdom traditions with modern culture and is nonsectarian in its approach.

Shambhala International; http://www.shambhala.org

According to the Shambhala tradition, there is a natural source of radiance and brilliance in the world, which is the innate wakefulness of human beings. There are over 100 Shambhala Centers in the United States and worldwide. At the heart of each Shambhala Center is the meditation hall, where students practice the discipline of meditation. At each Shambhala Center, meditation instruction is offered, along with weekend and weekly meditation programs.

Shambhala Mountain Center; http://www.shambhalamountain.org

Located in the Colorado Rockies, Shambhala Mountain Center offers programs on Buddhist meditation, yoga, and other contemplative disciplines. The center is a place where one of the basic truths of Buddhism—that people can be profoundly open to the wisdom of the present moment—is always readily available. It is a nonsectarian facility where the insights of Buddhism can mix with other traditions of human transformation and be applied to educational, cultural, artistic, and business disciplines.

Spirit Rock Center; http://www.spiritrock.org
　　Spirit Rock Meditation Center, in Woodacre, California, is dedicated to the teachings of the Buddha as presented in the vipassana tradition. The practice of mindful awareness, called Insight or Vipassana Meditation, is at the heart of all the activities at Spirit Rock. The center hosts a full program of ongoing classes, and daylong and residential retreats.

Transcendental Meditation (TM); http://www.tm.org
　　TM is one of the most widely practiced forms of meditation in the West; somewhere between 2 million and 5 million individuals have been taught the technique. Numerous research studies have been performed to investigate its efficacy. TM has its origins in the Vedic tradition of India and was introduced to the West by the Maharishi Mahesh Yogi. The site includes a search engine to locate teaching resources for those interested in learning more about TM, as well as an extensive bibliography.

REFERENCES

Achterberg, J., Dossey, L., Gordon, J. S., et al. (1994). Mind-body interventions. In *Alternative medicine: Expanding medical horizons. A report to the National Institutes of Health on alternative medical systems and practices in the United States* (pp. 3–43). Washington, DC: U.S. Government Printing Office.

Aftanas, L. I., & Golocheikine, S. A. (2002). Non-linear dynamic complexity of the human EEG during meditation. *Neuroscience Letters, 330,* 143–146.

Alexander, C. N. (1994). Transcendental meditation. In *Encyclopedia of psychology* (2nd ed., p. 545). New York: John Wiley and Sons.

Alexander, C. N., Langer, E. J., Newman, R. I., Chandler, H. M., & Davies, J. L. (1989). Transcendental meditation, mindfulness, and longevity: An experimental study with the elderly. *Journal of Personality and Social Psychology, 57,* 950–964.

Alexander, C. N., Schneider, R. H., Staggers, F., Sheppard, W., Clayborne, B. M., Rainforth, M., et al. (1996). Trial of stress reduction for hypertension in older African Americans: 2. Sex and risk subgroup analysis. *Hypertension, 28,* 228–237.

Alexander, C. N., Swanson, G. C., Rainfort, M. V., et al. (1993). Effects of the TM program on stress reduction, health and employee development: A prospective study in two occupational settings. *Anxiety, Stress and Coping, 6,* 245–261.

Alferi, S. M., Antoni, M. H., Ironson, G., Kilbourn, K. M., & Carver, C. S. (2001). Factors predicting the use of complementary therapies in a multiethnic sample of early-stage breast cancer patients. *Journal of the American Medical Women's Association, 56,* 120–123.

Arnis, R. (1989). *A different Christianity: Early Christian esotericism and modern thought.* Gainesville, GA: Praxis Press.

Astin, J. A. (1997). Stress reduction through mindfulness meditation: Effects on psychological symptomatology, sense of control, and spiritual experiences. *Psychotherapy and Psychosomatics, 66,* 97–106.

Astin, J. A., Pelletier, K. R., Marie, A., & Haskell, W. L. (2000). Complementary and alternative medicine use among elderly persons: One-year analysis of a Blue Shield Medicare supplement. *Journals of Gerontology Series A-Biological Sciences and Medical Sciences, 55,* M4–M9.

Baime, M. J., & Baime, R. V. (1996). Stress management using mindfulness meditation in a primary care general internal medicine practice. *Journal of General Internal Medicine, 11*(S1), 131.

Bair, P. (1998). *Living from the heart: Heart rhythm meditation for energy, clarity, peace, joy, and inner power.* New York: Three Rivers Press/Random House.

Beck, A. T., Rush, A. J., Shaw, B. F., & Emery, G. (1979). *Cognitive therapy of depression.* New York: Guilford Press.

Becker, D. R., & Shapiro, D. (1981). Physiological responses to clicks during Zen, Yoga and TM meditation. *Psychophysiology, 18,* 694–699.

Begley, S. (2001a, May 7). Religion and the brain. *Newsweek, 50*–57.

Begley, S. (2001b, May 7). Searching for the God within. *Newsweek, 59.*

Benhard, J. D., Kristeller, J., & Kabat-Zinn, J. (1988) Effectiveness of relaxation and visualization techniques as an adjunct to phototherapy and photochemotherapy of psoriasis. *Journal of the American Academy of Dermatology, 19,* 572–574.

Benson, H. (1976). *The relaxation response.* New York: Avon Books.

Benson, H. (1982) The relaxation response: History, physiological basis and clinical usefulness. *Acta Medica Scandinavica, 660*(Suppl.), 231–237.

Benson, H. (1985). *Beyond the relaxation response.* New York: Berkeley Books.

Benson, H. (1996), Mind over maladies: Can yoga, prayer and meditation be adapted for managed care? Interview by Jim Montague. *Hospitals and Health Networks, 70,* 26–27.

Benson, H. (1997). The relaxation response: Therapeutic effect [Comment]. *Science, 278,* 1694–1695.

Benson, H., Kotch, J. B., & Crassweller, K. D. (1977). The relaxation response: A bridge between psychiatry and medicine. *Medical Clinics of North America, 61,* 929–938.

Benson, H., Lehmann, J. W., Malhotra, M. S., Goldman, R. F., Hopkins, J., & Epstein, M. D. (1982). Body temperature changes during the practice of g Tum-mo yoga. *Nature, 295,* 234–236.

Benson, H., Malhotra, M. S., Goldman, R. F., Jacobs, G. D., & Hopkins, P. J. (1990). Three case reports of the metabolic and electroencephalographic changes during advanced Buddhist meditation techniques. *Behavioral Medicine, 16,* 90–95.

Bishop, A., & Scurlock, N. D. (1992). A community health program for the elderly. *Caring, 11*, 50–54.

Bogart, G. (1991). The use of meditation in psychotherapy: A review of the literature [Review]. *American Journal of Psychotherapy, 45*, 383–412.

Branin, J. J. (2001). The role of memory strategies in medication adherence among the elderly. *Home Health Care Services Quarterly, 20*, 1–16.

Brinson, S. V., & Brunk, Q. (2000). Hospice family caregivers: An experience in coping. *Hospice Journal, 15*, 1–12.

Brown, D., Forte, M., & Dysart, M. (1984). Visual sensitivity and mindfulness meditation. *Perceptual and Motor Skills, 58*, 775–784.

Brown, K. W., & Ryan, R. M. (2003). The benefits of being present: Mindfulness and its role in psychological well-being. *Journal of Personality and Social Psychology, 84*, 822–848.

Carlson, L. E., Ursuliak, Z., Goodey, E., Angen, M., & Speca, M. (2001). The effects of a mindfulness meditation-based stress reduction program on mood and symptoms of stress in cancer outpatients: 6-month follow-up. *Supportive Care in Cancer, 9*, 112–123.

Carpenter, J. T. (1977). Meditation, esoteric traditions—contributions to psychotherapy. *American Journal of Psychotherapy, 31*, 394–404.

Carrington, P., Collings, G. H., Jr., Benson, H., Robinson, H., Wood, L. W., Lehrer, P. M., Woolfolk, R. L., & Cole, J. W. (1980). The use of meditation—relaxation techniques for the management of stress in a working population. *Journal of Occupational Medicine, 22*, 221–231.

Cason, A., & Lindbergh, R. (2001). *Circles of care: How to set up quality home care for our elders.* Boston: Shambhala.

Castillo, R. J. (1990). Depersonalization and meditation. *Psychiatry, 53*, 158–168.

Caudill, M. A., Friedman, R., & Benson, H. (1987). Relaxation therapy in the control of blood pressure [Review]. *Bibliotheca Cardiologica*, 106–119.

Clarke, E. (2001). Role conflicts and coping strategies in caregiving: A symbolic interactionist view. *Journal of Psychosocial Nursing and Mental Health Services, 39*, 28–37.

Collett, M. (1999). *At home with dying: A Zen hospice approach.* Boston: Shambhala.

Corby, J. C., Roth, W. T., Zarcone, V. P. J., & Kopell, B. S. (1978). Psychophysiological correlates of the practice of Tantric Yoga meditation. *Archives of General Psychiatry, 35*, 571–577.

Craven, J. L. (1989). Meditation and psychotherapy [Review]. *Canadian Journal of Psychiatry–Révue Canadienne de Psychiatrie, 34*, 648–653.

Deckro, G. R., Ballinger, K. M., Hoyt, M., Wilcher, M., Dusek, J., Myers, P., Greenberg, B., Rosenthal, D. S., & Benson, H. (2002). The evaluation of a mind/body intervention to reduce psychological distress and perceived stress in college students. *Journal of American College Health, 50*, 281–287.

Deepak, K. K., Manchanda, S. K., & Maheshwari, M. C. (1994). Meditation improves clincoelectroencephalographic measures in drug-resistant epileptics. *Bio-feedback Self Regulation, 19*, 25–40.

DelMonte, M. (1987). Constructivist view of meditation. *American Journal of Psychotherapy, 41*, 286–298.

DelMonte, M. M. (1989). Meditation, the unconscious, and psychosomatic disorders. *International Journal of Psychosomatics, 36*, 45–52.

Dillbeck, M. C., & Orme-Johnson, D. W. (1987). Physiological differences between transcendental meditation and rest. *American Psychologist, 42*, 879–881.

Domar, A. D., Noe, J. M., & Benson, H. (1987). The preoperative use of the relaxation response with ambulatory surgery patients. *Hospital Topics, 65*, 30–35.

Ducharme, F., & Trudeau, D. (2002). Qualitative evaluation of a stress management intervention for elderly caregivers at home: A constructivist approach. *Issues in Mental Health Nursing, 23*, 691–713.

Eisenberg, D. M., Delbanco, T. L., Berkey, C. S., Kaptchuk, T. J., Kupelnick, B., Kuhl, J., et al. (1993). Cognitive behavioral techniques for hypertension: Are they effective? *Annals of Internal Medicine, 118*, 964–972.

Elias, A. N., & Wilson, A. F. (1995). Serum hormonal concentrations following transcendental meditation—potential role of gamma aminobutyric acid. *Medical Hypotheses, 44*, 287–291.

Epstein, M. (1995). *Thoughts without a thinker.* New York: Basic Books.

Esch, T., Stefano, G. B., Fricchione, G. L., & Benson, H. (2002). Stress in cardiovascular diseases [Review]. *Medical Science Monitor, 8*, RA93–RA101.

Evers, W., Tomic, W., & Brouwers, A. (2001). Effects of aggressive behavior and perceived self-efficacy on burnout among staff of homes for the elderly. *Issues in Mental Health Nursing, 22*, 439–454.

Farrow, J. T., & Hebert, R. (1982). Breath suspension during the transcendental meditation technique. *Psychosomatic Medicine, 44*, 133–153.

Fields, R. (1981). *How the swans came to the lake: A narrative history of Buddhism in America.* Boulder, CO: Shambhala Publications.

Fox, M. (1988). *The coming of the cosmic Christ.* San Francisco: Harper.

Fox, M. (2000). *One river, many wells: Wisdom springing from global faiths.* Los Angeles: J. P. Tarcher.

Freal, J. E., Kraft, G. H., & Coryell, J. K. (1984). Symptomatic fatigue in multiple sclerosis. *Archives of Physical Medicine and Rehabilitation, 65*, 135–138.

Gaylord, C., Orme-Johnson, D., & Travis, F. (1989). The effects of the transcendental meditation technique and progressive muscle relaxation on EEG coherence, stress reactivity, and mental health in black adults. *International Journal of Neuroscience, 46*, 77–86.

Glaser, J. L., Brind, J.L., Vogelman, J. H., Eisner, M. J., Dillbeck, M. C., Wallace, R. K., et al. (1992). Elevated serum dehydroepiandrosterone sulfate levels in practitioners of the Transcendental Meditation (TM) and TM Siddhi programs. *Journal of Behavioral Medicine, 15*, 327–341.

Goldberg, R. J. (1982). Anxiety reduction by self-regulation: theory, practice, and evaluation [Review]. *Annals of Internal Medicine, 96*, 483–487.

Goleman, D. (1976). Meditation and consciousness: An Asian approach to mental health. *American Journal of Psychotherapy, 30*, 41–54.

Goleman, D. (1991). A Western perspective. In D. Goleman & R. Thurman (Eds.), *MindScience: An East–West dialogue* (p. 4). Boston: Wisdom Publications.

Gould, K. L., Ornish, D., Kikeeide, R., et al. (1992). Improved stenosis geometry by quantitative coronary arterography after vigorous risk factor modification. *American Journal of Cardiology, 69*, 845–853.

Grossman, P., Niemann, L., Schmidt, S., & Walach, H. (2004, July). Mindfulness-based stress reduction and health benefits: A meta-analysis. *Journal of Psychosomatic Research. 57*(1), 35–43.

Harte, J. L., Eifert, G. H., & Smith, R. (1995). The effects of running and meditation on beta-endorphin, corticotrophin-releasing hormone and cortisol in plasma, and on mood. *Biological Psychology, 40*, 251–265.

Helpard, H., & Meagher-Stewart, D. (1998). The "kaleidoscope" experience for elderly women living with coronary artery disease. *Canadian Journal of Cardiovascular Nursing, 9*, 11–23.

Herzog, H., Lele, V. R., Kuwert, T., et al. (1990–1991). Changed pattern of regional glucose metabolism during yoga meditative relaxation. *Neuropsychobiology, 23*, 182–187.

Hess, T. M., Auman, C., Colcombe, S. J., & Rahhal, T. A. (2003). The impact of stereotype threat on age differences in memory performance. *Journals of Gerontology Series B–Psychological Sciences and Social Sciences, 58*, 3–11.

Hines, S. C., Babrow, A. S., Badzek, L., & Moss, A. (2001). From coping with life to coping with death: Problematic integration for the seriously ill elderly. *Health Communication, 13*, 327–342.

Infante, J. R., Peran, F., Martinez, M., Roldan, A., Poyatos, R., Ruiz, C., Samaniego, F., & Garrido, F. (1998). ACTH and beta-endorphin in transcendental meditation. *Physiology and Behavior, 64*, 311–315.

Jacobzone, S. (2000). Coping with aging: International challenges. *Health Affairs, 19*, 213–225.

Jevning, R., Wallace, R. K., & Beidebach, M. (1992). The physiology of meditation: A review. *Neuroscience and Biobehavioral Reviews, 16*, 415–424.

Jevning, R., Wilson, A. F., & Davidson, J. M. (1978). Adrenocortical activity during meditation. *Hormones & Behavior, 10*(1), 54-60.

Kabat-Zinn, J. (1982). An outpatient program in behavioral medicine for chronic pain patients based on the practice of mindfulness meditation: Theoretical considerations and preliminary results. *General Hospital Psychiatry, 4*, 33–47.

Kabat-Zinn, J. (1990). *Full catastrophe living: Using the wisdom of your body and mind to face stress, pain, and illness.* New York: Delta.

Kabat-Zinn, J. (1992). Psychosocial factors: their importance and management. In I. S. Ockene & J. K. Ockene (Eds.), *Prevention of coronary heart disease* (pp. 300–333). Boston: Little, Brown.

Kabat-Zinn, J. (1993). Mindfulness meditation: Health benefits of an ancient Buddhist practice. In D. Goleman & J. Gurin (Eds.), *Mind–body medicine* (pp. 262–263). Yonkers, NY: Consumer Reports Books.

Kabat-Zinn, J. (1996). Mindfulness meditation. In Y. Haruki, Y. Ishii, & M. Suzuki (Eds.), *Comparative and psychological study on meditation* (pp. 161–170). Amsterdam: Euboron.

Kabat-Zinn, J., Lipworth, L., & Burney, R. (1985). The clinical use of mindfulness meditation for the self-regulation of chronic pain. *Journal of Behavioral Medicine, 8*, 163–190.

Kabat-Zinn, J., Massion, A. O., Kristeller, J., Peterson, L. G., Fletcher, K. E., Pbert, L., Lenderking, W. R., & Santorelli, S. F. (1992). Effectiveness of a meditation-based stress reduction program in the treatment of anxiety disorders. *American Journal of Psychiatry, 149,* 936–943.

Kabat-Zinn, J., Ohm Massion, A., Herbert, J. R., & Rosenbaum, E. (1998). Meditation. In J. Holland (Ed.), *Textbook of psycho-oncology.* New York: Oxford University Press.

Kaplan, A. (Ed.). (1997). *Sefer yetzirah: The book of creation.* Boston: Red Wheel/Weiser.

Kaplan, K. H., Goldenberg, D. L., & Galvin-Nadeau, M. (1993). The impact of a meditation-based stress management program on fibromyalgia. *General Hospital Psychiatry, 15,* 284–289.

Keenan, J., Keenan, L. K., & Kasimow, H. (Eds.). (2003). *Beside still waters: Jews, Christians, and the way of the Buddha.* Boston: Wisdom Publications.

Kennedy, R. B. J. (1976). Self-induced depersonalization syndrome. *American Journal of Psychiatry, 133,* 1326–1328.

Khalsa, D. S. (1998). Integrated medicine and the prevention and reversal of memory loss [Review]. *Alternative Therapies in Health and Medicine, 4,* 38–43.

Koertge, J., Weidner, G., Elliott-Eller, M., Scherwitz, L., Merritt-Worden, T. A., Marlin, R., et al. (2003). Improvement in medical risk factors and quality of life in women and men with coronary artery disease in the Multicenter Lifestyle Demonstration Project. *American Journal of Cardiology, 91,* 1316–1322.

Ko-I Bastis, M. (2000). *Peaceful dwelling: Meditations for healing and living.* Tokyo: Charles E. Tuttle.

Kraaij, V., Pruymboom, E., & Garnefski, N. (2002). Cognitive coping and depressive symptoms in the elderly: A longitudinal study. *Aging and Mental Health, 6,* 275–281.

Kristeller, J., & Hallett, C. B. (1999). An exploratory study of a meditation-based intervention for binge eating disorder. *Journal of Health Psychology, 4,* 357–363.

Kutz, I., Borysenko, J. Z., & Benson, H. (1985). Meditation and psychotherapy: A rationale for the integration of dynamic psychotherapy, the relaxation response, and mindfulness meditation. *American Journal of Psychiatry, 142,* 1–8.

Kutz, I., Caudill, M., & Benson, H. (1983). The role of relaxation in behavioral therapies for chronic pain. *International Anesthesiology Clinics, 21,* 193–200.

Kutz, I., Leserman, J., Dorrington, C., Morrison, C. H., Borysenko, J. Z., & Benson, H. (1985). Meditation as an adjunct to psychotherapy: An outcome study. *Psychotherapy and Psychosomatics, 43,* 209–218.

Langer, E. (1989). *Mindfulness.* Cambridge: Perseus Books.

Lansbury, G. (2000). Chronic pain management: A qualitative study of elderly people's preferred coping strategies and barriers to management. *Disability and Rehabilitation, 22,* 2–14.

Lantz, M. S., Buchalter, E. N., & McBee, L. (1997). The Wellness Group: A novel intervention for coping with disruptive behavior among [corrected] elderly nursing home residents [Erratum appears in *Gerontologist, 37*(5), 687]. *Gerontologist, 37,* 551–556.

Lazar, S. W., Bush, G., Gollub, R. L., Fricchione, G. L., Khalsa, G., & Benson, H. (2000). Functional brain mapping of the relaxation response and meditation. *Neuroreport, 11,* 1581–1585.

Lehmann, D., Faber, P. L., Achermann, P., Jeanmonod, D., Gianotti, L. R., & Pizzagalli, D. (2001). Brain sources of EEG gamma frequency during volitionally meditation-induced, altered states of consciousness, and experience of the self. *Psychiatry Research, 108,* 111–121.

Levy, B. R., Jennings, P., & Langer, E. J. (2001) Improving attention in old age. *Journal of Adult Development, 8*(3), 189–182.

Longaker, C. (1997). *Facing death and finding hope: A guide to the spiritual care of the dying.* New York: Doubleday.

Luskin, F. M., Newell, K. A., Griffith, M., Holmes, M., Telles, S., DiNucci, E., et al. (2000). A review of mind/body therapies in the treatment of musculoskeletal disorders with implications for the elderly [Review]. *Alternative Therapies in Health and Medicine, 6,* 46–56.

Luskin, F. M., Newell, K. A., Griffith, M., Holmes, M., Telles, S., Marvasti, F. F., Pelletier, K. R., & Haskell, W. L. (1998). A review of mind-body therapies in the treatment of cardiovascular disease: 1. Implications for the elderly [Review]. *Alternative Therapies in Health and Medicine, 4,* 46–61.

Luskin, F., Reitz, M., Newell, K., Quinn, T. G., & Haskell, W. (2002). A controlled pilot study of stress management training of elderly patients with congestive heart failure. *Preventive Cardiology, 5,* 168–172.

MacLean, C. R., Walton, K. G., Wenneberg, S. R., et al. (1994). Altered responses of cortisol, GH, TSH and testosterone to acute stress after four months' practice of transcendental meditation (TM). *Annals of the New York Academy of Sciences, 746,* 381–384.

Majumdar, M., Grossman, P., Dietz-Waschkowski, B., Kersig, S., & Walach, H. (2002). Does mindfulness meditation contribute to health? Outcome evaluation of a German sample. *Journal of Alternative and Complementary Medicine, 8,* 719–730.

Massion, A. O., Teas, J., Hebert, J. R., Wertheimer, M. D., & Kabat-Zinn, J. (1995). Meditation, melatonin and breast/prostate cancer: Hypothesis and preliminary data. *Medical Hypotheses, 44,* 39–46.

Mathias, C. J. (1991). Management of hypertension by reduction in sympathetic activity. *Hypertension, 17,* 69–74.

McEvoy, R. M., Frumkin, L. R., & Harkins, S. W. (1980). Effects of meditation on brainstem auditory evoked potentials. *International Journal of Neuroscience, 10,* 165–170.

Merton, T. (1996). *Contemplative prayer.* New York: Image Books, Doubleday.

Michaels, R. R., Parra, J., McCann, D. S., & Vander, A. J. (1979). Renin, cortisol, and aldosterone during transcendental meditation. *Psychosomatic Medicine, 41,* 50–54.

Miller, J. J., Fletcher, K., & Kabat-Zinn, J. (1995). Three-year follow-up and clinical implications of a mindfulness meditation-based stress reduction inter-

vention in the treatment of anxiety disorders. *General Hospital Psychiatry,*
17, 192–200.

Mills, P. J., Schneider, R. H., Hill, D., et al. (1990). Beta-adrenergic receptor sensitivity in subjects practicing transcendental meditation. *Journal of*
Psychosomatic Research, 34, 29–33.

National Institutes of Health. (1995, October 16–18). *Integration of behavioral*
and relaxation approaches into the treatment of chronic pain and insomnia:
National Institutes of Health technology assessment statement. Bethesda,
MD: Author.

Newberg, A., Alavi, A., Baime, M., Pourdehnad, M., Santanna, J., & d'Aquili, E.
(2001). The measurement of regional cerebral blood flow during the complex cognitive task of meditation: A preliminary SPECT study. *Psychiatry*
Research, 106, 113–122.

Nhat Hanh, T. (1987). *The miracle of mindfulness: An introduction to the practice of meditation.* Boston: Beacon Press.

Nhat Hahn, T. (1995). *Living Buddha, living Christ.* New York: Riverhead.

Orme-Johnson, D. (1995). Summary of scientific research on Maharishi's
Transcendental Meditation and TM-Siddhi Program. *Modern Science and*
Vedic Science, 6(1).

Ornish, D. (1998). Avoiding revascularization with lifestyle changes: The
Multicenter Lifestyle Demonstration Project [Review]. *American Journal of*
Cardiology, 82, 72T–76T.

Ornish, D., Brown, S. E., Scherwitz, L. Z., et al. (1990). Can lifestyle changes reverse atherosclerosis? *Lancet, 336,* 129–133.

Ornish, D., Scherwitz, L. W., Doody, R. S., Kesten, D., McLanahan, S. M.,
Brown, S. E., et al. (1983). Effects of stress management training and dietary
changes in treating ischemic heart disease. *Journal of the American Medical*
Association, 249, 54–59.

Ostateski, F. (1994). Stories of lives lived and now ending. *Inquiring Mind, 10*(2).
Retrieved from http://www.zenhospice.org/html/what/stories_0494.html

Panjwani, U., Gupta, H. L., Singh, S. H. et al. (1995). Effect of Sahaja yoga practice on stress management inpatients of epilepsy. *Indian Journal of*
Physiology and Pharmacology, 39, 111–116.

Perlmutter, M. (1988). Cognitive potential throughout life. In J. E. Birren, V. L.
Bengtson, & D. E. Deutchman (Eds.), *Emergent theories of aging.* New
York: Springer.

Perlmutter, M., & Hall, E. (1992). *Adult development and aging* (2nd ed.). New
York: John Wiley and Sons.

Persinger, M. A. (1993). Transcendental meditation and general meditation are
associated with enhanced complex partial epileptic-like signs: Evidence for
"cognitive" kindling? *Perceptual and Motor Skills, 76,* 80–82.

Puentes, W. J. (2001). Coping styles, stress levels, and the occurrence of spontaneous simple reminiscence in older adult nursing home residents. *Issues in*
Mental Health Nursing, 1922, 51–61.

Puryear, H. B., Cayce, C. T., & Thurston, M. A. (1976). Anxiety reduction associated with meditation: Home study. *Perceptual and Motor Skills, 42,*
527–531.

Reibel, D. K., Greeson, J. M., Brainard, G. C., & Rosenzweig, S. (2001). Mindfulness-based stress reduction and health-related quality of life in a heterogeneous patient population. *General Hospital Psychiatry, 23,* 183–192.

Riskin, L. L. (2002, Spring). The contemplative lawyer: On the potential contributions of mindfulness meditation to law students, lawyers, and their clients. *Harvard Negotiation Law Review,* 1–10.

Robichaud, L., & Lamarre, C. (2002). Developing an instrument for identifying coping strategies used by the elderly to remain autonomous. *American Journal of Physical Medicine and Rehabilitation, 81,* 736–744.

Rochford, E. B. (2003). Interfaith encounter and religious identify: Sociological observatioins and reflections. In H. Kasimow, J. P. Keenan, & L. P. Keenan (Eds.), *Beside still waters: Jews, Christians, and the way of the Buddha.* Boston: Wisdom Publications.

Rosenberg, L. (2001). *Living in the light of death: On the art of being truly alive.* Boston: Shambhala.

Rosenzweig, S., Reibel, D. K., Greeson, J. M., Brainard, G. C., & Hojat, M. (2003). Mindfulness-based stress reduction lowers psychological distress in medical students. *Teaching and Learning in Medicine, 15,* 88–92.

Sakyong Mipham Rinpoche. (2003). "Meditation Instruction", Shambhala International Web site, http://www.shambhala.org/meditationinstruction.html.

Sarvimaki, A., & Stenbock-Hult, B. (2000). Quality of life in old age described as a sense of well-being, meaning and value. *Journal of Advanced Nursing, 32,* 1025–1033.

Sawatzky, J. E., & Fowler-Kerry, S. (2003). Impact of caregiving: Listening to the voice of informal caregivers. *Journal of Psychiatric and Mental Health Nursing, 10,* 277–286.

Saxe, G. A., Hebert, J. R., Carmody, J. F., Kabat-Zinn, J., Rosenzweig, P. H., Jarzobski, D., Reed, G. W., & Blute R. D. (2001). Can diet in conjunction with stress reduction affect the rate of increase in prostate specific antigen after biochemical recurrence of prostate cancer? *Journal of Urology, 166,* 2202–2207.

Schacter-Shalomi, Z. (1995). *From age-ing to sage-ing: A profound new vision of growing older.* New York: Warner Books.

Schimmel-Spreeuw, A., Linssen, A. C., & Heeren, T. J. (2000). Coping with depression and anxiety: Preliminary results of a standardized course for elderly depressed women. *International Psychogeriatrics, 12,* 77–86.

Schmall, V. L. (1995). Family caregiver education and training: Enhancing self-efficacy [Review]. *Journal of Case Management, 4,* 156–162.

Schneider, R. H., Alexander, C. N., Salerno, J. W., Robinson, D. K., Jr., Fields, J. Z., & Nidich, S. I. (2002). Disease prevention and health promotion in the aging with a traditional system of natural medicine: Maharishi Vedic Medicine. *Journal of Aging and Health, 14,* 57–78.

Schneider, R. H., Nidich, S. I., Salerno, J. W., Sharma, H. M., Robinson, C. E., Nidich, R. J., & Alexander, C. N. (1998). Lower lipid peroxide levels in practitioners of the Transcendental Meditation program. *Psychosomatic Medicine, 60,* 38–41.

Schneider, R. H., Staggers, F., Alexander, C. N., et al. (1995). A randomized control trial of stress reduction for hypertension in older African Americans. *Hypertension, 26,* 820–827.

Sharma, H. M., & Alexander, C. N. (1996). Maharishi ayurveda: Research review. *Complementary Medicine International, 3*(2), 17–28.

Shapiro, D. H. J. (1982). Overview: Clinical and physiological comparison of meditation with other self-control strategies. *American Journal of Psychiatry, 139,* 267–274.

Shapiro, D. H. J. (1992). Adverse effects of meditation: A preliminary investigation of long-term meditators. *International Journal of Psychosomatics, 39,* 62–67.

Shapiro, D. H. J., & Giber, D. (1978). Meditation and psychotherapeutic effects: Self-regulation strategy and altered state of consciousness. *Archives of General Psychiatry, 35,* 294–302.

Shapiro, S. L., Bootzin, R. R., Figueredo, A. J., Lopez, A. M., & Schwartz, G. E. (2003) The efficacy of mindfulness-based stress reduction in the treatment of sleep disturbance in women with breast cancer: An exploratory study. *Journal of Psychosomatic Research, 54,* 85–91.

Shapiro, S. L., Schwartz, G. E., & Bonner, G. (1998). Effects of mindfulness-based stress reduction on medical and premedical students. *Journal of Behavioral Medicine, 21,* 581–599.

Silberberg, D. S. (1990). Non-pharmacological treatment of hypertension. *Journal of Hypertension, 8*(Suppl.), S21–S26.

Smith, K. D. (1997). *The role of chronic disease and cognitive functioning on the labor force withdrawal process: Insight from retirement expectations.* Unpublished doctoral dissertation. Johns Hopkins University, School of Hygiene and Public Health, Baltimore.

Smith, K. D. (1999). *Cognitive competence and retirement from complex jobs: Is there a link?* Paper presented at the International Symposium on Restructuring Work and the Life Course, Toronto.

Smith, K. D. (2000, May). Older workers' cognitive ability: Is it all in their heads? *NCOA Networks, 1*–2.

Smith, W. P., Compton, W. C., & West, W. B. (1995). Meditation as an adjunct to a happiness enhancement program. *Journal of Clinical Psychology, 51,* 269–273.

Speca, M., Carlson, L. E., Goodey, E., & Angen, M. (2000). A randomized, wait-list controlled clinical trial: The effect of a mindfulness meditation-based stress reduction program on mood and symptoms of stress in cancer outpatients. *Psychosomatic Medicine, 62,* 613–622.

Standish, L. J., Greene, K. B., Bain, S., Reeves, C., Sanders, F., Wines, R. C., Turet, P., Kim, J. G., & Calabrese, C. (2001). Alternative medicine use in HIV-positive men and women: Demographics, utilization patterns and health status. *AIDS Care, 13,* 197–208.

Steele, C. M. (1997). A threat in the air: How stereotypes shape intellectual identity and performance. *American Psychologist, 52,* 613–629.

Stein, J. (2003, August 4). Just say om. *Time,* 48–56.

Stone, S. C. (2001). *At the eleventh hour: Caring for my dying mother.* Lake Junaluska, North Carolina, Present Perfect Books.

Sudsuang, R., Chentanez, V., & Veluvan, K. (1991) Effect of Buddhist meditation on serum cortisol and total protein levels, blood pressure, pulse rate, lung volume and reaction. *Physiology and Behavior, 50,* 543–548.

Szekely, B. C., Turner, S. M., & Jacob, R. G. (1982). Behavioral control of L-dopa induced dyskinesia in Parkinsonism. *Biofeedback Self Regulation, 7,* 443–447.

Tacon, A. M., McComb, J., Caldera, Y., & Randolph, P. (2003). Mindfulness meditation, anxiety reduction, and heart disease: A pilot study. *Family and Community Health, 26,* 25–33.

Taylor, D. N. (1995). Effects of a behavioral stress-management program on anxiety, mood, self-esteem, and T-cell count in HIV positive men. *Psychological Reports, 76,* 451–457.

Teasdale, J. D., Segal, Z., & Williams, J. M. (1995). How does cognitive therapy prevent depressive relapse and why should attentional control (mindfulness) training help? *Behaviour Research and Therapy, 33,* 25–39.

Teasdale, J. D., Segal, Z. V., Williams, J. M., Ridgeway, V. A., Soulsby, J. M., & Lau, M. A. (2000). Prevention of relapse/recurrence in major depression by mindfulness-based cognitive therapy. *Journal of Consulting and Clinical Psychology, 68,* 615–623.

Thera, M. (1962). *The heart of Buddhist meditation.* New York: Samuel Weiser.

Tiefenthaler, U., & Grossman, P. (2002). Buddhist psychology's potential contribution to psychosomatic medicine: Evidence from a mindfulness program for fibromyalgia [Abstract]. *Psychosomatic Medicine, 64,* 141.

Toseland, R. W., Labrecque, M. S., Goebel, S. T., & Whitney, M. H. (1992). An evaluation of a group program for spouses of frail elderly veterans. *Gerontologist, 32,* 382–390.

Trungpa, C. (Ed.). (1976). *Garuda four: Foundations of mindfulness.* Berkeley, CA, and London: Shambhala.

Trungpa, C. (1987). Natural dharma. In S. Walker (Ed.), *Speaking of silence: Christians and Buddhists on the contemplative way.* Mahwah, NJ: Paulist Press.

Van Tilburg, E. (1991). Meditation and palliative care. *CHAC Review, 19,* 9–12.

Wallace, R. K. (1970). Physiological effects of transcendental meditation. *Science, 167,* 1751–1754.

Walsh, R., & Roche, L. (1979). Precipitation of acute psychotic episodes by intensive meditation in individuals with a history of schizophrenia. *American Journal of Psychiatry, 136,* 1085–1086.

Weinberger, R. (1991). Teaching the elderly stress reduction. *Journal of Gerontological Nursing, 17,* 23–27.

Whitney, K. S. (2002). *Sitting inside: Buddhist practice in America's prisons.* Boulder, CO: Prison Dharma Network.

Woolfolk, R. L. (1975). Psychophysiological correlates of meditation. *Archives of General Psychiatry, 32,* 1326–1333.

Zamarra, J. W., Schneider, R. H., Besseghini, I., et al. (1996). Usefulness of the transcendental meditation program in the treatment of patients with coronary artery disease. *American Journal of Cardiology, 77,* 867–870.

Zimber, A. (1998). Workload and stress in caring for the elderly: Status of research and research agenda. *Zeitschrift fur Gerontologie und Geriatrie, 31,* 417–425.

CHAPTER FOURTEEN

The Concept of Spiritual Well-Being and the Care of Older Adults

Amy L. Ai and Elizabeth R. Mackenzie

The field of health care is, in many ways, a microcosm of the culture in which it is embedded, and its problems parallel those found in society at large. Despite an incredibly sophisticated level of medical technology and an enormous budget devoted to the health sciences, many of the health statistics in the United States (US) fall far short of those in other developed countries. Furthermore, patients consistently complain about the "coldness" of physicians and the lack of humane treatment in the health care system. Perhaps at the core of these problems is the lack of an articulated sense of the spiritual dimensions of medicine. Larry Dossey, MD, writes, "We find ourselves in a society that is spiritually malnourished and hungry for meaning" (Dossey, 2005, p. 151). He speculates that one of the main reasons behind the popularity of holistic medicine is its practitioners' openness to speaking with patients about the meaning of illness and the spiritual dimensions of health. It is true that one of the main themes of holism is the importance of acknowledging mind and spirit in addition to the body. Empirical studies have shown a link between values, beliefs, and spiritual perspectives and the use of complementary and alternative medicine (CAM) therapies (Ai & Bolling, 2002, 2004; Astin, Pelletier, Marie, & Haskell, 2000). Similarly, Hufford (1997) points out that it is a characteristic of folk medical systems to consider the meaning of disease and suffering: "Seriously sick people very often ask moral or metaphysical questions about why they are sick" (p. 729). When physicians ignore the spiritual dimension of the illness and suffering of persons in their care, patients often feel dissatisfied, dismissed, and even dehumanized.

This chapter discusses the concept of spiritual well-being and spiritual growth in relation to the care of older adults. From the holistic perspective, spirituality is one of the three major components of the individual. We speak of mind, body, and spirit, and the holistic approach to health requires that we address all three dimensions in some way. *Spirituality* has been defined as "the personal quest for understanding answers to ultimate questions about life, about meaning, and about relationship to the sacred or transcendent, which may (or may not) lead to or arise from the development of religious rituals and the formation of community" (Koenig, McCullough, & Larson, 2001, p. 18). A related concept, *religion,* has been defined as "an organized system of beliefs, practices, rituals, and symbols designed (a) to facilitate closeness to the sacred or transcendent God, higher power, or ultimate truth/reality and (b) to foster an understanding of one's relationship and responsibility to others living together in a community" (p. 18). Because the human need for spirituality occurred a long time before the emergence of institutionalized religions, the concept of religion is logically subsumed under the notion of spirituality (Ai, Dunkle, Peterson, & Bolling, 1998). People have long based their spiritual well-being on their perceived relationship with something beyond themselves, often infinite or transcendent. For most Christians, this connection refers to one's relationship with God, Jesus, or the Holy Spirit (Koenig, 1999). In other traditions, this vital interaction could be associated with a great variety of concepts such as Mother Earth, a supreme being or creator, community, environment, nature, or the cosmos.

In 1975 the National Interfaith Coalition on Aging provided a widely used definition of *spiritual well-being* as "the affirmation of life in a relationship with God, self, community, and environment that nurtures and celebrates wholeness" (cited by Payne, 1990, p. 13). This concept defined some fundamental relationships underlying spiritual well-being. For this reason, it is a useful way to approach the topic of spirituality and health.

SOCIODEMOGRAPHIC AND CULTURAL CHANGES

Several sociodemographic and cultural changes may have important implications for the conceptualization and perception of spiritual well-being in the US at present. The first change stems from the global expansion in the number and proportion of the aged population. The average life span increased by 20 years over the second half of the 20th century. Within 30 years, a third of the total population in developed countries will be over age 60. The US stands at the forefront of this demographic change. Over the past 2 decades, its population has undergone an aging explosion, the fastest growing number of people being those over age 65, especially those over age 85. (US Census Bureau, 2004). In terms of population age worldwide, by 2040 the US will be a truly grey-haired member of the global family, with about 80 million senior citizens.

Successfully caring for the aging US population will be a major challenge for health care professionals in the 21st century. This task should include attention to the spiritual dimension of care for several reasons. First, spirituality is an important aspect of human well-being (Ai, 2000). This is especially true for older adults, who typically experience more loss and disability than other age groups. Today, a larger population of elderly and near-elderly persons not only deal with age-related losses, disabilities, lack of resources, and death of loved ones but also with skyrocketing costs of medical care, restraints imposed by managed care, and questions left unanswered by technological advances (Konrad, 1998). Research shows that among Americans, spiritual and religious beliefs and practices tend to increase when coping with negative life events and general unhappiness (Mattlin, Wethington, & Kessler, 1990; Poloma & Gallup, 1991; Viroff, Douvan, & Kulka, 1981; Wuthnow, Christiano, & Kuzloski, 1980). In other words, the kinds of negative stressors likely to be faced by older adults make it probable that they will turn to spiritual and religious resources to cope.

Second, both the loss of status associated with becoming old and the prospect of coming to terms with one's mortality render spiritual concerns, such as the meaning of life, especially salient for this age group. We live in a youth-oriented society that often ignores the elderly and views the inevitability of aging as something to avoid. In this context, it can be very helpful for older adults to attend to their spiritual well-being, nurturing the inner strength and sense of self-worth required to successfully manage the internal and external changes that come with becoming elderly.

Third, the baby boomers are aging, and this group has already demonstrated their special needs for spiritual care as a part of their overall well-being. Sociology of religion expert Robert Wuthnow (1998) has described the escalating fascination with spirituality, including Christian spirituality, among American boomers. There has been a shift among them from a spirituality anchored in a church or synagogue to a more independent spirituality in response to a complex, fluid, and unstable social environment. Following new ideas of spiritual freedom that arose in the 1960s and '70s, many seekers have attempted to form new languages of faith, new relationships to the sacred, and more private commitments.

For example, there has been a rapid growth in American Buddhism; at least 1 million Americans identified themselves as Buddhists a decade ago (Fields, 1998), and the number has undoubtedly increased since that time. Millions of people have been introduced to the Vedic underpinnings of Hinduism through the study of yoga and meditation. Spiritual beliefs and practices from a variety of traditions have found their way into the boomer generation worldview, and often have profound implications for health and well-being. Lastly, an impressive amount of data shows that religion and spirituality may promote both mental and physical health, suggesting that a sense of spiritual well-being may not only help persons cope with adversity, but may also contribute to overall health.

THE CONCEPT OF SPIRITUAL WELL-BEING IN RESEARCH

The concept of spiritual well-being is related to several other theological, psychological, and sociological constructs. For research purposes, the concept of spiritual well-being is designed to be inclusive of diverse spiritual traditions. The hope is to promote cross-faith dialogue and the use of this concept in scientific studies, especially those related to care for the aged. A working definition for spiritual well-being is as follows:

> [Spiritual well-being] lies at the very core of one's life-span journey with respect to ultimate concern about the meaning of life and a need for wholeness, transcendence, or enlightenment. Achieving [spiritual well-being] implies a sense of harmony, inner freedom, and peace in relationship to such infinite entity as God, community, nature, the environment, or the cosmos (Ai, 2000, p. 8).

Consistent with previous efforts among other scholars, the first sentence of this concept makes it explicit that spiritual well-being is associated with the inner resources or deep values of a person. As theologian Paul Tillich (1957) suggested, "Man, in contrast to other living beings, has spiritual concerns (p. 1). The first sentence also implies that spiritual well-being lies at the highest or the deepest level of an individual's well-being, given its motivational power, and is related to personal growth throughout life (Ellison, 1983; Ellor, 1997).

Two decades ago, Ellison (1983) pointed to the subjectivity and to the difficulties of operationalizing the early concept of spiritual well-being from the perspective of the behavioral sciences. Accordingly, a "spiritual well-being scale" was developed to measure the religious and psychosocial components of spiritual well-being. In this effort, Ellison addressed Moberg's (1979) two facets of spiritual well-being: a sense of well-being in relationship to God, and a sense of life purpose and life satisfaction. Thus, the second sentence of this concept addresses two components, *spiritual* and *well-being*, but uses more global language to include the rooting spiritual well-being in various spiritual relationships. First, in general, the central theme of the concept *spiritual* "refers to what transcends materialism or exceeds preoccupation with self-maintenance" (Conn, 1999, p. 86). Accordingly, spirituality is seen to occur in different societies, cultures, communities, and historical periods under this generic definition, through different religious traditions or spiritual beliefs and practices that nourish human well-being. Thus, pathways to spiritual well-being may vary greatly. The need to be "spiritual" could be expressed in "self-transcendence through God's pervasive presence" and "love-giving for one another" in light of Christian spirituality or in "a sense of unity with the cosmos" from more secular perspectives (Conn, 1999). It could also develop in the "communal struggle," most notably observed in African American spirituality (Smith, 1999).

The second component of this concept refers to well-being. Here, the choice of descriptions—"harmony, inner freedom, and peace"—is based on three reasons. First, as indicators of spiritual well-being, these terms are shared by a great many traditions, both spiritual and religious. Second, they reflect the positive side of life, including an achievable reality for most disadvantaged populations, and of persons who face death, fatal illness, or irreversible disabilities. Third, the sense of spiritual well-being extends beyond tangible material satisfaction, physical health, momentary happiness, and psychological wellness, though it is not entirely separable from other dimensions of life. The concept of spiritual well-being is distinct from that of psychological well-being. Psychological well-being is a concept embraced in the social sciences. In psychological research, it is related to certain measures, such as self-esteem, life satisfaction, psychological adjustment, or healthy affect. Spiritual well-being, in contrast, is a concept rooted in both the social sciences and the humanities. A humanities approach tends to be related to one's outlook as well as attitudes concerning some fundamental questions with respect to the finite nature of human life and the relationship of a person to the infinite or transcendent nature of the universe or God.

Further, spiritual well-being is distinct from another concept related to psychological well-being, subjective well-being. Subjective well-being, as a concept in quality of life research, focuses on happiness and related psychological factors, such as stress dispositional influences, adaptation, goals, and coping strategies (Diener, Suh, Lucas, & Smith, 1999). Its various components involve life satisfaction, pleasant affect, and morale. Yet the spiritual dimension in measuring well-being has been largely ignored by psychologists studying the pathways to well-being (Ellison, 1983). Spiritual well-being, in contrast neither emphasizes nor denies a human need for happiness. Rather, it stresses the aspect of well-being related to a more profound motive, such as the search for ultimate meaning and purpose in life, that transcends negative impacts of distress, physical handicaps, and human suffering. For people who face more stressful life events, such as the aged, a sense of well-being may not be measurable in terms of happiness or by an absence of illness. In this light, spiritual well-being may be especially applicable in assessing the quality of life of older adults.

SPIRITUAL WELL-BEING AND SPIRITUAL GROWTH

Like spiritual well-being, spiritual growth is another concept closely linked with care for the aged. Spiritual well-being reflects an aspect of quality of life, whereas spiritual growth indicates a process toward spiritual well-being. Spiritual growth can be encouraged by experiencing spiritual well-being or by the motive to achieve spiritual well-being. Both are crucial for the aged populations, because they are relatively less associated with physical functioning. In addition, both have something to do with facing adversity, yet the relationships between them may not be completely straightforward. An infant may sense spiritual well-being but not be in a process of conscious striving for spiritual growth, whereas a dying person may not immediately sense spiritual well-being in terms of a journey toward spiritual growth.

Compared with younger populations, the aged often face negative stressors that are difficult to control. Adverse conditions challenge people's existing outlooks and attitudes concerning their images of self, relationships with others, and life goals, notably in a society where personal autonomy, independence, and sense of control are highly valued. An awareness of one's mortality and of limitations in one's capacities may thus pave the way to a new journey in one's life. In this journey, people need to be able to explore and to reconstruct a new sense of the meaning of life in the presence of adversity or diminished capacity. The aged have a strong need to learn how to accept or to cope with pain, dependency, and their own mortality, while simultaneously enjoying what life still has to offer. For many persons, an acute awareness of the ephemeral nature of life can actually increase one's sense of joy.

SPIRITUAL GROWTH AND NORMATIVE DEVELOPMENT

There has been no coherent theory concerning spiritual growth over the life span. Developing the theory in the future demands not only research evidence drawn from a perspective of developmental psychology; it requires also an interdisciplinary team effort. However, it may be worthwhile to distinguish the concept of spiritual growth from that of normative development available in present psychological theories. The process of spiritual growth and normative psychological development tend to differ from each other in several ways.

First, to some extent the two concepts have different orientations and central tasks. Developmental theories in the tradition of individual psychology mainly address questions about the maturity of an individual's *self-identity* and *healthy personality* (Erikson, 1959). The concept of spiritual growth, on the other hand, leads to an inquiry not only about personality or a sense of *I* but also about *interactive relationality* with various layers of other entities as *a part of self,* as implied by Moberg's (1971) account. In his later study of psychosocial theory, Erikson and colleagues (Erickson, Erickson, & Kivnick, 1986, p. 52) also came to recognize the need in old age for "the spiritual personality" and a shared sense of "we" within a communal state of mutuality. This more advanced idea of psychosocial development seems to come close to the concept of spiritual growth. In addition, the theme of psychosocial development, in terms of human capacity, is largely based on increasing personal mastery of tasks or control of situations in ever developing stages (Erikson, 1959). The emphasis of spiritual growth, in contrast, lies in adaptation or adjustment through alteration or affirmation of one's consciousness and belief system through interaction with a much larger system and acceptance of the self as only a part of it.

Second, spiritual growth is not directly associated with biological determinants in one's developmental journey, such as psychosexual stages presented in Freudian thought or genetic accounts for personality development. However, a basic level of human consciousness and intellectual development sets the necessary foundation for spiritual growth. The spiritual world of each individual is constructed within various sociocultural and ideological contexts. Given its complexity, spiritual growth may not follow a universally ordered sequence as presented in Piaget's (1971) stages of cognitive development or in Kohlberg's (1973) model of moral development. One of the goals of scientific studies is to reveal various aspects of universal law, including some aspects of human nature that are relatively free of confining personal values or ideologies. For many psychologists, the main building block of scientifically structured form is comprised of a developmental norm related to successive chronological stages. Spiritual growth, however, may not fit a universal schema concerning its diverse ideological contexts. It is based on constructing and reconstructing personal experiences related to basic beliefs and practices that cannot be entirely mastered through one chronological sequence. One implication of this perspective is that one could have a sense of approaching spiritual well-being even without reaching a highly mature level of development in all dimensions of the *self* or even within a deteriorated stage of mind, such as that in Alzheimer's disease.

Finally, spiritual growth may not need a prerequisite completion of stage-related achievement or hierarchical task fulfillment, in general, as was proposed in Erikson's (1959) early psychosocial theory and in other development theories as well. In a smooth journey of normal development, a healthy earlier life and its corresponding problem-solving success are certainly conducive to a person's spiritual growth in later life. For instance, a sense of trust and hope established in one's infancy may lay the foundation for one's religious faith in later life. However, given the impact of adversity in such development, spiritual growth could be in the form of a spiral instead of a straight line. In fact, spiritual growth could come in the form of a quantum leap, as the result of witnessing or experience intense suffering. It is never too late for spiritual awakening, though paths to a sense of heightened spirituality can vary considerably.

SPIRITUAL AWAKENING AND COPING IN ADVERSITY

Unusual circumstances and adverse situations can open the gate to sudden awakening or enlightenment in spiritual growth. The meaning of life tends to be reexamined in the face of crises, particularly those of severe illness and disability (Idler, 1995), and at the end of life conceived as a part of the normal aging process (Erikson et al., 1986). Because the current generation of older Americans is predominantly Christian, for most of them religious faith is an important part of their spiritual life, and using religion to cope is common among them. People's religiousness at a late age is likely to be based on a journey moving along the path of lifelong faith, particularly when the prospect of death has drawn near.

Idler (1995) found that a high association between poorer health and religiousness was due to the needs for comfort and social support among people in the midst of crises. Rehabilitating clients pointed to spiritual awakening resulting from a sudden illness such as a stroke or an injury. Many of them experienced new meanings of life, gratitude for being alive, strengthened faith, and growing peace and encouragement. Despite physical disability and disfigurement, they saw the beauty of their inner growth and spirituality. In other words, this transcending approach led them to engage more in a spiritual self and to better cope with stressful events (Idler, 1995).

From a more secular perspective, shared among some social and medical scientists in different fields dealing primarily with aging and religion, turning to spirituality for one's personal growth under these drastic conditions may have other protective benefits. Through seeking support or control from the divine or a corresponding higher power, one will fend off self-blame and prevent desperation in a sense of lost control in facing serious distress (Heckhausen & Schulz, 1995). By admitting to limitations of self, an individual will give up some obsessive striving to control an uncontrollable situation and open up to different goals under stress (Pargament, 1997). Faith, through the practice of private prayer, provides a cognitive and emotional resource accessible to the sick or disabled (Koenig, 1993). Religious coping was classified as an emotional-focused coping strategy that reduces frustration and restores hope among the aged (Koenig, George, & Siegler, 1988). Studies with large sample sizes have explored the relationship between religious involvement and functional disability among the aged (Idler & Kasl, 1997a,b). The results showed that religious involvement facilitates health practices or lifestyle in terms of higher levels of physical activities, less alcohol use, and less smoking.

Mackenzie and colleagues (2000) theorized that older adults with a strong subjective sense of receiving support from a higher power or transcendent being may enjoy better health due to the stress-buffering effect that support of any kind (e.g., social support) is known to provide. Their qualitative study of 41 older adults found that subjective feelings of well-being were intimately bound up with experiencing a personal connection to a transcendent being (e.g., God). A subsequent pilot study of a prayer intervention found that regular participation in prayer reduced anxiety and mild depression in this population (Rajagopal, Mackenzie, Bailey, & Lavizzo-Mourey, 2001). Ai and colleagues (Ai, Peterson, Rodgers, & Tice, 2005; Ai, Peterson, Tice, Bolling, & Koenig, 2004) showed that in middle-aged and older patients undergoing open heart surgery, the use of private prayer for coping contributed to optimism, hope, and a sense of internal control. They also found that over time protection of positive religious coping styles for post-operative global functioning and vitality in these patients (Ai, Peterson, Bolling, & Rodgers, in press; Ai et al., under review). In fact, numerous studies in the past decade suggest a connection between spirituality and health. These range from epidemiological research that shows a correlation between attendance at religious services and decreased mortality (Oman & Reed, 1998), to a study on intercessory prayer and postsurgical health outcomes of cardiac patients (Harris et al., 1999). Although there are mixed findings suggesting the need for more sophisticated research (Ai et al., in press), practically spirituality may contribute to one's ability to cope with loss and promote health by encouraging healthy behavior, connecting with congregations, or supporting positive emotions (Levin, 1996).

PROFESSIONAL ATTENTION TO THE
SPIRITUAL NEEDS OF THE AGED

To encourage spiritual well-being among the aged, the spiritual needs of this population have to be recognized and satisfied. Traditionally, spiritual well-being, spiritual growth, and spiritual needs are not areas of concern for mental health professionals but are left to be dealt with by clergy. Increasingly, however, health care professionals are becoming interested in the spiritual needs of their clients (Millison & Dudley, 1992). Given the mounting evidence on the importance of spirituality and faith in health and well-being, spiritual professional care needs to be advocated, especially among mental health professionals. This form of spiritual care does not mean a form of quasi-pastoral care performed by health care professionals. Rather, the spiritual well-being of populations for which they provide care should be adequately addressed in a professionally appropriate manner. Clearly, diverse ideologies exist among professionals, not just medical chaplains, health care providers, and patients. Hence, professional education should enhance training in a way that enables helpers to be attentive and responsive to multiple spiritual needs among the aged.

To assist the spiritual well-being of the aged, mental health professionals should walk in their shoes to best understand their spiritual needs. Although many health care professionals receive no training in understanding patients' and clients' belief systems, there are aspects of the clients' spiritual life with which they can offer immediate help. For instance, to make life worth living, they could help the aged person remove the negative stereotype of dependence and build a positive sense of life in the face of difficulties. Unconditional love is an essential spiritual need for many within Christian and Jewish populations (Koenig, 1994). The faith in God's love for God's people unconditionally makes a person feel accepted, valued, and cared for, thus enhancing the individual's spiritual growth and sense of spiritual well-being. Among Buddhists, compassion from Buddha or among his believers is valued as high as unconditional love by Christians, though the two concepts may not be identical. It has been suggested that loving kindness (or *metta*), a concept from Buddhism, can be cultivated through meditation and applied in the clinical setting for the purposes of practicing a more humane medicine (Aung, 1996). To nonreligious aged people in crisis, unconditional love and compassion may be equally important in the process of spiritual nourishment. Both concepts could be addressed in forming professional ethics of care. In practice, mental health professionals could express deep concern for, provide emotional comfort to, and simply listen to the spiritual wishes of the aged with patience, respect, and supportive reflection.

Professionals may also take a more responsive position in facilitating people's efforts, as they struggle through adverse events, by expressing an understanding of their distress-related spiritual needs. For instance, physical illness and disability tend to evoke feelings related to loss, isolation, rejection, and alienation. For both religious and nonreligious aged people, having faith in something that can promise ultimate security will help them to "tolerate deeply troubling skepticism" and to deal with serious survival questions at this stage (Erikson et al., 1986, p. 228). Turning to religion or maintaining one's lifelong faith, for instance, will sometimes provide important comfort to many older people (Erikson et al., 1986). In health crises, people with mainstream religious beliefs will need to sense a belonging to God to cope with the difficulties that they face. For others, a connection to the transcendent through nature, humanitarianism, or some other appropriate path can help them to manage the crisis. In these situations, health care professionals can lend their support and validation of people's use of these protective coping methods to assist their patients.

THEORIES OF SPIRITUALITY AND RELIGION THAT MAY FACILITATE CARE

Research has already documented patients' wish for health care staffs' being heedful of their religious needs (Sodestron & Martinson, 1987). However, many health care providers are neither religious nor trained to respond to the religious and spiritual concerns of their patients and clients (Sherril & Larson, 1987; Taylor & Amanta, 1994). How can we bridge the gap between the demands for professional care regarding spirituality and the lack of awareness of spiritual issues among health care professionals? Some social science theories have elaborated extensively on spirituality and religion, especially in terms of interventions. Two examples that stand out in this regard are psychology of religion and coping (Pargament, 1997) and transpersonal psychology (Strohl, 1998), the application of which could help professionals become more competent to address their patients' spiritual needs.

Pargament's Theory of Religious Coping

Pargament (1997) challenged conventional views in both psychology and religion. He believed that health care professionals and others in the caring professions should receive training in religious issues, including education on the potential influence of their own beliefs on the process of caring for clients. In bridging the worldviews and practices of the two sides, they could be equipped by the wealth of religious traditions in helping people to cope with their limitations and seeking beyond the self for answers to serious questions that arise in crises. Pargament's work does not center on the particular needs of the aged. Yet, based on intensive research, he concluded that people who seek religious coping tend to be members of less powerful groups, including the poor, elderly, minorities, women, and the disenfranchised (Pargament, 1997). Many of them see themselves and others in a larger field of spiritual forces and tend to face many negative life events, such as serious illness, loss of loved ones, and social injustice. In these crises, religion becomes an available and compelling way of coping that pertains to their spiritual well-being and maintains inner strength. Pargament's (1997) core theory offers an anatomy of connections between religion and coping. Going beyond the stereotype of religious coping, which views it as a passive approach, he pointed to many facets and determinants, situational, cultural, and personal. Through in-depth analysis, he elaborated evaluative and practical issues with respect to both positive and negative patterns of religious coping. Specific forms of coping, such as spiritual support, benevolent religious reframing, or expressing anger at God, tend to be associated with different outcomes of adjustment (Pargament, 1997). According to Pargament, health care professionals need to understand these potential patterns to provide effective spiritual care.

Transpersonal Psychology

Transpersonal theory can be traced back to many psychological traditions, particularly humanistic psychology, and has been grounded philosophically on a convergence between ancient Asian thought, including Buddhism, and modern science (Strohl, 1998). Jung (1917/1953) first used the term *transpersonal* as a synonym for *collective,* as it was conjoined with *unconscious.* Maslow (1968) named transpersonal psychology as the "Fourth Force" psychology, following the sequence of "First Force" (psychoanalytic), "Second Force" (behavioral), and "Third Force" (humanistic) psychologies. In the 1960s, Maslow and other leaders of humanistic psychology came to realize the limits of notions related to conventional ego boundaries and the need to include the transcendent human capacities in psychological theory (Strohl, 1998). Influenced by ancient Eastern philosophies, he brought a spiritual dimension into his concept of "self-actualization" (Maslow, 1968; Strohl, 1998). After 25 years of evolution, transpersonal psychology is defined as a theory "concerned with the study of humanity's highest potential, and with the recognition, understanding, and realization of unitive, spiritual, and transcendent stages of consciousness" (Lajoie & Shapiro, 1992, p. 91).

Accordingly, transpersonal perspectives highlight spiritual growth and levels of human functioning beyond ego or personal self. This theory inherits openness to diverse aspects of spirituality and opens the way to incorporating types of nontraditional methods other than the "talk therapy" common in clinical practice. Transpersonal counseling addresses the impacts of belief systems and other aspects of consciousness in self-healing and growth. Focusing on expanding human qualities, the intervention aims at enlightenment, freedom, liberation, and transcendence of self to a sense of interconnectedness with all of existence. With an awareness of the limits in intellectual and analytical approaches, transpersonal psychology uses traditional and many nontraditional approaches to growth and change, including meditation, prayer, imagery, relaxation, and other mind–body or spiritual methods. As such, it may contribute to bridging the gap between the need of serving the spiritual well-being of patients and a lack of spiritual focus in the health care professions.

CONCLUSION

As researchers parse out all the varying theoretical dimensions to be found in the concept of spiritual well-being, where does that leave the health care professional who wishes to include a spiritual component in his or her care for older adults? One of the first things professionals can do is become aware of the role that religion or spirituality plays in the lives of their patients. To respect the patient's privacy, this discussion can be initiated by simply asking, "Would you like me to discuss spirituality and health with you?" Or one can mention a particular book or article on the topic one has read recently and observe the response. Initiating such a dialogue will likely increase the bonds of trust between provider and patient as well as reveal important information that can help with caring for the whole person. Another way to support the spiritual well-being of patients is to work in concert with clergy, family, and others to address their spiritual needs. Finally, it is important for health care professionals to be mindful of their own spiritual well-being as they witness the successes and challenges, the healings and sufferings of those in their care. Professionals who can connect with their own spirituality as they care for others, are best prepared to address issues related to spiritual well-being and spiritual growth in their practice.

RESOURCES

Books

Koenig, H. G., McChulough, M. E., & Larson, D. B. (2001). *The handbook of religion and health*. New York: Oxford University Press.

Thorson, J. A. (Ed.). (2000). *Perspectives on spiritual well-being and aging*. Springfield, IL: Charles C. Thomas.

Web Sites

www.spiritualityhealth.com
A magazine devoted to the exploration of the body and soul connection

www.gwish.org
George Washington University's Institute for the Study of Spirituality and Health

www.dukespiritualityandhealth.org
Duke University's Center for the Study of Religion, Spirituality, and Health

www.healthy.net/wellness/spirituality/
HealthWorld Online's offering on the topic

www.experiencefestival.com/spirituality_and_health
A "new age" oriented Web site on the topic

www.elca.org/health/spiritual.html
An evangelical Christian view of spirituality and health

REFERENCES

Ai, A. L. (2000). Spiritual well-being, spiritual growth, and spiritual care for the aged: A cross-faith and interdisciplinary effort. *Journal of Religious Gerontology, 11*(2), 3–28.

Ai, A. L., & Bolling, S. F. (2002). The use of complementary and alternative therapies of middle-aged and older cardiac patients. *American Journal of Medical Quality: Official Journal of the American College of Medical Quality, 17*(1), 21–27.

Ai, A. L., & Bolling, S. F. (2004). Complementary and alternative care for the hearts of middle-aged and older patients. *Evidence-Based Integrative Medicine, 1*(4), 261–268.

Ai, A. L., Dunkle, R. E., Peterson, C., & Bolling, S. F. (1998). The role of private prayer in psychosocial recovery among midlife and aged patients following cardiac surgery. *The Gerontologist, 38*(5), 591–601.

Ai, A. L., Peterson, C., Bolling, S. F., & Rodgers, W. (2006). Depression, faith-based coping, and short-term post-operative global functioning in adult and older patients undergoing cardiac surgery. *Journal of Psychosomatic Research, 60*(1), 21–28.

Ai, A. L., Peterson, C., Rodgers, W., & Tice, T. N. (2005). Effects of faith and secular factors on health locus of control in middle-aged and older cardiac patients. *Aging and Mental Health, 9*(5), 470–481.

Ai, A. L., Peterson, C., Tice, T. N., Bolling, S. F., & Koenig, H. (2004). Faith-based and secular pathways to hope and optimism subconstructs in middle-aged and older cardiac patients. *Journal of Health Psychology, 9*(3), 435–450.

Ai, A. L., Peterson, C., Tice, T. N., Rodgers, W., Seymour, E. M., & Bolling, S. F. (under review). Faith-based coping, optimism, and fatigue symptoms in cardiac patients.

Astin, J. A., Pelletier, K. R., Marie, A., & Haskell, W. L. (2000). Complementary and alternative medicine use among elderly persons: One-year analysis of a Blue Shield Medicare supplement. *Journal of Gerontology: Medical Science, 55A*, M4–M9.

Aung, S. K. (1996). Loving kindness: The essential Buddhist contribution to primary care. *Human Health Care International, 12*(2), E12.

Conn, J. W. (1999). Spiritual formation. *Theology Today, 56*, 86–97.

Diener, E., Suh, E. M., Lucas, R. E., & Smith, H. (1999). Subjective well-being: Three decades of progress. *Psychological Bulletin, 125*, 276–302.

Dossey, L. (2005). What does illness mean? In Schlitz, Amorok and Micozzi (Eds.), *Consciousness and healing.* St. Louis: Elsevier.

Ellison, G. W. (1983). Spiritual well-being: Conceptualization and measurement. *Journal of Psychology and Theology, 11*, 330–340.

Ellor, J. W. (1997). Spiritual well-being defined. *Aging and Spirituality, Newsletter of ASA's Forum on Religion, Spirituality and Aging, 9*, 1–2.

Erikson, E. (1959). *Childhood and society.* New York: W. W. Norton.

Erikson, E., Erikson, J., & Kivnick, H. (1986). *Vital involvement in old age.* New York: W. W. Norton.

Fields, R. (1998). Divided dharma: White Buddhist, ethnic Buddhists, and racism. In C. S. Prebish & K. K. Tanaka (Eds.), *The faces of Buddhism in America* (pp. 196–206). Berkeley: University of California Press.

Harris, W. S., Gowda, M., Kolb, J. W., Strychacz, C. P., Vacek, J. L., Jones, P. G., et al. (1999). A randomized controlled trial of the effects of remote intercessory prayer on outcomes in patients admitted to the coronary care unit. *Archives of Internal Medicine, 159*, 2273–2278.

Heckhausen, J., & Schulz, R. (1995). A life-span theory of control. *Psychological Review, 102*, 284–304.

Hufford D. J. (1997). Folk medicine and health culture in contemporary society. *Complementary and Alternative Therapies in Primary Care, 24*, 723–741.

Idler, E. L. (1995). Religion, health, and nonphysical sense of self. *Social Forces, 74*, 683–704.

Idler, E. L., & Kasl, S. V. (1997a). Religion among disabled and nondisabled persons: 1. Cross-sectional patterns in health practices, social activities, and well-being. *Journal of Gerontology: Social Sciences, 52B*, S294–305.

Idler, E. L., & Kasl, S.V. (1997b). Religion among disabled and nondisabled persons: 2. Attendance at religious services as a predictor of the course of disability. *Journals of Gerontology: Series B: Psychological Sciences and Social Sciences, 52B,* S306–S316.

Jung, C. G. (1953). Two essays on analytical psychology. In G. Adler, M. Fordham, & H. Read (Eds.), R. F. C. Hull (Trans.), *The collected works of C. G. Jung* (vol. 7). New York: Pantheon Books. (Original work published 1917.).

Koenig, E. (1999). Keeping company with Jesus and the saints. *Theology Today, 56,* 18–28.

Koenig, H. G. (1993). Religion and hope for the disabled elder. In J. Levin (Ed.), *Religion in aging and health.* Thousand Oaks, CA: Sage.

Koenig, H. G. (1994). Spiritual needs of physically ill elders. In *Aging and God: Spiritual pathways to mental health in midlife and later years* (pp. 283–295). New York: Haworth Pastoral Press.

Koenig, H. G., George, L. K., & Siegler, I. C. (1988). The use of religion and other emotion-regulating coping strategies among older adults. *The Gerontologist, 28,* 303–310.

Koenig, H. G., McCullough, M. E., & Larson, D. B. (2001). *The handbook of religion and health.* New York: Oxford University Press.

Kohlberg, L. (1973). Continuities in childhood and adult moral reasoning revisited. In P. B. Baltes & K. W. Schaie (Eds.), *Life-span developmental psychology* (pp. 179–204). New York: Academic Press.

Konrad, T. R. (1998). The patterns of self-care among older adults in western industrialized societies. In M .G. Ory & G. H. Defriese (Eds.), *Self-care in later life.* New York: Springer.

Lajoie, D. H., & Shapiro, S. I. (1992). Definition of transpersonal psychology: The first twenty-five years. *Journal of Transpersonal Psychology, 24,* 79–98.

Levin, J. S. (1996). How religions influence morbidity and health: Reflections on nature history, salutogenesis, and host resistance. *Journal for the Scientific Study of Religion, 27,* 90–104.

Mackenzie, E. R., Rajagopal, D. E., Meibohm, M., & Lavizzo-Mourey, R. (2000). Spiritual support and psychological well-being: Older adults' perception of the religion and health connection. *Alternative Therapies in Health and Medicine, 6*(6), 37–45.

Maslaw, A. (1968). *Toward a psychology of being* (2nd ed.). New York: Van Nostrand/Reinhold.

Mattlin, J. A., Wethington, E., & Kessler, R. C. (1990). Situational determinants of coping and coping effectiveness. *Journal of Health and Social Behavior, 31,* 103–122.

Millison, M., & Dudley, J. R. (1992). Providing spiritual support: A job for all hospice professionals. *The Hospice Journal, 8,* 49–66.

Moberg, D. O. (1971). *Spiritual well-being.* Washington, DC: University Press of America.

Oman, D. & Reed, D. (1998). Religion and mortality among community-dwelling elderly. *American Journal of Public Health, 88,* 1469–1475.

Pargament, K. I. (1997). *The psychology of religion and coping.* New York: Guilford Press.

Payne, B. P. (1990). Spirituality and aging: Research and theoretical approaches. *Generations, 14,* 11–14.

Piaget, J. (1971). *Insights and illusions of philosophy* (W. Mays, Trans.). New York: World, Meridian Books.

Poloma, M. M., & Gallup, G. H., Jr. (1991). *Varieties of prayer: A survey report.* Philadelphia: Trinity Press International.

Rajagopal, D., Mackenzie, E., Bailey, C., & Lavizzo-Mourey, R. (2002). The effectiveness of a spiritually-based intervention for relieving subsyndromal anxiety and minor depression in older adults. *Journal of Religion and Health, 41*(2), 153–166.

Sherril, K. A., & Larson, D. B. (1987). Adult burn patients: The role of religion in recovery. *Southern Medical Journal, 81,* 821–825.

Smith, A., Jr. (1999). Reaching back and pushing forward: A perspective on African American spirituality. *Theology Today, 56,* 44–58.

Sodestron, K. E., & Martinson, R. (1987). Patients' spiritual coping strategies: A study of nurse and patient perspectives. *Oncology Nursing Forum, 14,* 41–46.

Strohl, J. E. (1998). Transpersonalism: Ego meets soul. *Journal of Counseling and Development, 76,* 397–403.

Taylor, E. J., & Amanta, M. (1994). Midwifery to the soul while the body dies: Spiritual care among hospice nurses. *American Journal of Hospice and Palliative Care, 11,* 28–35.

Tillich, P. (1957). *Dynamics of faith.* New York: Harper & Row.

Viroff, J., Douvan, E., & Kulka, R. A. (1981). *The inner American: A self-portrait from 1957 to 1976.* New York: Basic Books.

U.S. Census Bureau. Retrieved from http://www.census.gov/prod/2004pubs/04statab/pop.pdf

Wuthnow, R. (1998). *After heaven: Spirituality in America since the 1950s.* Berkeley: University of California Press.

Wuthnow, R., Christiano, K., & Kuzloski, J. (1980). Religion and bereavement: A conceptual framework. *Journal for the Scientific Study of Religion, 19,* 408–422.

CHAPTER FIFTEEN

Therapeutic Gardens

Jack Carman

People have maintained a connection with nature throughout time. This goes back to when people wandered the land in search of food or could read the weather signs of an approaching storm. Even now, our everyday world is shaped by what is happening outside our home. We depend on nature for our food, clothing, medicine, and the roof over our head. We may need a raincoat to go to the store because it is raining or boots because it is snowing. We enjoy a bumper crop of tomatoes because of the right amount of sun and moisture this season. Our vacation at the beach or the mountains was perfect this year because it was sunny every day. Not a day goes by that the natural world does not affect us.

Our connection with nature does not change just because we grow older. Whatever the age, we are affected by the sun, trees, sky, and all of the various elements we know to be nature. Have you ever stopped to enjoy a sunset and marvel how the sky is lit up with such magnificent colors? Maybe you have opened a window to listen to a summer rain shower as the water bounces off the leaves of a tree. What person has not tried to catch a snowflake on his tongue, or looked for an elusive four-leaf clover in a field of grass?

Current research validates our intuitive sense that our involvement with nature positively affects our lives. Research psychologist Roger S. Ulrich (1984a,b, 1992) has shown that we recover sooner, take less pain medication, and have a more positive outlook on our personal health when we have a view of nature. His study of recovery from gallbladder surgery showed that patients who had a view of trees from their hospital window "had shorter postoperative stays, had fewer negative evaluative comments, took fewer moderate and strong analgesic doses, and had lightly lower scores for minor postsurgical complications" (Ulrich,

1984a, p. 421). This work is now being used to improve the design of hospital buildings, allowing patients to have a view of nature from their hospital beds. As professionals, we need to look for ways to give residents and patients access to nature in all types of health care facilities.

Ulrich has conducted research in other settings to show how a view of nature reduces levels of stress. One study involved college students who had completed a difficult exam, naturally increasing levels of anxiety. The students were divided into two groups, one viewing nature scenes and the other urban scenes. Ulrich (1984b) found that the emotional states of the individuals who had viewed the slides of vegetation were significantly improved. In contrast, the students who had watched the urban images felt somewhat worse after the slide viewing. These results are significant in that they indicate the need to increase visual access of nature for older adults residing in senior communities, consequently improving their quality of life. Not only would the levels of stress be reduced for the residents, but staff and caregivers could also benefit from well-designed gardens and pleasant views. As a result, we are compelled to create more natural exterior settings and reduce the visual impact of parking lots, trash containers, utilities, heating and air conditioning equipment, and other man-made objects. Designers of senior residences would be wise to include "home-like" outdoor environments that resemble a person's yard. Ulrich's research found that "people consistently express a preference for natural scenes rather than 'built' environments" (Ulrich, 1984b, p. 20).

We all enjoy nature in a variety of ways. It can be through activities such as gardening, planting vegetables, cutting flowers to offer to a friend, or maybe even pulling weeds. Other activities may not be as physical and can involve more passive pastimes, such as bird watching, taking a walk on a woodland path, or sitting on a bench watching others pursue more active involvement. These activities are pleasurable, whether active or passive, and can elicit the release of a chemical called endorphin, a natural mood elevator and painkiller. The brain releases endorphins into the bloodstream, which produces a state of relaxation in the body and mind (McGrath, 1996).

Knowing all of this places a greater level of importance on the creation of therapeutic outdoor environments. The garden is an ideal place to get away from one's cares. If you have ever been under stress or have had a bad day, the garden can be a familiar place to escape. Gardening is also a source of quiet fascination. According to Rachael Kaplan (1973), gardening "calls on the basic informational processes that humans do so well," and "not only permits, but actually invites recognition, prediction, control and evaluation." It is a "nature based activity, and nature per se has been shown to be the object of preference."

In the field of environmental psychology, nature has been described as a "positive distraction" (Ulrich, 1992). Nature, which encompasses trees, plants, and water, in the natural environment, does not ask us any questions or judge us. The natural world accepts us for who we are. This involvement can be as simple as sitting on a bench and watching a bird in a birdbath or noticing a butterfly traveling from flower to flower or a child taking a dog for a walk. Creating and enjoying these special environments can have a restorative effect on us all. That is why it is important to design and develop these gardens as a place of respite for older adults, as well as for their caregivers.

As we age, the ability to do all of the things we have done throughout our lives may be reduced. There may be a need for more reliance on others for help, which in turn means less control over our lives. When you can eat, where you can go, how you get from place to place, and other everyday needs are very often managed by others in a senior care facility. Having the ability to maintain control over our environment is important. Designing environments so that a person is able to remain more independent can improve health and increase social interaction (Ulrich, 1992). One of the ways this can be accomplished is to provide access to the outdoor environment, both visually and physically. The interior environment should be arranged so that a person can see outside from the bedroom or living room area. Physical access to garden areas should be easy to get to and well labeled, so that a person can go outside whenever he or she chooses. The gardens should be stimulating as well as interesting.

People, especially older adults, do not want to give up the things that they have enjoyed throughout their lives. Maintaining a connection with familiar elements and surroundings is important to us all. A study by Talbot and Kaplan (1991) found that older adults listed nature, gardens, and the ability to access the outdoors among the most important elements in their lives. The study revealed that older adults "consider access to nature near their homes to be very important." As one of the participants in the study described, "I love being retired, so that I can be outdoors . . . as you get older these things become more important" (p. 123).

Helping older adults to maintain a connection with nature is very important. The creation of accessible and functioning exterior environments is an integral part of every senior community. The development of outdoor spaces entails design of specific areas and the selection of the garden elements. Surface materials for walks, enclosures for safety and security, and furnishings that allow comfortable usage are a few of the primary considerations. Outdoor areas should be designed to include a variety of activities that make the garden fun for everyone. Raised planters in varying heights should be included to allow a person in a wheelchair or a walker access to plants and soil. The addition of bird-feeders and birdbaths can be entertainment throughout the year. It is important to incorporate the help of a landscape architect who is experienced in working with seniors and understands the requirements of creating exterior spaces for older adults.

The design of the garden should reflect the cultural vernacular of the region, which will assist those using the outdoor areas. The residence may be located in a marine or agricultural part of the country. The use of an old waterman's boat or some farm implements, for example, would be important elements in a residence located near these settings. Becoming familiar with what people have had in their yard will help re-create their special place. Encouraging families to bring a favorite plant to their new home will help residents feel as if their surroundings are truly home. Seeing a favorite shrub, such as a hydrangea or an azalea, can help to create a sense of familiarity. If it is not possible to transplant a plant into the garden, arranging to have a similar shrub or tree planted will be the next best thing. This in turn becomes an activity and a reason to visit the garden to see how a particular plant is growing. Encouraging families to start a vegetable garden in a portion of the main garden is another way to get help create the connection between familiar settings and to encourage familial interactions.

Familiar garden elements are an important aspect of the garden because they increase the likelihood that people will use it. Every aspect of the garden design needs to relate to the intended use of the garden. For example, although gazebos are commonly believed to be something that should be included, not many people actually have a gazebo in their backyard. They may have had a summerhouse or tool shed, rather than a gazebo. If a gazebo is contemplated, it should be designated for specific activities and outfitted with a ceiling fan, movable chairs, electrical outlets, and screens, in order to obtain the most function out of this architectural element. Ultimately, the goal is to select a garden structure that meets the program's needs. The questions to ask are How many people are involved in an activity? Are tables and chairs needed? What is the proximity of the gazebo to the building? It may also be possible to accommodate the program's requirements using a canopy or pergola, rather than a gazebo, saving money in the process.

Safety is one of the prime considerations in the design of an outdoor garden area. Eliminating the need for steps whenever possible is important to reduce the likelihood of falls. Pathways should be smooth and limit the number of control joints, while still being constructed properly. Material such as concrete is an economical walking surface. Tinting the concrete will help reduce glare and make it easier for an older adult to navigate the garden safely. Other options include the use of recycled rubberized material that is used on playground and running track surfaces. This application can, however, be double the cost of concrete or asphalt.

One of the big deterrents to the use of the garden is access. Many times the inclusion of a garden is an afterthought to the design of a senior residence. Gardens and usable outdoor areas should be part of the initial concept plan. Easy access into the garden and views of the garden from within the building are primary factors in the successful use of the garden. Staff will have a greater level of comfort when they can see from the interior of the residence a resident who is in the garden. Large windows that look out onto the garden are another consideration. Signs, garden elements, and other visual cues will help a person find the garden more easily. The garden will be used more frequently once residents are familiar with access to and the location of the garden. It should have markers that help persons navigate throughout the area. The plantings should be designed to permit good views into and within the garden.

Developing outdoor gardens is the first half of the process. Creating programs that allow residents to participate in outdoor areas is the continuation of the process. Gardens are for people to enjoy, both visually and physically. There should be areas for residents to grow herbs, flowers, vegetables, and other favorite plants. Families should be encouraged to participate in garden activities when they visit. It is a good excuse to ask residents to visit the garden and see how the plants that they have been growing and tending are doing. A flagpole, watering can, clothesline, and other familiar outdoor elements allow individuals to interact with the garden. Bending, stretching, and reaching during garden activities are helpful in maintaining good health. It is possible to schedule many of the activities that are programmed within in the garden, including reading groups, painting, woodworking, and photography and exercise classes. The activities schedules for exterior environments are only limited by weather and creativity.

Another important aspect of the garden is the interaction of people in the garden. The garden is an excellent means of subtly encouraging people to socialize. A crucial part of the design process is to consider the ways in which people can interact. The location of a bench or grouping of tables and chairs may cause the users of the garden to converse more frequently. The garden is a great place to meet friends, entertain visitors, or just observe other people. Incorporating a climbing structure or other play equipment in the garden area will encourage visiting children to use the garden. The sound of children playing and laughing is a pleasant experience for everyone, especially older adults. A garden is a perfect place to create settings where children and older adults have the opportunity to interact in a familiar environment.

Special care needs are a part of the development of a therapeutic garden. This should involve a landscape architect who is experienced in working with and understands the physical, social, and psychological needs of older adults. The landscape architect can assist with designing a universally accessible outdoor area and coordinating the various elements that comprise a therapeutic garden. Along with the landscape architect, the design team needs to be comprised of a gerontologist, administration, residents, and caregivers. A gerontologist will be able to evaluate the overall residence and surrounding gardens to ensure that they functionally meet the needs of the elderly residents. Staff members who are involved in the day-to-day care of older adults, such as activity professionals, physical therapists, and nursing staff, will be able to complete the picture of how the garden can best be programmed and designed. Most important in this process, whenever possible, are the residents themselves. The involvement of the residents will help them to take ownership of the garden and make the garden a success and thrive.

A horticulture therapist should be involved to assist in the development and implementation of specific therapeutic gardening–related programs for older adults. According to Steven Davis, "Horticultural therapy is a process through which plants, gardening, activities and the innate closeness we all feel toward nature are used as vehicles in professionally conducting programs of therapy and rehabilitation" (quoted in Simson & Strauss, 1998). A horticultural therapist works with older adults to develop specific therapeutic programs that will improve quality of life, general well-being, and mood (Mackenzie et al., 2000). These programs can be developed through the utilization of exterior and interior gardens. Indoor areas are especially important for maintaining programs and activities in off-seasons, such as the winter months. "Gardening—like many other physical activities—has been found to affect body shape, bone strength, muscle strength, skeletal flexibility, motor fitness, cardiopulmonary fitness and metabolic fitness" (Mackenzie et al., 2000, p. 69).

According to the American Horticultural Therapy Association (AHTA) Web site, "People with physical or mental disabilities benefit from gardening experiences as part of [horticultural therapy] programs, and they learn skills, adaptations, and gardening methods that allow for continued participation at home" (www.AHTA.org). Everyday tasks, such as potting a plant, arranging flowers in a vase, pruning and watering plants, and weeding, have been shown to improve physical, social, psychological, and spiritual well-being. The addition of stimulating activities and exercise will help produce a renewed interest in events that an older adult might have possibly enjoyed earlier in life. One research study indicated that the second most popular leisure activity for the elderly was gardening and raising plants, following socialization (Rothert & Daubet,

1981). Gardening and socializing are two activities that blend well together and can lead to an overall increase in quality of life for anyone, but most especially institutionalized older adults.

Simple gardening tasks and activities can be accomplished with a raised planting bed with grow lights. Raised planters come in a variety of shapes and sizes. Some key features to remember when specifying a planter is the overall size and accessibility. Seat planters, approximately 18 inches in height, can be used by people to sit on the edge of the planter to work in the planting bed. Planters, approximately 24 inches in height, can be used by a person in a wheelchair. And planters that are 30 inches in height are most readily accessed by a person using a walker or other assisted mobility device. The section below the planter box itself should be an open space, between the legs of the planter, for use by a person in a wheelchair.

The success of a particular program depends on having the right tools and equipment, as much as it does on having the right person to coordinate the activities. There are adaptive tools available today through various catalogues that help make a gardening task physically easier and more enjoyable (refer to Resources). Hats to shade a person's eyes from the sun, sunscreen to protect the skin from sunburn, and gloves to keep hands clean are a few of the necessary items on an equipment list.

It is important to start slowly and build up interest and excitement with new activities. There are many basic activities that can generate participation and are easy to start. Bird watching is currently the second most popular leisure activity in the United States, the first being gardening. People delight in spotting a particular bird and telling others what they have seen. A thistle birdfeeder will attract colorful house and gold finches to the feeders all year long, depending on the region of the country in which the garden is located. The selection of specific birdfeeders will attract those birds that are "invited" to visit the garden and limit unwanted birds. There are several resources for birding information, including the National Audubon Society and the Cornell Lab of Ornithology. Local bird experts can also be found by contacting birdwatching clubs, universities, and stores, such as Wildbirds Unlimited and the Wild Bird Center.

CONCLUSION

Anyone can begin to create a therapeutic garden by remembering the basic ingredients. First, create a program that is of interest to the residents. Second, assemble a design team comprised of administration, staff, residents, and design professionals to create a garden that reflects the needs of the residents. Third, pick therapeutic gardening activities that are simple and offer the greatest opportunity for success. Once created, the most important element is to evaluate the effectiveness of the programs that have been created for the therapeutic garden. The measurement of success will be determined by how well the people who participate in the various activities utilize all of the opportunities the garden has to offer. One of the most obvious ways to determine the success of the garden is by the smiles on the faces of the people in it.

RESOURCES

Associations

Alzheimer's Association, 225 N. Michigan Ave., Suite 1700, Chicago, IL 60601-7633; telephone: (800) 272-3900; fax: (312) 335-1110; Web site: www.Alzheimer'sAssociation.org

American Horticultural Therapy Association (AHTA), 909 York St., Denver, CO 80206; telephone: (303) 370-8087; fax: (303) 331-5776; Web site: www.AHTA.org

American Society of Landscape Architect–Therapeutic Garden Design Professional Interest Group, 636 Eye St. NW, Washington, DC 20001-3736; telephone: (202) 898-2444; fax: (202) 898-2444, Web site: www.ASLA.org

Chicago Botanic Garden–Enabling Garden; 1000 Lake Cook Rd., Glencoe, IL 60022; telephone: (847) 835-5440; Web site: www.Chicago BotanicGarden.org

Cornell Lab of Ornithology, Cornell University, Ithaca, NY 14850; telephone: (800) 843-BIRD (800-843-2473); Web site: cornellbirds@cornell.edu

National Audubon Society, 700 Broadway, New York, NY 10003; telephone: (212) 979-3000; fax: (212) 979-3188; Web site: National AudubonSociety.org

Catalogues

Access with Ease—tools and assisted devices; (800) 531-9479

AdaptAbility—garden games and products; (800) 288-9941; www.adaptability.com

Droll Yankees—birdfeeders and products; (800) 352-9164; www.drollyankees.com

Duncraft—birdfeeders and products; (800) 593-5656; www.duncraft.com

FlagHouse—tools and games; (800) 793-7900; www.flaghouse.com

Gold Violin—garden products; (877) 648-8465; www.goldviolin.com

Additional Readings

Brawley, E. C. (1997). *Designing for Alzheimer's disease.* New York: Wiley Press.

Cooper Marcus, C., & Barnes, M. (1999). *Healing gardens: Therapeutic benefits and design recommendations.* New York: Wiley Press.

Gerlach-Spriggs, N., Kaufman, R. E., & Warner, S. B., Jr. (1998). *Restorative gardens: The healing landscape.* New Haven, CT: Yale University Press.

Kaplan, R., Kaplan, S., & Ryan, R. L. (1998). *With people in mind: Design and management of everyday nature.* Washington, DC: Island Press.

Rawlings, R. (n.d.). *Healing gardens.* Minocqua, WI: Willow Creek Press.

Rothert, E. A., Jr., & Daubert, J. R. (1981). *Horticultural therapy for nursing homes, senior centers, retirement living.* Chicago: Chicago Horticultural Society.

Shoemaker, C. A. (2002). *Interaction by design—bringing people and plants together for health and well-being.* Ames: Iowa State Press.

Simson, S. P., & Straus, M. C. (1998). *Horticulture as therapy—principals and practices.* Binghamton, NY: Food Products Press/Haworth Press.

Wells, S. E. (1997). *Horticultural therapy and the older adult population.* Binghamton, NY: Haworth Press.

Wou, J. (1997). *Accessible gardening—tips and techniques for seniors and the disabled.* Stackpole Books.

REFERENCES

Kaplan, R. (1973, June). Benefits of gardening. *Environment and Behavior.*

Mackenzie, E. R., Agard, B., Portella, C., Mahangar, D., Barol, J., & Carson, L. (2000). Horticultural therapy in long-term care settings. *Journal of the American Medical Directors Association,* 69–73.

McGrath, V. (1996, September). The healing power of the garden. *Landscape Design,* 8–12.

Rothert, E. A., & Daubert, J. R. (1981). *Horticultural therapy for nursing homes, senior centers, retirement living.* Chicago: Chicago Horticultural Society.

Simson, S. P. & Straus, M. C. (1998). *Horticulture as therapy—principles and practices.* Binghamton, NY: Food Products Press/Haworth Press.

Talbot, J. F., & Kaplan, R. (1991). The benefits of nearby nature for elderly apartment residents. *International Journal of Aging and Human Development, 33*(2), 119–130.

Ulrich, R. S. (1984a, November/December). The psychological benefits of plants. *Garden,* p. 19.

Ulrich, R. S. (1984b, April 27). View through a window may influence recovery from surgery. *Science,* p. 421.

Ulrich, R. S. (1992, September/October). How design impacts wellness. *Healthcare Forum Journal,* 23–25.

CHAPTER SIXTEEN

The Eden Alternative: Nurturing the Human Spirit in Long-Term Care

Sandy Ransom

The Eden Alternative™ is a management and design philosophy that transforms long-term care organizations into warm, caring environments: places where elders are given control over their own lives and staff members are empowered to make decisions regarding their work life. The Eden Alternative™ began through the vision of William Thomas, MD, when he took a job as medical director of a small nursing home in upstate New York in the early 1990s. Dr. Thomas's words describe his initial journey into long-term care:

> I am a doctor: More specifically, I am a nursing home doctor. I provide medical care for people who live in long-term care institutions and my work fascinates me. It holds all of the challenge and variety one usually associates with the more glamorous specialties. My work as a geriatrician, however, has also led me to reflect upon the enormous impact that design and operation of a long-term care facility has upon residents. Nowadays, I spend about half of my time in clinical practice and the other half thinking, teaching and writing about a new way of designing and operating long-term care facilities. We call this approach The Eden Alternative™.
>
> I began my work in long-term care in 1991 and began my career as a rather reluctant recruit. I took the job as medical director and sole physician at a local nursing home initially because it was close to my home and I could ride my bicycle to work. About the only good thing

I can say for myself at that time is that my ignorance left me free of the cobwebs that can entangle those more familiar with conventional routines and policies. As I settled into my new practice I became troubled by the yawning gap between the diagnosis and treatments I provide my patients' bodies and the afflictions that so troubled their spirits. I soon saw that I had no pill that could remove the sting of loneliness, no injection that could lift a person from the depths of helplessness and no lotion that could soothe the ache of boredom.

I began to see that genuine caring and medical treatment were very different things. All my years of medical education and training had left me with a deeply flawed understanding of what it means to take care of another human being. Before I came to work in the nursing home, I believed that Care = treatment + empathy. In other words if I was skilled with the methods of diagnosis and treatment and I spiced those skills with a gentle bedside manner I was doing my job. In truth, real caring is something both more simple and more difficult. Caring = helping another person to grow. Lonely, helpless, and bored people cannot grow. We have an obligation to provide them with companionship, opportunities to give care, variety, and spontaneity just as we provide them with food, water, and shelter. (Thomas, 1997)

When Dr. Thomas recognized loneliness, helplessness, and boredom as afflictions of the human spirit, he set out to eliminate them by creating a "human habitat" within the institution of the nursing home. He hypothesized that changing the environment and the management philosophy of the nursing home would affect the quality of life for the elders living there and the quality of work life for the staff. Through a grant from the New York State Health Department, a human habitat was created within the existing walls of the nursing home, and thus, the prototype for future Eden Alternative homes was established. Dr. Thomas, along with his wife and project director, Judith Meyers Thomas, developed a set of principles that form the basis of the Eden Alternative, regardless of its setting.

THE EDEN ALTERNATIVE: 10 PRINCIPLES

The Eden Alternative's core philosophy is based on 10 principles:

1. The three plagues of loneliness, helplessness, and boredom account for the bulk of suffering among our elders.
2. An elder-centered community commits to creating a human habitat where life revolves around close and continuing contact with plants, animals, and children. It is these relationships that provide the young and old alike with a pathway to a life worth living.

3. Loving companionship is the antidote to loneliness. Elders deserve easy access to human and animal companionship.
4. An elder-centered community creates the opportunity to give as well as receive care. This is the antidote to helplessness.
5. An elder-centered community imbues daily life with variety and spontaneity, by creating an environment in which unexpected and unpredictable interactions and happenings can take place. This is the antidote to boredom.
6. Meaningless activity corrodes the human spirit. The opportunity to do things that we find meaningful is essential to human health.
7. Medical treatment should be the servant of genuine human caring, never its master.
8. An elder-centered community honors its elders by deemphasizing top-down bureaucratic authority, seeking instead to place the maximum possible decision-making authority into the hands of the elders or into the hands of those closest to them.
9. Creating an elder-centered community is a never-ending process. Human growth must never be separated from human life.
10. Wise leadership is the lifeblood of any struggle against the three plagues. For it, there can be no substitute.

WHY DO WE NEED THE EDEN ALTERNATIVE?

Long-term care facilities, as they exist today, are institutions patterned after hospitals. In all the hubbub of treatments and therapies, the fact that the people who live there deserve control over their own lives and have a right to live a life worth living is frequently lost. People are not meant to live in "facilities." The Eden Alternative is a response to the spiritual death created by prolonged institutionalization. People, especially the frail, cannot thrive in such places; indeed, they wither and die. Elders, regardless of degree of mental or physical infirmity, should live in life-affirming places that are more like gardens and less like institutions. The Eden Alternative teaches people how to change not only the physical environments of their facilities, but also the social environments in their organizations.

Here are some of the ideas that form the foundation of the Eden Alternative:

- Loneliness is the pain we feel when we want, but do not have, companionship. Elders blossom when they have access to companionship with other living things. Organizations that follow the

Eden Alternative principles address this issue by providing close and continuing contact with plants, animals, and children. Many animals, of many species, live within the building(s); children of all ages are present on a near daily basis; and the external community embraces the home.

- Helplessness is the pain we feel when we always receive care but never have the opportunity to give care. The Eden Alternative offers elders opportunities to provide care by assisting in the care and maintenance of the human habitat. The relationships that are formed help them balance their emotional and spiritual lives.
- Boredom is defined, in Eden terms, as the pain we experience when our lives are lacking in variety and spontaneity. Institutions excel in creating conformity, compliance, and routine; they are not good at fueling the spark of spontaneity that can make a life worth living. The Eden Alternative teaches people how to ignite that spark.

The Eden Alternative is concerned with the well-being of the caregivers as well as the needs of the elders. People who work in the field of long-term care receive far less pay then their true worth. Hands-on staff work is incredibly difficult, both physically and emotionally. The mainstream media's perspective on long-term care typically focuses on isolated instances of abuse. Although these events are tragic, they detract attention from the thousands of individuals who choose to honor and care for the frailest in our society. The current long-term care industry forces these dedicated people to work in a broken system, a system that continues to offer a product that consumers do not want. Contemporary long-term care facilities tend to be autocratic, hierarchical institutions that remove caregivers and elders from the decision-making process. The Eden Alternative challenges people to change their organizational cultures by aligning them with two fundamental ideas:

1. Decisions belong with the elders or as close to the elders as possible. In a traditional nursing home setting, a top-down bureaucracy exists: Staff workers do not take initiative to perform their duties, but instead wait for and receive direction from their superiors. In Eden Alternative homes, staff members form work teams, and each team accepts responsibility for management of its own work. Team members make their own schedules and their own assignments. People within the work teams make appropriate decisions and resolve issues through team meetings and conflict resolution. Also, in many nursing homes, there is distinct delineation of duties by department. This often causes conflict, resulting in attitudes that create "That's not my job" scenarios. As duties

and responsibilities are shared among team members, a cooperative work environment is cultivated.

2. Do unto your employees as you would have your employees do unto the elders. This is the Eden Alternative Golden Rule. An organization that gives love, respect, dignity, tenderness, and tolerance to the members of its staff is more likely to have staff that treats elders with these same qualities.

The Eden Alternative is a not-for-profit organization that supports a network of teachers and mentors throughout the world. It is dedicated to helping people who want to transform their institutions into human habitats that are dedicated to helping people grow.

GREEN HOUSES

The Green House Project was developed by and has drawn its philosophical foundation from the Thomases pioneering work with the Eden Alternative. It is based on the notion of growing Eden from the ground up. The model provides the frail elder with an environment that promotes autonomy, dignity, privacy, and choice while continuing to meet the practice standards of a skilled nursing facility. It is an intentional community for elders and those who work with elders. It is organized as a true *home*, and it places necessary clinical services within a holistic, habilitative, social context. Whereas the medical, institutional model encourages dependence and mitigates the perceived failings of elders, the overall design and implementation of the Green House encourages the pursuit of an elderhood oriented on continued growth.

The Green House design is a radical new approach to residential long-term care for elders founded on the idea that physical and social environments in which we deliver long-term care can and should be

- Warm: addresses the necessary social climate and size of the home. The Green Houses themselves are small (6- to 10-person) community homes where people requiring skilled nursing services live and receive the care they need. The houses fit the character of the geographic areas and neighborhoods in which they are built. Interior warmth is established through a floor plan, which is centered on a hearth, personal furnishings, decor, and, most importantly, the people. Small numbers of caregivers (Shahbazim) share ongoing responsibilities for the elders, each other, and the house. Each Green House provides a staffing ratio far above that provided in conventional, facility-based organizations.

- Smart: makes uses of the latest technology to assist in providing services. The use of technology that ensures safety, promotes quality of care, rigor in record keeping, and community and family involvement links with a sophisticated health care delivery network that ensures quality, provides expertise, and delivers office and ancillary support.
- Green: refers to essential connections to the living world.

The work of the Eden Alternative has shown that people find great pleasure in the company of animals, the laughter of children, and the growth of green plants. Contact with the living world is a major factor in both quality of life and improved clinical outcomes. The Green Houses give elders, staff, families, and the community at large multiple opportunities for life-affirming connections.

The Green House model offers a high-quality, safe, cost-effective alternative to institutionalization for frail and disabled people who require skilled care.

The first Green Houses opened in May 2003. The following is an excerpt from *The Green House Project Newsletter* (http://thegreenhouse-project.com/, 2003).

ELDERS MOVE INTO FIRST GREEN HOUSES

Ten happy elders who were living at The Cedars Health Center, a skilled nursing facility in Tupelo operated by United Methodist Senior Services of Mississippi [UMSSM], moved into the first Green Houses in the nation May 3, 2003. The first house is named the Laney House, after the oldest elder living there. Ten elders moved into the second house, named the Paige House, on May 10th. One elder, who has normally been withdrawn and not usually verbal, sat down in the hearth area after arriving at the Laney House, and was heard to say, "My, it is good to be home again after all this time away."

"One only has to spend a few minutes in a Green House to recognize that it is the right answer to a broken system and is a good thing," said Steve McAllily, president and CEO of UMSSM, which operates the Green Houses. "The elders are stronger, more vibrant and more content than ever; their families are more involved in their lives. The staff members have circled themselves around the elders and feel much better about themselves and their work."

"This is just the beginning of a new type of long-term care, one that allows elders to be free of the plagues of loneliness, helplessness and boredom," said Dr. William Thomas, president and founder of The Eden Alternative in Sherburne, New York. "We are so proud of the Shahbazim (those who staff the Green Houses in Tupelo). They have spent countless hours learning how to make life in a Green House not just good enough, but as close to perfect as it can be."

THEY'RE HAPPY AND EATING AS NEVER BEFORE

"The expressions on the elders' faces when they first entered the house affirmed a hundred times over that this is the right thing," said Alan Brown, vice president and COO of UMSSM. "They are happy and eating as never before."

"It is so nice not to be in a cold hospital environment; working in the Green House is like home. When I walk through the door, the smell of breakfast is in the air. The table is set. The coffee is on and we're waiting for the elders to wake up," said Matt Belue, a Tupelo Green House Shahbaz. (Shahbaz is the term that Dr. Thomas uses for a specialized worker within the Green House.) "One at a time, the elders come into the kitchen and sit at the table and there is laughter and conversation." UMSSM staff also report that one Green House resident, who had not been seen reading and who did not dress herself while at The Cedars, has been dressing herself and one day sat down and read the Bible.

We are beginning to see some evidence of the expected outcomes. We hoped that the scale of the house would enable elders to be less wheelchair dependent, and seven out of the ten elders who arrived in wheelchairs are able to navigate the house without the chairs, there have been encouraging weight gains, increased appetites and lots of laughter, said Project Director Jude Rabig. The Shahbazim have been working successfully in their self-managed work teams, and they are collaborating with the clinical support team very effectively.

RESEARCH RESULTS

The initial research project, funded by the New York State Health Department, compared an "Edenizing" facility to a traditional nursing home with similar demographics over a period of 3 years. Results of this study, conducted by Dr. Thomas, included a 50% decrease in the infection rate, a 71% drop in daily drug costs per elder, and a 26% decrease in nurse's aide turnover (Thomas, 1999).

A second project, funded by the Texas Long-Term Care Institute, was conducted over a 2-year period (1996–1998) involving six facilities in Texas. Beds in the participating facilities totaled 734. A task force of academicians, providers, and consumers developed the conceptual model for Texas. Sandy Ransom, director of the institute, served as principal investigator for the project.

Outcomes were analyzed within each home, individually, and cumulatively among all participating homes. A summary of significant findings follows.

Cumulative Findings

60% decrease in behavioral incidents
57% decrease in stage I–II pressure sores
18% decrease in restraints
11% increase in census
48% decrease in staff absenteeism
11% decrease in employee injuries

Outstanding Outcomes within Individual Facilities

Facility A

80% decrease in decubitus ulcers
49% decrease in restraints

Facility B

62% decrease in urinary tract infections

Facility C

58% decrease in restraints

Facility E

35% decrease in polypharmacy (resident on 5 or more medications)
76% decrease in contractures
96% decrease in decubitus ulcers
67% decrease in resident complaints
86% decrease in behavior incidents (Ransom, 2000)

Informal findings from Bringing Eden Alternative to Michigan (BEAM) yield a few more recent examples. Each bulleted item represents a separate home (www.edenealt.com, 2003):

- 75% decrease in staff turnover, 60% decrease in absenteeism
- 104% to 42% decrease in staff turnover over 1 1/2 years. Agency use for the same period of time dropped from $60,435.00 to $247.00

- Turnover CNA (Certified Nursing Assistant) 1998: 87.26%; 2002: 22%
- Turnover of 72% in 1997; 17% in 2001.
- Turnover all staff: 1996: 78%; 2002: 9.5%
- Prevalence of falls: 94% in 1998; 41% in 2001

After all the data have been collected, all the numbers counted, and all the analyses computed, there remains the fact that real human lives are involved. Some things just cannot be quantified. A radiant smile on the face of an elderly woman who lights up in the presence of a cat cannot be counted. The increase in the presence of laughter in the hallways cannot be counted. The witnessing of two hearts touching as an elder and a child share jellybeans cannot be counted. It is this humanness—this intangible feeling that one senses in a true Eden Alternative™ home—that really matters. Thus, the stories about the individuals whose lives have meaning, individuals who have reasons to get up in the morning—that is the true value of the Eden Alternative™. The language of community is shared through stories, or narratives. The stories that follow impart tiny pieces of how that *community* is returned to the people in these narratives, the staff and elders who live and work in these nursing homes. Real names are not used.

STORIES:
THE HEART OF THE EDEN ALTERNATIVE

Sue Ann, a quiet 82-year-old who had not been able to communicate effectively for a number of years, was sitting in the lobby when Sam (the home's little dog) ran into the lobby and started entertaining everyone sitting there. He raced around chasing his tail, jumped onto the sofa, leaped across a chair, and had everyone laughing so hard that tears were flowing. The harder they laughed, the wilder Sam's antics grew until he just stopped in midleap and plopped himself in front of Sue Ann's wheelchair. Sue Ann, grinning widely, pointed at Sam as if to say, "Look, he came to sit by me!" Sue Ann's son, while later telling the nurses how much his mother enjoyed Sam, tearfully shared a very moving moment with them. Sue Ann had actually verbalized to her son, "I've always loved you, but I may not show it."

Joan wandered continuously about the home. She looked sad and lost. Frequently she would break into tears for no discernible reason. A nurse's aide discovered one day that Joan's face burst into a beaming smile whenever she saw a cat. Thereafter, anytime Joan started crying, one could see the nurse's aides searching through the halls for a cat for Joan to hold, and Joan required fewer and fewer antipsychotic medications.

Lillian was one of those people who drive staff to distraction. She complained constantly to anyone who walked in the building. She accused staff of serving her poisoned food. She reported bogus complaints to the state regulatory agency, which necessitated visits to the home by state officials. She was very unhappy. After the Eden Alternative™ became well established in the home and Lillian knew that her words and feelings were important to the staff, she was elected president of the resident council and became the self-proclaimed "greeter" to visitors. She gave many tours to visitors of all ages and was photographed for a national publication in *her home*.

Mary had been living in the Alzheimer's unit for many months and, as reported by her family, had talked only "nonsense" for several years. One afternoon, the local fifth-grade class made its weekly visit to the home. On that particular day, the group was preparing the garden for spring planting. Mary had had much experience gardening before her illness and gravitated toward the children, who seemed somewhat at a loss as to exactly how to work in the garden. Mary picked up a hoe and handed another hoe to the child nearest her, while other children found additional hoes to use. As Mary began working, she clearly articulated to the children how to turn the soil. The children were openly attentive and very interested in learning this new skill as they listened intently to Mary's instructions.

Rick, a live-in parrot, seemed to squawk extra long and loud when the elders were going to their morning exercise class. Just to see what would happen, Rick was allowed out of his cage one morning and was taken into the exercise room. He looked around, found a perch, quieted down, and began flapping his wings as the elders raised their arms in rhythm with the music. Rick became a regular at the exercise class, and, strangely enough, more and more elders became interested in exercising.

Perhaps the most poignant story to be told has been repeated at all the homes involved in the Texas study, the story of the cats. The cats in these Eden Alternative™ homes somehow know which elders are terminal. They take up a death watch during the last 2 to 3 days of a person's life. In one home, the "Angel Kitty" will stay with a dying resident and will not leave the room until the person has passed away. In another home, the cats take turns staying with the person. When one cat leaves, another is waiting to enter the room, and several animals participate in this vigil. Susanne, dying of cancer and never fond of animals, remained in her bed during her last days. She remarked to the staff, "I am so comfortable. I want you all to know how comforting it is to me to have this cat stay with me at this time in my life."

> In the words of one 95 year old Elder: "You tell them that this is a dang good place! There is never a dull moment around here with the animals and the children. I'd be six feet under if it wasn't for this home!"

Remarkable stories about employee responses to the Eden Alternative™ and changes in their lives further enrich the model. One such account involves a nursing assistant who, after several years as an exceptional caregiver, began a pattern of missing work on her scheduled weekends. Barbara, a single mom, was attempting to hide from her problems through drinking binges that resulted in severe hangovers. Not only was this detrimental for the elders, but it placed hardships on her coworkers. After an especially stressful weekend, Barbara's work team gathered and, after considerable debate, voted her "off the team." Barbara voluntarily resigned. Several months later, Barbara approached the administrator and asked to be reinstated on her team. The administrator informed Barbara that she would have to take her request to the work team. Barbara met with the team and explained that she had extricated herself from an abusive relationship, had received professional help with her drinking problem, and believed that she "had her life together." The team members agreed to allow Barbara a trial period on the team. That trial period is now a year in the past, and Barbara is currently a stellar team member and a shining role model that new employees look up to. As one administrator in the Texas study stated, "The Eden Alternative is really about growing people. I have seen incredible growth with some of my staff members" (Ransom, 2000, p. 58).

CONCLUSION

An entire book could be written about the response of staff and elders to changes brought about by the Eden Alternative™. Issues continue to surface within communities where old ways are entrenched and innovative leaders initiate change. Some residents, families, or staff members may not like animals, children, or plants. Some people resist and resent changes in management styles. Not all elders appreciate or are overtly influenced by the Eden Alternative™. However, some lives are changed profoundly. For these persons, whether staff, visitors, families, or elders, the meaning added to their lives has no measure. Life becomes, once again, worth living.

RESOURCES

Books

Haleigh's Almanac: Eden Alternative training aanual. (2002). San Marcos: Texas Long-term Care Institute, Texas State University—San Marcos.

Thomas, W. H. (1999). *The Eden Alternative handbook: The art of building human habitats.* Sherburne, NY: Summer Hill Co.

Thomas, W. H. (1999). *Learning from Hannah: Secrets for a life worth living.* Acton, MA: VanderWyk & Burnham.

Thomas, W. H. (1999). *Life worth living: How someone you love can still enjoy life in a nursing home.* Acton, MA: VanderWyk & Burnham

Videotapes

Action Pact, Inc. (Producer). (2000). *The ten principles of Eden: "The Learning Circle" Training Video Series.*

The Eden Alternative. (Producer). (1997). *Life worth living: Eden Alternative in action—an introduction to the principles and practices of the Eden Alternative.*

Electronic Media, Ohio University Southern Campus. (Producer). (2000). *It's better tolLive in a garden.*

Contacts

Eden Alternative, Inc., 742 Turnpike Rd., Sherburne, NY 13460; telephone: (607) 674-5232; fax: (607) 674-6723; Web site: www.edenalt.org, http://thegreenhouseproject.com; e-mail: info@edenalt.com

Texas Long-term Care Institute, Texas State University–San Marcos, 601 University Dr., San Marcos, TX 78666; telephone: (512) 245-8234; fax: (512) 245-7803; Web site: http://ltc-institute.health.txstate.edu; e-mail: LTC-Institute@txstate.edu

REFERENCES

Ransom, S. (1998). The Eden Alternative in Texas. *Texas Journal on Aging, 1*(1), 8–13.

Ransom, S. (2000). *Eden Alternative: The Texas project.* San Marcos: Texas State University–San Marcos.

Thomas, W. H. (1996). *Life worth living: How someone you love can still enjoy life in a nursing home.* Acton, MA: VanderWyk & Burnham.

Thomas, W. H. (1997, January/February). The Eden Alternative. *Spectrum.*

Thomas, W. H. (1999a). *Eden Alternative handbook: The art of building human habitats.* Sherburne, NY. Summer Hill Co.

Thomas, W. H. (1999b). *Learning from Hannah: Secrets for a life worth living.* Acton, MA: VanderWyk & Burnham.

Index